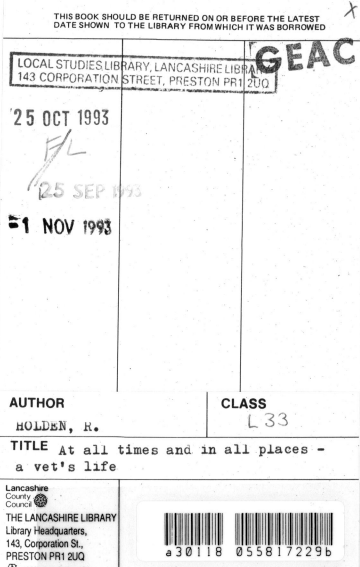

AUTHOR

HOLDEN, R.

CLASS

L 33

TITLE At all times and in all places -
a vet's life

At all Times and in all Places—a Vet's Life

At all Times and in all Places
–a Vet's Life

by

Richard Holden

The Pentland Press Ltd.
Edinburgh Cambridge Durham

05581722

Typeset by Print Origination (NW) Ltd, Liverpool
Printed and bound by Antony Rowe Ltd., Chippenham,
Wiltshire, SN14 6LH

To Miss Eileen Slinger

Acknowledgements

To Mr W. B. Slinger MRCVS for advice and
for kindly reading the manuscript and to
Miss K. Cross and Mrs D. Bainbridge for typing it.

I

Richard was waiting to cross the road which was busy with traffic, most of it horse drawn, but there were some motor cars and lorries. The horses interested him, and he was always thrilled when he saw one of the Express Parcels delivery vans belonging to the Railway Company being driven at a fast canter, with sparks flying from the horse's shoes as they struck the granite sets, and heard the noise from the iron bound wheels.

After he had crossed the road, he walked past the tall iron gates which opened onto the Carriage Drive through the Park. Soon he turned into the drive which led to the stone built Jacobean Grammar School, to which he had won a scholarship when he was eleven years old. His sister Mary was two years younger, and she was precocious musically, starting to try to play their Steinway piano when she was five years old, so their father obtained a professional teacher for her. She made such rapid progress that now she was in much demand to play at concerts in aid of the Church or the British Red Cross, but especially at her school in Droughton. The family lived in a terraced Victorian house which was very large, having ten rooms, and the road was in a pleasant area on the outskirts of the town.

Droughton, a very ancient town, with charters going back to the early thirteenth century, had been almost drowned by the tide of the Industrial Revolution; the mediaeval centre, Norman church, and adjoining seventeenth century houses had been rapidly surrounded by streets of poor houses built for the influx of workers to the various industries which had developed. There was the iron and later the steel production; cotton spinning and weaving; huge engineering complexes; soap and linoleum factories; a jam works, and numerous trades. The two reasons for this industry were nearness to a large coalfield, and the small port of Droughton which had since been greatly enlarged. The skyline was crowded with two hundred factory chimneys from which the smoke darkened the sky, blackened the buildings, and made the industrious housewives wash their lace curtains every fortnight and the steps at the front of their houses every day. When the window sills and the steps had been washed, they were donkey stoned cream or white, and they stood out vividly against the soot-blackened brickwork.

It was when the winter came and the sulphurous fogs developed that the old people died from chest infections; traffic was reduced to a crawl; the railways almost stopped operating, and the candles, gas lights, and oil lamps burned all the day hardly seen in the dirty gloom. Tom Bradshaw, Richard's

1

uncle, indirectly helped to create this smoke and fog, because he was a coal merchant who had a stable of twenty Shire, and Shire-Clydesdale cross horses which pulled the heavily loaded lorries delivering the coal and coke for domestic use. He also owned four steam wagons which made bulk deliveries to the factories. These were invaluable on foggy days, because they had two large acetylene headlamps only about a foot above ground level which gave a brilliant light in front of the driver who, sitting high up, had a good field of vision as they chuffed along. Richard enjoyed riding on the steam wagon, filling the reservoir at the top of the headlamps with water and then, having turned on the tap and opened the front with its big glass lens, lighting the lamp; or dropping the hose with its wicker basket end over a roadside hedge into the stream so that the water level in the boiler could be raised. But the magnet which drew him to the coal yard was the stable and the horses, and he used to go there on his bicycle on Saturday mornings and help to water and feed and work in the tack room. He loved to climb up the ladder which was fixed to the wall into the loft above the stable. There with a pitchfork he would help to push the hay through the holes in the floor into the racks which were above the mangers in the stable below.

Victoria was Tom Bradshaw's sister. She had married Edward Holden and Richard Baden was their first child. Edward, now a civil servant, worked in the Ministry of Labour offices in Droughton and had achieved an executive position. One of his brothers, Ezra, was a farmer who lived eight miles away at Westend Farm near Weston village. The 160 acre farm was rented from the Squire whose estate included most of the village and the surrounding farms, but who was not very interested in them, leaving their administration to his farm manager while he was busy with his industrial pursuits in Droughton. Another of Edward's brothers, Dick, owned a large farm in the hills 25 miles away. The children were never happier than when they were taken to Westend farm, and could spend an afternoon among the cows, pigs, and poultry. Richard was soon in the stable where the farm horses were housed; he had two favourites: Dolly, a Shire mare, and Mollie: a bay half-bred hunter which pulled the trap. As he grew older he began with his parents' permission to spend a lot of his free time at the coal yard with his cousin Frank, or at the farm with his cousin John. The farm was only five miles away from his home, and he would cycle there and stay all Saturday, and sometimes over the weekend. Nevertheless his attendance at his classical school came first, but he had been allowed to drop Greek and was now studying chemistry. He was a day boarder, and popular, winning medals for his house (St. Wilfreds) and playing at right back in the school's football team. His ambition was to get into the first eleven, and get a sports blazer.

It was at the farm that he was happiest, working among the animals, helping to feed the horses, pigs, and poultry; or bringing up the cows for milking. Soon he had learnt the names of all the feeding stuffs, and of the breeds of the animals and poultry, and also of the wild flowers growing in the hedges and ditches. His uncle was a short, stocky, powerful man, who walked with a stoop—this latter was the result of carrying milk from the shippon to the dairy year after year. He used a wooden yoke which was laid across his shoulders, and at each end of the yoke hung a short chain which ended in a hook, to which were attached the buckets, each of which held four gallons of milk. He always wore a union flannel shirt, open at the neck; brown fustian breeches; long stockings; and clogs. Martha had knitted his waistcoat, over which he wore an old coat. His hat, used when milking the cows, was a brimless trilby, polished where it had been pressed against the cow's side. Though he employed two men, it was a life of endless work for Martha, Ezra, and their eighteen-year-old son John, who was a fair-haired, handsome, powerfully built young man, and everybody had to work including Richard when at Easter he stayed at the farm for two weeks.

Every morning at 5.30 the five males would walk into the dairy, each take a clean bucket off the shelf, and then cross the cobblestoned yard to the shippon. His uncle had taught him how to milk so having got a three legged stool he sat on it beside the fifth cow. With the bucket gripped between his legs and his head pressed against the cow's flank, he would seize the nearest teats and begin to milk. He was much slower than the others, and for the first week his arms and knees ached, so he was very pleased when his uncle praised his efforts. Little was said; a cow would be told to come over or stand still; or some comment made about the amount of milk given. The twittering sparrows would fly in and out, ignored by the cats drinking milk from the battered bowl. Richard watched for Sooty, the black cat with four white paws which he had adopted when she was a kitten; she often followed him about and was the only one allowed into the farm kitchen.

Every so often, one of the milkers would rise, hook two buckets onto the yoke, and walk across the yard to the dairy. This was not so easy to do; you had to hold the chains firmly to avoid spilling the milk which was then poured into the tank at the top of the cooler. From the tap in the tank the milk ran down its corrugated surface, which was cooled by the cold water flowing through the interior of the cooler. From the bottom the milk ran through the muslin-lined sieve into the ten-gallon can. When full this was dragged aside, and another took its place. In the winter they were left in the dairy even though the fire was alight under the boiler. Martha filled this with water every morning and laid the fire. Ezra set it alight in the morning so that there was plenty of boiling water for washing all the utensils and buckets used for milking. In the summer the full cans were put into the water trough, and covered with wet sacks to keep them cool until Mr Hodgson came to collect them, and he later retailed the milk in the town.

By eight o'clock the milking was finished; the horses had been watered and fed, the pigs fed, and all the milking utensils put in the big wooden tub full of cold water–this prevented the milk drying hard on them before they could be scalded. Then the five went in for breakfast, and they all had hearty appetites. Fried home-cured bacon, eggs, and bread were rapidly eaten and more sweet tea drunk, and some plates refilled. It was a cheerful meal with some banter but Martha kept order, though all the time she was wiping eggs clean, and putting them in the straw-lined bucket. When more tea was wanted Richard was surprised to see his aunt refill the tea caddy from the square three-ply wood box on the side of which was stamped in large black letters "Best Ceylon Tea", which she bought in bulk from the tea company. The collie Bracken and the cat Sooty were asleep on the peg rug in front of the big fire in the range, but even so the kitchen was not very warm owing to the fact that it faced north, had a cold, sanded flagged floor, and always had condensation running down the walls and window. Under that window was the long stone slopstone, at one end of which was the water pump. As the handle of the pump was pulled forwards and backwards water was pumped up into the huge tank, which was in a cupboard in the bedroom above. Richard once counted the 500 strokes he made so that there was enough water for a bath. The kitchen range was very big; in the centre was the deep grate which held the fire, to the left the oven with its heavy door which was held shut by a bar on which was a round knob. On the right of the grate was the boiler which had a lift-up lid, with a handle which was always very hot. Everyone in the house, on drawing off the boiling water through the brass tap on the front of the boiler, always had to fill it up again. More hot water was made by the copper boiler, at the back of the grate, which fed the cylinder underneath the tank in the bedroom overhead.

After breakfast the three men worked in the buildings. John would be up on the haystack cutting down through the hay with the big hay knife. Ezra would plunge his pitchfork into the hay, and carry it into the shippon, always dropping some on the way, which would be picked up later. In each stall in the shippon two cows were tied, and he would push his way between them and drop the hay. This he would then shake out, creating a fog of dust. Richard would sweep up the muck in the dung channel behind the cows, and soon learnt to be careful not to touch them with the brush in case they kicked him. When the dung had been swept into a heap, it was shovelled into a barrow. He soon realised why his cousin John was strong and had such bulging muscles. The loaded oak barrow was very heavy, and Richard struggled to get it moving, and then to trundle it across the cobbled yard and up the plank where it was emptied into the midden. When this was finished, the next work varied according to the weather and the time of year. At Christmas he watched the geese, turkeys, and hens have their necks wrung, and was taught to pluck, and then to draw and truss them. Some were put on the stone shelves, and the larger birds were hung in the pantry which was very cold because it faced north, and the top half of the window, which was covered with a piece of zinc mesh, was always open. A spell of warm weather at this time could lead to catastrophe—the carcases would begin to go bad, so plucking was left as late as possible. In the light from the two oil lamps hanging from the beam overhead, Ezra, Martha, John and Richard could be seen sitting in a shed in the evenings steadily plucking. In spite of being bandaged Richard's fingers became sore, so then he would have to truss and push the wooden skewers through the carcases to hold the wings and legs together. At the end of the evening the heaps of feathers were stuffed into sacks, to go ultimately to the manufacture of bedding.

Sometimes it was his job to feed the poultry. Ezra would go with Richard into the proven house, and he would tip bags of dry meal into an old iron bath, then add water and mix it with a big shovel, leaving Richard to fill the four-gallon buckets with the mash, and then to line some more buckets with straw. He would go to Dolly in the stable—she was his favourite—and sometimes get a body brush and a curry comb and groom her for a few minutes, until his uncle would come in and put on her harness and lead her out, back her between the shafts and lower them so that the chain lay in the metal channel of the saddle and she would be hooked on. The cart was loaded by Ezra, including a ten-gallon milk can full of water. Richard would get into the cart, would be given the reins and, feeling very pleased with himself, would drive out of the yard and across the fields to the poultry houses. There he would top up the water fountains, fill the troughs with mash, and collect the eggs and put them into the straw-lined buckets. Sometimes he found a dead hen and wondered why it had died, but his uncle did not know, and accepted the odd loss as normal. By this time, John would have arrived with the "baggin"—cheese sandwiches and hot tea in a small kit, and this was consumed before the fold units were moved onto fresh ground; and thus the morning's work ended. Again, some Saturdays when his uncle and aunt had gone to Droughton to stand the hen market, he would have to attend to the pigs which were housed in six sties built as one unit; the rear half was slate roofed, the front an open yard, and a four foot high opening led from the yard into the sty. In each yard was a long stone trough into which he poured the meal and water, with scraps from the kitchen. There were four sows, and he was always careful when he was feeding them, because one day one which had just farrowed came up behind him and tipped him over the door. He was not hurt, but began to appreciate the dangers always present when dealing with animals. He always carried a strong stick whenever, bent double, he shuffled into the sty to spread some clean straw. In the two end sties were the porkers, and they were a different proposition, playful and mischievous, and with a good turn of speed which he found out when he was trying to catch two which had escaped. They did not keep a boar, so when a sow was brimming, she was loaded into a cart, a net tied over her and she was taken to the boar on a farm in the village. Next to the pigs was a bull box; only Ezra and John went in to the shorthorn bull, which was led out twice a day on a divided chain, one spring hook clipped into the head chain, the other onto the nose ring; he was always quiet but very strong.

It was a cold Easter when Richard first went to Higher Hindshead which was farmed by his Uncle Dick but this did not distract him from enjoying the journey by train. His plaited bamboo suitcase was held together by a broad leather strap on which was a handle. On getting into the compartment he put this on the rack over his head, and then watched the changing scenery as the train gathered speed. Once over the river bridge the grimy canal and the rows of back-to-back houses were soon left behind, and the flat fields were gradually replaced by hills and pastures, and a tower or spire showed where a village was hidden in a fold in the hills. At his destination he was met by his uncle, and they climbed on to the trap; then the black horse set off at a fast trot. Aunty Alice greeted Richard warmly, and kissed him, and made him sit by the fire so that he could get warm after the long cold ride. Across the valley, snow was still on the highest hills, and in the fields near the farm a lot of sheep were grazing. When he awoke next morning, a faint light outlined the window, so he lit a candle to see his way across the room to the wash-stand. At that moment there was a knock on the door, and Alice entered carrying a ewer of hot water.

"Good morning, Richard, did you sleep well?"

"Yes, thank you, Auntie," he replied.

"That's good. Don't bother to make your bed and I'll call you when breakfast is ready."

At breakfast he realised that Dick and Alice must be better off than Ezra and Martha. He noticed especially the damask table-cloth, the china cups, saucers, and plates, the silver teaspoons, and the brocade curtains. The white ceiling reflected the bright morning light on the floral wallpaper and the bright red carpet, and through the open door he could see a well-furnished kitchen, where Tom the shepherd and Walter the labourer were eating. He had finished breakfast and was telling his aunt all the news when Dick came into the room. Six feet tall, he walked erect and briskly—in appearance very much the country gentleman. He wore a collar and tie, a tweed jacket and waistcoat, breeches, and brown leather leggings and boots. His weather-beaten face broke into a smile when he said:

"Come on, Richard, and see the idle life we sheep farmers lead—there's no getting up at five in the morning to milk the cows; we have only four and 7 o'clock is their time. It's very different from Ezra's."

As they walked into the farmyard, the sound of sheep bleating came from a big stone barn, and they went in and inspected the animals. At each side of a central passage were many pens made of hurdles tied together with baleing wire, each containing ewes and lambs.

"Lambing has just started and is going well," said Dick, "So we must walk round the sheep this morning. I bring them all down into the fields about a month before they are due to lamb; it's easier to feed them a bit extra, and to find them if the weather gets bad."

So his uncle explained things as they walked up the first field which from being level soon became steep, and Richard found his legs beginning to ache from the unaccustomed exercise, and his eyes from the sting of the bitter east wind, but Dick strode steadily on. Most of the sheep were grazing and there were a few lambs playing when Dick stopped and pointed out a ewe close to the stone wall and said that he thought she was in trouble. They soon caught her and found that though she was trying to lamb nothing was happening, so they marked her with a bright red paint stick. Later they found another ewe in trouble and marked her, and when they had walked all the sheep they rounded up these two, and walked them down the field and into the barn, where they were each put into a pen. Tom came in, carrying an old towel and a bucket of hot water to which a carbolic disinfectant had been added. Richard held the ewe and Tom, with his shirt sleeves rolled up, washed his hands, soaped them well and began to explore the ewe, and then said,

"It's a big lamb wrong way round; stop straining, you silly old fool; that's it, I've got one leg, now where's t'other? It's here," and as he withdrew his hand two little feet appeared protruding from the ewe's passage. Dick and Tom each got hold of a leg and began to pull, and the lamb's hindquarters appeared, the tail wagging; then with a rush the lamb was born.

"It's a big'un is that," commented Dick as Tom wiped the blood and mucus from its face.

"Aye, it is that, I don't think she'll have another, but I'll just feel to make sure."

Tom did so but she had no more, so she was released and began to lick the struggling lamb. They went into the second pen, and now Richard had to examine the little black-face ewe because Tom's hand was too big. He was worried that he might hurt the ewe, but the two experts advised him: "so there's a head and a leg; right, feel on the other side for the other leg." He found it and as he was trying to bring it forwards, the lamb moved and his hand closed on the foot. Working the head and legs through the opening hurt his fingers, and he had to pull very hard before the chest appeared. The lamb jerked as they pulled harder until finally it came flopping motionless onto the straw. It looked a gonner but Tom picked the lamb up by its hind legs and swung it to and fro. Liquid dripped from its nostrils and its tail twitched, so Tom laid it down and began to rub it with straw. It began to breathe and move.

Dick said, "We were lucky there, with Richard having a small hand; we were just in time." On re-examination there were no more; years later he often remembered those words when he had delivered his first lamb, and how pleased he had been.

The farm consisted of 30 acres of arable and about 100 of grass; the rest was the steep hillside grazing and moorland extending a mile and a half up the valley, and Richard enjoyed the varied work which had to be done to maintain it in good heart. One morning he was at one of the outbarns loading a cart with muck, and though he had a small fork he found it very heavy work. Walter brought a big bay gelding from the stable, attached him to the cart and together Richard and he continued to load it, and then went to one of the arable fields. The horse knew what to do without any commands being given, and walked on about eight paces and then stopped. Using drop forks, they pulled off a small heap of muck. At once the horse walked on the right distance and stopped, more muck was pulled off, and this was repeated until the cart was empty. They did two trips and it was lunch time, and in the afternoon they went back to muck knocking. Walter, using a big fork, could throw and scatter the manure evenly, steadily and rhythmically working along the line of heaps, but Richard, using a smaller fork, found it very hard work, and soon tired, so Walter sent him to find Tom who was repairing a stone wall damaged by sheep getting over. Using a batter rule he was rebuilding a length of a dyke (as these walls were called), but Richard sorted the stones into heaps of the same size. Some of the square blocks of millstone grit he could not lift and he began to appreciate the enormous amount of hard labour required to build a mile of dyke. Before dark he went with Tom to walk the sheep, and again in the morning, but Dick usually did it at midday.

In the big outbarn he helped to feed the store cattle, forking the hay through a hole in the loft floor down into the passage below. The cattle had been loosed out into the yard to drink at the stone trough which was fed by a spring running down the hillside. From a clamp he loaded mangolds into the root chopper while Walter turned the wheel, and then the chopped roots were given to the tied-up cattle and the hay fed. In the small shippon on the farm four Jerseys were tied up. It was a breed he had never seen before, and he loved their gentleness and docility, after the struggles to tie up and milk some of the younger Shorthorns and Ayrshires at Westend.

Walter looked after the few pigs and poultry, and Richard helped him groom the horses, but his main interest was the sheep and he learnt a lot working with his uncle and Tom. Soon he could trim an overgrown foot or skin a ewe's dead lamb and tie the skin onto an orphan and get the ewe to take it. He could turn up a sheep and hold it while Tom clipped away dirty, matted wool hiding the udder, could draw milk from each teat, and once found a blind teat which caused one of the twin lambs to be fostered onto another ewe which had lost her lamb. He learnt patience trying to foster a lamb or getting a dozy one to suck; he was shown a ewe with the dreaded garget, an inflammation which caused the udder to go black and the ewe to die. His uncle did not know what brought it on but said that he would cut off the dead cold teat, and a few times the ewe would slowly recover, to be cast with the broken-mouthed in the autumn. He never bought any sheep, saying that buying them was a quick way to get trouble. He bought a tup some years but only from someone he knew and could trust; and even then kept it isolated in a little paddock far away from the flock, until he was sure it was healthy.

In the short time he had been at the farm Richard had begun to feel very much at home and said so to his uncle, who informed him that he was not surprised, seeing the family had its roots in the valley going back 250 years; it was bred in the Holdens. Alice and Dick gave him an open invitation to go back any time he was able, and he was a little sad to leave them when he boarded the train to return home. He had become curious about many things: would the ewe have died if he had not had a small hand, and what had caused these dreaded diseases his uncle talked about? Braxy and hoose; screw cows and picked ones; dysentery and foot rot and gid. But he had to forget these things for the moment; both his mother and his father impressed on him the importance of getting his Matric. at school, as the way of getting to college and a job with better pay and chances of promotion. His father had retired from the Army with the rank of RSM, and was now an established civil servant with a position in the labour exchange.

His salary and Army pension enabled them to live well in a pleasant Georgian house called Bowland situated on the outskirts of the town. Richard's sister Mary was passing one examination after another for piano playing, and would obviously become a concert pianist in time. Though it was a classical school, science subjects were taught and now, back in school, Richard worked hard studying chemistry, mathematics, English, French and Latin and the other subjects in the curriculum.

On the first Saturday after his return from Higher Hindshead he went shopping with his mother, and they walked to the end of the road where they lived and waited at the tram stop for the arrival of the tramcar, heralded by the squealing noise of the steel wheels on the steel rails as it came round the corner. If it was late, it was always a bumpy ride down Cannon Hill to the centre of the town, and well worth the penny it cost, especially if it were a wet day. Arriving in the centre they went at once to the old market where stalls were erected on the flags outside the church every Saturday. In this old part of the town the streets were very narrow, and on Saturdays they were crowded, but they soon found Ezra and Martha behind their stall which was covered with white sheeting. On it were buckets of eggs; half-pound and one pound blocks of white butter; cartons of cream; two big cheeses, one strong and one mild in flavour; dressed chickens; home-made egg custard tarts;

bunches of dried mint, sage and thyme; and spring flowers in a vase. They chatted for a few minutes and bought eggs, cheese, butter, and a chicken. As they walked up Church Street they could see many horses, some with nose bags on, all tied to the rings which were in the wall at the entrance to Hartley's garage. The centre area was filled with carts and traps, their shafts pointing to the sky. The "Garage" repaired all sorts of agricultural machinery, and at the rear was a smithy with horses waiting outside to be shod. The carriage department repaired wagons and carts and also "horse-less carriages". Nearby was the "Farmers Supply Store", really a huge warehouse selling everything from a plough to a shovel: rope; stack sheets; Stockholm tar and creosote; lamps and lamp oil. Next door to it was the saddler's shop where two men could be seen sitting at a bench under the window stitching girths and collars. Across the road was the veterinary chemists, then the finest confectioner's in the town, and many other shops all full of customers, and on the corner the Blue Bell Hotel. It must have been a very pleasant country town before it was completely hemmed in by shoddy houses, industrial premises, and huge mills. Connecting High Street, Church Street, Watergate, Stanfordgate and Bridge Street were many courts, weinds, and lanes, surviving mediaeval roads just wide enough to allow one cart to pass through. They walked through one and arrived at the covered market where they bought meat and fruit. The High Street was dominated by the Victorian Gothic Town Hall which had a 120-foot-high clock tower; the building of sandstone was now begrimed with soot and dirt. They finished shopping at the large grocer's store which was on the opposite side of the road, and then went upstairs into the restaurant where Ted was waiting for them, and they had coffee before walking to the tram for the return home.

The next Saturday Richard cycled to Westend, feeling a little guilty because he had not spent the holiday there. A bucket of eggs stood on an old white-wood table beside the gate which led into the farmyard, together with some blue paper bags which were held down by a 2lb iron weight, and a basin in which were some coppers left by people when they had taken eggs. Inside the gate, Leo the guard dog was standing, firmly attached by a strong chain to a barrel. He was the result of the Squire's chow-chow bitch being mated with the Airedale from the Post Office, and because he had a mane of gingery-coloured hair had been given the name Leo. Ezra always took him for a walk all around the farm in the evening, to assure himself that the stock was all right, that the oil lamps had been extinguished, and the doors and gates closed. He was a heavy strong dog and could knock a person over if he leapt up at them; he also was a good fighter and hated cats, but was devoted to Ezra and followed him closely whenever he was loose. His aunt and uncle had gone to market so Richard helped finish the milking, and then gave John an account of the time spent at Higher Hindshead. He had learned that the farm had belonged to Alice's brother, who had made it over to his sister a short time before he suddenly died of pneumonia. Dick had been the manager of a sheep farm in Scotland when he married Alice, and when she inherited the thriving farm they soon moved there and lived in some style, helped by the big bank balance left to her by her careful brother. He had heard his uncle Ezra say it was getting near rent day, so it came as no surprise to learn that his uncle rented Westend from the Squire, who was a poor landlord and did little to maintain the farms which made up his estate.

He found Dolly much bigger, and John told him that she was in foal and due about the second of June, but he still scrambled onto her back and rode her down the green lane to turn her out in the evenings. He was happy to be back here because he and John were becoming good friends, and he was pleased that he was allowed to wash up after milking, to clean out the stables and pigs, and to help feed the cattle. When the first Saturday in June arrived he was excited waiting for Dolly to foal, and was told the signs to watch for; and the three of them took it in turns to watch her all day and all night, but nothing had happened when he set off home on the Sunday evening. She foaled at six o'clock on the Monday morning–it was a colt, and the afterbirth was thrown onto a hedge for luck. He was disappointed to miss the event, but each weekend he spent time handling the foal and gaining its confidence until finally he slipped a halter over its head, and soon could lead it about.

Richard had done well at school, coming top of his class in three subjects, so at home there were discussions about his future. He told his parents that he wanted to work with livestock, and the idea of becoming a farm manager formed in his mind, so it was decided that he should obtain his Matric., and then attend an Agricultural College. During the summer holidays he drove Lofty, a very big bay Shire gelding, an old horse which moved slowly, but was still very strong, and which could pull a fully-loaded hay wain or manure cart with ease. They were so busy on the farm that it was all work and bed. For weeks Mr Hodgson did not want the milk, so cheese had to be made and Richard helped in every way that he could. This was much appreciated by his aunt and uncle, who showed it by giving him potatoes or cabbages, and eggs and cream to take home. At hay and harvest time his father came and helped, and with John and Richard made a good team. This extra help was invaluable at harvest as Ezra had an accident.

This is how it happened. After putting sheaves of corn in stooks, they were all finishing odd jobs round the buildings, and John was in the barn sharpening a scythe when his father walked past carrying a bucket of food for the bull, closely followed by Leo. Some minutes later he heard his father give a scream; the dog was barking furiously, and the bull bellowed. Grabbing pitchforks, John and the men raced towards the bull box, and at that moment the bull came out with Leo clinging to his bleeding muzzle. Running into the box he found his father sprawled in a corner, ashen-faced and still. For an instant John was petrified by fear that his father was dead, but as he knelt by his side his father said in a weak voice, "John, get me up." As he tried to lift him, Martha came running in, alerted by the noise and seeing the bull run past the kitchen window, and between them they all carried Ezra to the house, groaning at every movement.

Martha said, "Richard, on your bike quick up to the post office, and get them to ask Dr Derham to come as quick as he can because Ezra has been hurt by the bull."

Martha wrapped a blanket round her husband, and then gave him the whiskey and water he had asked for. The initial shock began to wear off, and he slowly explained that as he had put the bucket down he had noticed a piece of broken metal tie chain on the floor. In the split second he appreciated the fact that the bull was loose, it swayed sideways and then lunged at him.

"He knocked me into the corner and I couldn't move as he had winded me, then he came at me with his head down, but his horns stopped him getting at me. It was lucky I left the door open because Leo was in in a flash, biting his legs. He kicked him off and shuffled back to have another go at me, but as he dropped his head Leo had him by the nose, and he couldn't shake him off and charged out of the box."

"Thank God Leo was there," said Martha.

"Aye, I am sure he saved my life."

When the doctor arrived, his examination revealed a broken collar bone, and three broken ribs on the left side of the chest. His ribs and collar bone were bandaged and his left arm supported by a sling.

"You have been very lucky, Ezra Holden," said the doctor, "I am certain you are not hurt inside, it's just your collar bone and ribs, and they are going to be very painful for some time. This medicine will ease the pain, follow the instructions on the label, and don't knock that arm. Sleep sat up in that big chair for the next few nights, and I'll come and see you in a week."

The men helped John catch the bull, which was led back to the box, and tied up using two neck chains. There was a lot of comment as to the fate of the bull; some said he should be killed at once, but it was decided that as he was usually quiet to handle and had a good pedigree, he would be kept. Each time Leo was allowed in to see his master, Sooty was locked in the front room; he just ignored Bracken.

Richard stayed at the farm for another fortnight and learnt a lot about cheese-making, and turned the handle of the cream separator until his arms ached. The separated milk was fed to the calves, pigs and chickens, but he was relieved when Mr Hodgson began to collect the milk again and cheese-making ceased, while his uncle was steadily getting better.

The autumn term passed quickly, and when Richard arrived at the farm on the Saturday before Christmas John had plenty of work for him. Soon he had been four times to the village to various houses delivering orders for turkeys, geese, chickens, eggs, butter and cream, and when he went home he had a huge turkey securely tied onto the carrier of his bicycle. So when Christmas day arrived Ted and Richard were in the front room of Bowland greeting their guests as they arrived–Ezra, Martha and John, the Healds, and the Bradshaws. Outside it was bitterly cold, with snow lying deep, but this room decorated with holly and ivy was very warm; a big fire was burning brightly in the grate, so they soon thawed out and began to gossip and joke, to talk about the presents they had received, and to wait for lunch. Soon Victoria came into the room and said, "Come on, all of you, everything is ready," and they all trooped quickly into the dining room, and seated themselves round the very old oak refectory table. Ted said Grace, and then while the ladies served the soup he and Tom Bradshaw filled every glass with homemade elderberry wine, the youngsters getting only half a glass. When the soup had been eaten, Ted went into the kitchen and returned carrying the very large turkey on a meat dish; the well-roasted bird was greeted with cries of "That looks good!" and "Well done Vicky!" He put it on the sideboard, and after sharpening the knife on the steel, began quickly to carve. Soon all the plates were piled high with meat, roast and boiled potatoes, brussels sprouts, and stuffing, while the cranberry sauce and gravy boat were passed along the table. Finally, when all the ladies were seated, Ted, standing at the top of the table, raised his glass and said,

"Here's a Happy Christmas to all of us, and may we have a prosperous New Year."

They all raised their glasses and drank the toast, and in after years Richard often recalled the memory of all the smiling faces as he looked along the table, and the feeling of happiness he experienced in that magical moment.

In spring he went to Higher Hindshead. He was greeted with open arms by his aunt and uncle and thoroughly spoiled, but he helped on the farm in every way he could. He gave them all the news of Westend and of Ezra's accident, and Dick looked at Alice and said,

"I wonder if Martha let Harry and Jane know about it, they're not much at writing letters at Westend." Richard had heard the names mentioned at home and, being curious, asked where they lived.

"They live near each other in Alresford down south. Your Uncle Harry is a cattle dealer in a fair way of business. We don't often see him, but he and your Aunty Jane always come to weddings and of course funerals; he put us in touch with Tom when we wanted a shepherd."

Richard asked about his cousins, and why wasn't his own father farming, and how did he become a soldier?

Dick said, "Yes, you have three cousins: two boys and a girl. Your dad joined the Army after your grandfather died. Under his will our home Elm Bank Farm, quite a bit of land, and a lot of property he owned in the village, as well as rows of houses in Linfield which your grandmother had left at her death were sold and the proceeds divided equally among the four of us. But your father being the eldest claimed he should have inherited the farm and cut up a bit rough, and in the end when he got his share he went into the Army. My sister, your Aunt Jane, went to live near Henry, but she has not married yet and works in the cathedral in Winchester."

In this way Richard learned that farming was in his blood, and accounted for its great attraction for him and his love for horses and cattle. He enjoyed being here and promised that he would come back in the summer.

It was on a Saturday morning at Westend that he felt the first awakening of interest in the disease of animals. It was late spring, the overnight rain had ceased, and now the sky was cloudless and the sun hot as he rode on his bike up the green road that led to the farthest field. John was hereabouts repairing the hedge where the cows had broken through a few days before, and in a basket strapped onto the carrier of the bike was the midmorning snack for the two of them. This "baggin" as it was called was bread and cheese sandwiches, and with it was a kit of hot tea and two pint mugs. Suddenly John appeared in the distance, running towards him, and shouting,

"Go and get Dad, quick; there are two cows blown in the six acre."

Richard put the basket down and rode back as fast as he could to the farm where he shouted the message to his uncle.

"Hell, we've got to move fast; wait a sec," he said and rushed into the house, reappearing with a knife in his hand; then into the shippon and came out pushing bottles into his pockets.

"Off quick," he said, mounting on the back step of the bike. Richard strained every muscle to get going across the yard, and then pedalled fast up the track, meeting the herd coming towards them.

"Keep going," said his uncle and then there was John in the small field. Ezra was off the bike quickly and ran to the side of the cow which was very swollen. "Nose her, John," and the cow bellowed and blew froth and saliva all over him, and Richard saw that his uncle was holding a knife in the cow's side, from which a foul-smelling gas whistled as it escaped.

"Hold her nose, Richard; John, drench t'other one, here's the bottle; she's not too bad." Richard watched the cow going down rapidly, and finally his uncle withdrew the knife; there was very little blood.

"Now, hang onto her horns, Richard," he said as he uncorked a bottle, seized the cow's nose, pulled the head up and pushed the bottle into her mouth. The cow gulped and coughed, then belched and the smell of turpentine was strong. The three of them pushed her into a sitting position, as the other cow began slowly to walk away.

"She's a good deal better already," said Ezra. "Richard, take your bike, and quietly walk her home." When they arrived at the buildings she walked in, and into her stall. Martha had tied the others up in their places, and now tied up the sick one and said,

"You watch her, Richard, while I bring you some tea."

This latter was very welcome as it was almost lunch time. Slowly the cow became normal, drank water from a bucket, repeatedly belched, and passed copious amounts of watery dung. Martha said, "I think she'll do now," and as they walked out of the shippon, they saw the other cow almost her normal size walking towards them. She was tied up, and carbolised oil poured into the wound. She was given a drink of water but nothing to eat. When they were having their meal Richard asked,

"Uncle, what made the cows ill?"

"Wet grass," said Ezra.

"But Uncle, they always eat wet grass when it's raining and they don't blow up then."

"I know that, Richard, but I don't know what started it this morning. The vet might be able to tell you; anyway I must get some more blown drinks off Day's man, or at the chemists on Saturday."

Richard was puzzled by the events of the morning and could not understand why only two cows had blown up, when all of them had got into the six-acre. On this morning the idea of becoming a veterinary surgeon was born.

That evening Richard took Leo for a walk on a leather lead. After being tied up all day the dog enjoyed these outings, sniffing at all the trees, and investigating the ditch bottoms. Richard was looking at the wild flowers at the side of the road, when Leo suddenly took off, so quickly that Richard stumbled and fell but grimly clung onto the lead and was dragged along the road and then into the hedge by Leo, who had seen a cat. Not being able to get through the hedge, the dog stopped and barked furiously. Richard got to his feet, scolding the dog, and surveyed his bleeding hands torn by the gravel on the road. His trousers were torn at the knee, but it did not worry him because they were old ones he used for work. When he arrived back at the farm, it was dusk, and Ezra was crossing the yard carrying a lighted oil lamp.

"What's happened to you, Richard?"

"Oh, Leo chased a cat, pulled me off my feet, and dragged me along the road," said Richard.

"Let me have him. I'm glad you hung onto him otherwise we would have had to look for him half the night; go and get your hands washed and then come with me," said Ezra.

When Richard had rejoined him, Ezra said, "I am going to have a look at Dolly, she's been a bit colicky tonight, though she is not due for a week yet."

They soon found her in the field, and watched her for some time, because she kept looking round at her flank. Once she pawed the ground with a fore foot, then shook herself, and walked nearer to the men.

"What's the matter, old lady?" said Ezra, patting her neck, and then stroking her muzzle. She stood quietly for some time, and finally he said, "I think it's the foal kicking, she seems easier now. We'll leave her for a bit, and you can get to bed but I'll sleep for an hour or two in the kitchen and then come and have another look at her."

She was normal on the Sunday when Richard went home. The following Saturday his first question to John was, has she foaled yet?

"No, but she is very near it," he replied. The mare was grazing in the field near the house, and she could be watched from the kitchen window, but nothing happened all day; so it was decided that the men would keep watch on her all night. At five o'clock John shook Richard awake, so he quickly dressed and went to the field to watch Dolly. It was a lovely cool morning, and as all was quiet he brought a chair from the house, and in comfort resumed his duty. Later the mare lay down and suddenly strained; he immediately ran to the house shouting,

"Come on, she has started."

When they got back to her the mare was on her feet, and over the next few minutes, strained several times, and walked round slowly in a circle. After she had made more attempts to foal, Ezra said, "It won't be long now," and Richard could see a shiny bluish white lump swelling up beneath the mare's tail, but in spite of more expulsive efforts over the next few minutes nothing else happened, though she repeatedly got up and down. John joined them and his father said,

"There's something wrong. It should be here by now. Richard, get on your bike up to the post office, and tell them to get Mr McAllister to a mare that can't foal, as quick as you can."

Richard was on his bike and away in a flash; he was really fond of Dolly, and was puzzling in his mind what could be wrong. The message delivered, he cycled back rapidly as he did not want to miss anything, but felt a twinge of fear when he saw his aunt and the two men walking across the yard. "Has she had it?" he shouted, but was unprepared for the body blow delivered by his aunt as she turned towards him, tears running down her face, and said in a quiet voice, "No she's dying." They trooped into the kitchen.

"Why is she dying?" asked Richard.

Raising his arms in a helpless sort of way Ezra said, "Because the damned foal is somehow coming through the wrong hole, and she's in a bloody mess!"

Speechless, Richard slowly drank the mug of tea, and looking at the clock realised that only an hour had passed since he had begun watching Dolly.

"He's coming," said John, going to the door, "And he's fairly shifting."

The engine of the Douglas motor-bike died away, and the rider pulled off his glasses and asked, "Where is she?"

"In the field," said John, leading the way.

"And I have got the water, soap and towel," said Ezra, "And Richard, bring that big leather bag."

When he got to her, he was not prepared for the tragic sight the mare presented behind. The two passages were torn into one, through which two bloody twisted legs protruded amid a mass of shiny grey intestine.

"Mr Holden, I'm sorry, but there's no hope for her," said the vet.

"I thought as much," said Ezra, "Put her out of her misery quick."

Richard went and stroked Dolly's head, then set off back to the house with his aunt close behind. He heard the vet say: "Behind the wall, you two," followed by the crack of the pistol shot. Assembled in the kitchen, more tea was drunk and Mr McAllister asked if Dolly had been insured for foaling.

"Yes," said Ezra quietly.

"Right, give me the forms and I'll fill them in when I've had a look at her at Whiteside's. I'll tell them on my way back," said the vet.

Bob Whiteside was the local knacker, a big pleasant man, indispensable in this area with so much livestock. Richard, very calm now, took a silent vow to become a veterinary surgeon, and went up to the bedroom, choking back the tears.

The next few weeks were spent studying difficult areas of the subjects he had to take in the examinations, and revising as much as he could, but he was glad when they were all over and he could get back to Westend for the weekend. He was glad to see them all, and found plenty to do because one of the men had left, but felt intensely sad for a moment when he went to bring old Lofty from the stable, and saw the empty stall where Dolly used to stand. John told him how Ezra had spent half a morning at the cheese merchant's extolling the merits of his cheese, and how finally he had got paid a farthing a pound more, making $3\,^3/_4$ pence a pound.

On Monday he drove the pony and trap to Droughton to the warehouse, and helped to unload the cheeses, and had to make another trip to complete the emptying of the pantry at the farm. Coming back along the straight road which passed the farm, he tickled the pony with the point of the umbrella. He was amazed at the speed she could move, and decided to ask Ezra if he could ride her in the field that night. Permission granted, he found he could stay on riding bareback, though it made his legs ache, but his uncle told him to persevere if he wanted to be a good rider. For this advice he was very grateful in later years, when he could ride any horse, however fractious it might be. For getting his Matric. with two distinctions his father bought him a second-hand saddle at the shop in Church Street. Using this present he rode Mollie regularly, and found out she could jump when she went flying over a drainage trench John had dug at the top end of the long pasture where the ground was getting boggy.

The need was for a second heavy horse for the general farm work, and Ezra went to a Shire horse sale and bought a five-year-old black Shire gelding. He was lively and powerful, and soon proved his stamina at harvest, and especially on the day when Richard drove him to the railway sidings in Droughton to get five tons of coal for the winter. He strode up the hill on the way back to the farm making light of the load he was hauling. Richard admired him and was proud to be seen driving him, and thought he was not called Chieftain for nothing. At the farm he tipped the coal at the end of the cart shed, loosed the horse and let him drink at the trough. When one of the cats ran behind him he kicked at once, and after he was unharnessed and tied up in his stall he kept stamping his hind feet.

Richard went to Hindshead to spend the rest of the school holidays, just in time to help clip the last few sheep using hand clippers under Tom's guidance. He told Richard not to blame himself when one of the sheep he had clipped became ill and died two days later. "We always lose some after clipping and dipping." These losses were accepted as normal, but he was disappointed when Dick and Tom did not know the reason for them; there seemed to be so many deaths among stock which were mysterious. In the evening he gave his aunt and uncle all the news from Westend: the death of Dolly, what a powerful horse Chieftain was, and how he was riding Mollie. Ezra, he said, had had a good hay time, and also sold his cheese well, and when Dick asked him what was he was going to do, he said he wanted to be a vet and so must go back to school, and try to get a scholarship.

"So you have got it all worked out; which college would you like to go to?" asked Dick.

"I don't know, but Mr McAllister went to one in Scotland, Ezra told me," replied Richard.

"Maybe, but it's a long way from home, and your mother wouldn't like that, I'm sure. But there's at least one in England, I'll ask our vet the next time I see him."

This occurred sooner than expected. They were having breakfast one day when Tom knocked on the diningroom door, entered, and said that a beast was dead up the field.

"Damn! That's a bad do," said Dick, "I was thinking of selling some now they are so fit. What do you think it is?"

"I don't really know," said Tom, "But in case it is blackleg I've moved the rest into Longshaw."

"Right, Tom, you can't do anything else, so you get your breakfast and I'll go and get a message to the vet," said Dick.

This was Mr Brookman, a fair-haired man of medium height and with a pleasant manner, who arrived riding a Red Indian motor-bike.

"What's this? You have lost one of your cows, Mr Holden?"

"No," replied Dick, "It's a good store beast Tom found dead this morning."

"Right, I'll have to take a blood sample to find out." said the vet.

He unstrapped the box, and a small case from the back of the bike. When they reached the animal Richard was very interested, and watched the vet make a little cut with a small scalpel in the skin of the ear, put a drop on to a glass slide, and then spread a thin film with the scalpel. He lit a spirit lamp and carefully dried the blood film over the flame, and then passed the scalpel through the flame. Back at the farm he prepared the slide, and examined it using a microscope. Looking up, he said,

"It is blackleg, so it can be moved."

"No, I think I will bury it," said Dick.

"Well, I wouldn't. It's a difficult germ to get rid of if it gets into the soil; get it moved, then pour paraffin over the spot where it died and set fire to it, afterwards lime it well, and fence it off."

Dick said he would and then introduced his nephew, saying "Richard here wants to be a vet." Over a cup of tea, Mr Brookman gave him a lot of useful information, and told him about the two colleges in England, in London and Liverpool. He also answered his questions about blackleg, and told him also about the dreaded anthrax.

"But mainly concentrate on chemistry, and learn all you can about looking after livestock, and knowing all the breeds. Can you ride a horse? Yes? That's essential, because you will have to ride all sorts to test them for soundness...but I must be off." With that he began to run, pushing the motor-bike until the engine started; then he leapt on and rode away.

John and Richard became firm friends, and spent some of their free time together in the village where John was a member of the cricket club, and could be counted on to knock up a good score when batting at No. 3 on a Saturday afternoon. After the match in the evening John would spend an hour with the team in the Bull's Head in Weston. That Christmas all the families converged on Westend for the lunch; it was a sunny day, though cold, and all enjoyed the traditional meal, the banter and the happiness. Afterwards simple presents were given to the young people and carols were sung accompanied by Mary Holden on the piano, but all too soon they set off for home well wrapped up against the frost of the early evening.

Wednesday 19 July was a glorious sunny day, so Ezra, John and the hired man were out early in the fields turning the hay. After the midday meal, Lofty and Chieftain pulling the hay wains were driven to the first field, and steadily all worked together loading the warm, dry, fragrant hay onto the wagon until it was piled high. Then Ezra and the man drove it back to the farm where it was off-loaded into a bay in the Dutch barn. Martha, carrying a big wicker basket with a broad handle which contained kits of cold sweet tea, cheese and cake, joined them for the return journey. They all helped John load, and with Richard went to the farm. On their return in the middle of the afternoon they ate their snack in the shade of an oak tree, and then continued to load until 5 o'clock when both carts came back, leaving Martha and the labourer with Bracken to round up the cows, and drive them in for milking. When this was finished and a meal had been eaten, they returned to the field and worked for another two hours and were all glad to ride up with the last loads of the day. Soon the horses were loosed out and they were quickly at the watering trough where they drank their fill.

Then Ezra led Lofty into the stable, followed by John leading Chieftain; the harness was removed and hung on the big brackets which were attached to the heel post at the end of each stall. The horses began to eat noisily and John got a broom and started to sweep the droppings along the channel behind them, Ezra picked up a shovel and stood watching him. As John swept, he touched a strap which was hanging down and the headcollar fell behind Chieftain. As he bent down to pick it up the horse kicked him on the side of the head. John, uttering a cry, fell back against the wall; Ezra dropped the shovel, grabbed him by the shoulders and dragged him along the floor clear of the horses, shouting, "John, John, has he hurt thee badly?" but as he dropped to his knees beside his son he saw the right eye and forehead were already a bloody pulp; blood was pouring from his nose and staining his golden hair, while his breathing was getting more stertorous. At once he gathered John in his arms, hoisted him onto his shoulders and staggered out of the stable shouting at the top of his voice, "Martha!" She met him at the kitchen door, with Richard close behind her. They gently laid John on the long settee, and she ran and brought a blanket saying, "What are we going to do?"

"Do? why, drive like hell to fetch Dr Derham while you stay here with him," and with that he ran across to the stable. Richard was transfixed with fear as he looked at John, but very soon they heard the trap rattle across the yard, Ezra shouting "Get up with thee!" and the crack of the whip.

Martha knelt down beside her son and softly said, "Can you hear me, Johnny, speak to me please, please speak to me." As there was no response, she stroked his hair, then seeing the blood on her hand began to sob and moan.

"Oh God, spare my Johnny, please save him," and her sobbing became louder.

Thus Ezra and the doctor found them when they hurried in and all three, almost holding their breath, watched anxiously as the examination was made carefully and gently, until the doctor rose to his feet, and one look at his face confirmed their worst fears.

Hesitantly Martha asked, "He isn't going to die is he?"

Dr Derham put his arms around her shoulders and said, "Yes."

She slumped forwards and began to cry hysterically, "Oh, not again." Ezra and the doctor supported her and lowered her into the old armchair and stood there trying to comfort her. A little later when they looked at John they saw his breathing had stopped, a reflected ray of the setting sun briefly illuminated his face, and an intense silence filled the room.

Richard was dazed by what he had just seen; it was the first time he had seen a dead person, and with his emotions in turmoil he opened the door, mumbled that he was going home, and went outside. The cool evening breeze steadied him and he jumped out onto his bike and rode home as fast as he could. Having put his bike in the garden shed, he opened the kitchen door to find his mother finishing baking. She looked at him and said,

"Richard, whatever's the matter?"

He said nothing but walked into her arms, and suddenly the dam burst, and he sobbed out the tragic story. She made him sit down in the living room and, opening the door which led into the hall, she called Ted and Mary to come at once. This they did and soon learned the reason for her brusque command. While they sat talking to Richard she made some sandwiches and brewed some tea, and brought the meal in on a tray.

"Mum, I don't want anything," said Richard.

"Maybe you don't," said Victoria, "But you are going to have something to eat, and then get out of those dirty clothes, and go and have a bath, and go to bed, my boy."

Feeling very miserable, Richard started to eat, and his father said:

"You wouldn't think lightning would strike the same place twice; it's absolutely dreadful for them."

"Yes," replied his mother, "It's unbelievable; we must go over first thing in the morning."

"What do you mean about lightning?" asked Richard.

"Well, of course you don't know, but their first baby was called John and when he was eleven months old he died of TB of the brain, caught from their best cow. It took your aunt a long time to get over it, and that's why they idolised their second baby, again a boy so he had to be called John too. I am sorry your pal died, but from what you have told us I think he would have been paralysed had he lived and that can be horrible. I can tell you because I have seen them in the Military Hospital," said Ted.

Richard finished his tea and did as he had been told, but it was a long time before he finally cried himself to sleep.

Early next morning Ted rode off on his bike, arriving back about an hour later. He was in command and announced that he had ordered a taxi to take them to the farm at 9 o'clock, but Mary had an exam. for the next grade for piano playing in ten days time, so she would stay home and practise. Richard had to get the big suitcase off the top of the wardrobe in his bedroom, and put into it his and his father's working clothes and boots.

"I called at the coalyard and told your Tom, Vicky: he was speechless; now let's get breakfast over and we can get going," said Ted.

"But what about your work?" asked Vicky.

"Don't worry, I called at Mr Leonard's and told him the position and he gave me compassionate leave at once," replied Ted.

They went to Westend at 9 o'clock, and found the curtains at every window drawn together. All was quiet. As they walked into the kitchen Martha came into the room and in a low voice greeted them and asked them to go on into the diningroom. Vicky put her arms around her and kissed her, saying how sorry she was, and Martha began to cry so they remained behind. In the diningroom they found the Vicar, Knowles the village constable, and Walley the undertaker with Ezra, all seated round the table talking softly. Ted joined them. Richard went across to another group made up of the Healds, the Bartons from the next farm and Tom Seed, the hay and straw dealer. Soon he was telling them about the dreadful events of the night before. Vicky brought in a pot of tea, sugar and milk and the china, and all were grateful for the drink. Knowles announced that he thought the Coroner's inquest would be held on the next day, and after that the funeral could be arranged. Soon the visitors began to leave, but the Vicar took Ezra and Martha into the front room and comforted them until finally they prayed together for the blessing of God Almighty to be upon them.

Richard and Ted changed into their working clothes, and went into the shippon. They found Clegg the hired man, who told them that he and Bill Barton hadn't finished the milking until 9 o'clock, and only the pigs had been fed to try and stop them making such a noise. Now they set to with a will to try and get through the day's work. When Bill Barton came back at 5 o'clock they did the milking, and had just finished when the Walmsleys arrived. Over the evening meal the account of the accident was again given, and Ezra said that they knew that the horse would kick if anything went near or touched his hind legs, and Richard told how he had seen him lash out at one of the farm cats which had gone near him.

"In spite of that our John liked the horse because he was such a good looking powerful beast; that's why he always drove him. He'd been brought up with Shires and could handle the roughest of them, but I'm not keeping him; he's going in the morning. Bob Whiteside has got a horse slaughterer coming for him in the morning."

Whatever differences they had had in the past were now forgotten. Ted told Ezra that as soon as he had got the news he had been to his superior and had got leave at once so that he and Richard could stay and help at once. Ezra looked at his brother and said, "Thanks Ted"; his eyes filled with tears, and he got to his feet and quickly left the room. This brief show of emotion was followed by days when he was silent and grim-faced.

The quiet of the cloudy Thursday morning was broken by the tolling of the muffled passing bell of the centuries-old village church of St. Giles, and by the murmur of the people standing outside the lychgate, and lining the path to the church porch along which the Vicar began to walk slowly, saying the burial service. Behind him six members of the cricket team carried the wreath-covered coffin which was followed by Martha, supported by Ezra on one side and Bob Heald her brother on the other. Richard, holding Mary's hand, went with his parents into the church, and they and all the family were ushered into the pews by the two churchwardens carrying their silver-topped black wands. As the hymn "There's a friend for little children" was sung, many of the congregation were in tears, and again during the moving valedictory address given by the Vicar. It all seemed unreal to Richard as he walked across the graveyard in the pale sunshine, and he was in a dream-like state as he stood at the graveside, but when he threw a handful of soil onto the coffin he realised that his friend had gone forever, and the feeling of loss which surged through him reduced him to tears.

At the farm, lunch was held in the big front room, all the family sitting round two long trestle tables which were covered with white table-cloths, and loaded with food. Here he met his Uncle Harry and his Aunties Joan and Jane as well as his cousins; and of course Dick and Alice, the Healds and the Walmsleys, as well as distant relatives he did not know. Later in his memory of that day, one person stood out from them all—she was the Squire's younger daughter, a beautiful girl, with lovely large, grey eyes, and her dark hair tied with a big velvet bow. Her name, she told him, was Joan.

Working as a team Ezra, Ted, Clegg and Richard soon finished the hay time, and went on to get up the new potatoes, and to cut spring cabbage—the farm work went steadily on, all pulling their weight. One morning he went to the smithy riding Mollie and leading Lofty and met the smith, Tommy Towers, who soon found Richard a job blowing the forge bellows. While he was doing this he watched Tommy working, and began to appreciate the skill needed to practise this age-old craft. The smith obviously knew a lot about him and as they chatted Richard told him that he was hoping to be a vet, and would like to know more about horse shoeing.

"In that case, come here when you have got a spare hour and I'll show you how a shoe is made."

As her new shoes were already made, it was not long before Mollie was shod, and Lofty's loose shoe had been nailed on again, so he thanked Mr Towers and rode back to the farm. At lunch that day his father asked Richard if he would stay at the farm for two more weeks and help out.

"You see I have asked Mr McAllister if you can go with him on his rounds to see if you are going to like all that being a vet entails, and he said you can go in a fortnight."

Richard was thrilled and then said so. Then Ezra said,

"You must know, Richard, that your aunt and me are very fond of you, but we don't want to stand in your way; but we would like you to stay two more weeks, until Harry Gregson can come."

"Oh, Uncle, I will," replied Richard, and quickly learnt a lot more about farming, especially how tiring it is working from 5.30 a.m. until at least 6.00 p.m. seven days a week. He was well-fed, grew more muscular, and was almost six feet tall. One Sunday evening he went to Evensong with his aunt. Across the church he saw Joan sitting with her parents. She smiled at Richard, who soon learnt from Martha that she attended the Girls High School in Droughton; and that the Squire's wife was very wealthy, being the owner of a ladies fashion shop, called Matthews—one of the biggest in Droughton High Street.

Some days later Ezra said, "Harry Gregson should be coming tomorrow. He's a grand chap; he used to have his own farm but he had a lot of bad luck. When they were having their first baby, it was born dead and his wife died of fever three days after. He went to pieces, you couldn't blame him, so he sold up lock, stock and barrel and moved in with his unmarried sister. He kept the Bull going for a bit, and then he settled down, and now helps out. There's nowt he doesn't know about farming. You'll have seen him riding about on his motor-bike."

At 5.45 the next morning Ezra and Richard were drinking tea in the kitchen when the roar of the motor-bike engine died away, there was a knock on the door, and in walked Harry—a broad-shouldered middle-aged man of medium height. He was wearing spectacles; on his head he wore a flat cap, the front of his shirt was open, and his nose was flattened. Ezra said, "I'm glad to see you, Harry, will you have some tea?" This he did; Richard was introduced, and soon they were in the shippon milking the cows.

On Monday morning his father took Richard to Mr McAllister's house at 8.30; the vet obviously knew all about Westend and asked after his uncle and aunt. Later they went out and got into the Model-T Ford and spent the morning going round the stables treating sick horses; in the afternoon they did visits to farms. He enjoyed the fortnight, and was certain this was what he wanted to do, so that when he went back to school he was determined to do well and began to study with great determination. In ten months time, he would have to take the Higher School Certificate Examination, on the results of which his chances of getting a scholarship would depend. His sister, two years younger, was also working hard, to pass another examination for piano playing. Her piano was in the lounge, and she practised every night which distracted Richard, so he was given a big study bedroom at the back of the house. Besides all the usual bedroom furniture, there was a table, chairs and a glass-fronted bookcase. There was another distraction–one very wet November day he went to school on the tram and, seeing Joan, sat down beside her. She told him that she stayed in Droughton at her aunt's during the week as a day boarder and went home to Weston from Friday to Sunday night. He asked if he could walk her home occasionally, and soon they did this once or twice a week, and rapidly became friends; he began to consider her to be his girl, and to day-dream about her when he should have been studying.

At Christmas he went for a week to Westend, and helped in any way he could, because there was so much work to do. They were all glad to see him, and he was learning many skills: how to dress a chicken; how to draw the sinews out of a turkeys legs; how to cut hay from the stack; and at the smithy how to take off a horse's shoe.

One night he went with Harry to the village pub, the Bull's Head. It was a long low building, the Snug at one end and the Taproom at the other, and this was the room they entered. Inside there was a babel of voices; the air was blue with tobacco smoke, and the big fire burning in the Jacobean fireplace made the room very hot. Harry was well-known, and introduced Richard as "Yon Ezra Holden's nephew, a real handy lad", to some village men, and he began to talk to Willie Barton from the next farm. Soon, having got a beer each and found a seat, they sat drinking and talking in a group about horses, the Society's travelling stallion and cattle troubles—one man said that he had lost a new calved heifer with redwater. The conversation turned to the poor price for milk and eggs, and what would Ezra do? Harry was smoking twist in a clay pipe, and the smoke made Richard's eyes water. He had tried smoking a pipe previously, but disliked the taste of twist tobacco and did not attempt it again; so he sometimes smoked a Wild Woodbine cigarette. An hour soon passed, and it was pleasant walking the mile and a half back to the farm chatting non-stop, until finally Richard asked Harry how he got his nose broken. Harry laughed and said, "Boxing–I was in the Droughton club when I was younger."

"But you couldn't box wearing glasses," said Richard.

"Now, you are quite right, you see I had a lot of bad health. I got TB when I was a child and that's why I have these two big scars on my neck where the doctor lanced my glands. I was kept at home for years and missed a lot of schooling, but my mother fed me up and I grew into a strong lad; working on the farm at home helped a lot. So I was beginning to be a good boxer when I was about eighteen, when I went to see our Nellie, you know Bartons at the next farm, and caught measles off her kids. You see, I missed it with not going to school, at least so the doctor said, and it attacked my eyes and now I am short-sighted. But I can still spar a bit. Can you box, Richard?"

"No, I can't," replied Richard.

"Well I'll give you a few lessons, you should be able to defend yourself."

Harry was as good as his word; he brought two pairs of boxing gloves to the farm, and regularly after they had had their midday meal they would go into an empty bay in the Dutch barn, and he taught Richard the basics of the art of boxing. He found his reflexes were very good, that he had a powerful right, and soon became keen to be a good boxer.

At Easter he went about with Mr McAllister and began to find his way about the surgery which was at the back of the house. This was a huge room at one end of which there was a broad long table. Round the walls were three tiers of shelves on which were packets of powders, large medicine bottles, whiskey bottles with contents of varying colours, and many jars. Under the shelves were hampers, three-foot-high yellow glazed jars with labels he could not understand, and tins. In one corner was a cupboard on which was a label which read, "Poison–Keep Locked". A door led into an outer room which was bisected by a mahogany counter and in the wall-cupboards at each end were more packets of powders, bottles and jars. The door beyond the counter opened into the back street and moving it rang a large bell. It was here that the horse foreman from the stables in the town, and the farmers on market day, came to obtain all the medicines and dressings they needed. The first time Richard stood there watching Mr McAllister give out so many different things he realised how much there was to learn and in this mood went back to school for the crucial term.

When he sat his examinations in the summer he was quietly confident he had done well, but he became very anxious during the five weeks' wait for the results. During this time he spent two weeks at Hindshead, and Dick and Alice were very pleased to see him and get all the latest news from him. He arrived home in time to go with his family to the seaside for a week where they stayed in a private hotel. The weather was good and the two children were taught to swim by their father. When he was older Richard was sad to realise that this holiday had been a turning point in his life; it was the last holiday they spent as a family, and from then on he had to stand on his own feet and make his own decisions; because when the examination results were published he had won a scholarship.

The school hall filled up rapidly on the day of the Prize Giving. The masters wearing their black gowns found seats for all the relatives and friends of the prize-winners. When the Governors and the masters were seated on the stage at the end of the hall, the school orchestra began to play "Country Gardens" by Percy Grainger until the Mayor of Droughton, Alderman Wood, wearing his gold chain of office, was ushered in by the Headmaster followed by Professor Winston the guest speaker who would present the prizes. When the two dignitaries were seated, the hymn "Praise my soul the King of Heaven" was sung by the assembly, led by the school choir and accompanied by the orchestra and the organ. Suddenly Richard stopped singing, overcome by the emotion, and, swallowing vigorously, brushed the tears from his eyes. He never forgot that day in high summer, the excitement he felt; the beautiful hymn singing; the professor's speech, and then the Headmaster announcing that the school had obtained two State Scholarships and the roar of the applause that followed. They had been won by Harry Attwater and Richard Baden Holden. Harry had also won the Senior Classics prize which was given by the Corporation of Droughton, and Richard the Senior Science prize given by the School Governors. The Professor congratulated both of them, the Mayor presented the prize to Harry, and Dr Gordon, the Chairman of the School Governors, a scientist of great distinction, presented Richard with his prize. As he shook hands with Dr Gordon, Richard felt himself perspiring, his knees were shaking, and his mouth was so dry he found it difficult to say "Thank you".

Soon all the prizes were presented, the hymn "Lord dismiss us with Thy blessing" and the National Anthem were sung, and he found himself surrounded by his family and school friends, all patting him on the back and congratulating him. Later, as they all walked to the main road to the tram stop, Richard turned to look back at the grey stone building, acutely aware of his attachment to the place, and the intense pang of regret he felt at leaving it. He arranged to meet Joan later, and that evening they walked round the Beacon—a hill covered in gorse and bracken—probably more than three miles and talked of the future. She told him that she had got her Matric., and was leaving High School and going to college to take a course in Domestic Science, in Liverpool.

"I'm going there," said Richard, "So we will be able to see each other."

"But it will only be for two years, and then I will go to London," said Joan.

Richard told her that the veterinary course lasted for four years, and that he had written to the Secretary of the Board of Veterinary School applying for a place, that October. By now they had arrived at her aunt's house and he was invited in to meet her relatives who were polite but cool towards him. The house stood in its own grounds where there was a tennis court. It was beautifully furnished, and had a ballroom and a billiard room, and he quickly sensed that they thought he was socially a long way below them. Nevertheless he never forgot that thrilling moment when he kissed her for the first time when they said good night.

II

The Secretary of the Board of Veterinary Studies examined Richard's birth certificate, his Matriculation and Higher School certificates, and all the letters he had received concerning his scholarship, and informed him that they would be retained until after the meeting of the Board which would be held on 7 September. Richard took the booklet about the University Veterinary School and the course of studies held there, and various pamphlets, thanked the Secretary and spent the rest of the day exploring the university precincts and the centre of the city.

After he had been accepted as a student he went with his father and found a university approved lodging, which proved to be a fortunate choice because when the academic year began there were ten undergraduates staying there and three of them were veterinary students. He worked hard, studying botany, zoology and osteology but finding the chemistry and physics easy.

Quickly the first term was over, and during the Christmas vacation, he went to Westend, unprepared for Ezra's news: that he was giving up the tenancy of the farm on the next quarter day, and would have a sale of live and dead stock. Feeling a bit miserable that evening he went to the Bull's Head, just in time to buy the last ticket in the Cricket Club Raffle, and spent a happy hour with the team, Bill Barton and Harry Gregson, who all wanted to know how he was getting on in Liverpool.

The next evening he was talking to his aunt and uncle in the farm kitchen, when there was a knock on the door and in walked Harry Gregson, with a big smile on his face.

"Here, you're a lucky beggar; you've won the first prize," he said, handing Richard a big turkey. It was bedtime before he had finished plucking and dressing it.

The next evening he went with his mother to a Fur and Feather Whist Drive which was held in St. Thomas's Church Hall. Vicky won the first prize and it too was a turkey, so they decided to take it to her brother Tom Bradshaw; he and Winifred were delighted and invited them to lunch on Boxing Day. One night they went to hear the *Messiah* sung in church, and another night they went to the Carol Service where Mary was a soloist; finally all the family at 11 p.m. on Christmas Eve went to church for the first communion of Christmas. The church was lit by candles in the two great candelabra hanging from the ceiling, and other candles were on every window sill.

A few days later in the evening he went with Mr McAllister to the railway stables to treat a horse with colic. When they drove into the yard they were met by the horse foreman wearing the dark railway uniform and a peaked hat.

"Good evening Lewis," said Mr McAllister.

"Good evening," Lewis replied. "I've had to send for you, Sir, because it's big Silver; he started about 6 o'clock and we drenched him with some of your pink medicine, but he is no easier. I didn't want him cast in his stall so he is in No. 2 Box."

"Good," said the vet, and Richard, carrying the leather bag, followed them into the gas-lit box. The horse, sweating on his neck and flanks, was sitting upright and wisps of vapour were rising from him. They made the horse rise and Mr McAllister using his stethoscope listened to both flanks.

"Nothing much there, I'm afraid, but the medicines have eased the spasms and we must dose him now to get his bowels moving."

Richard opened the bag and the vet took out a big tin drenching bottle, and a laxative drink and a stimulant drink which he poured into the bottle and then filled it to the top with water. He and Richard climbed up into the manger while Lewis got a pole which had a hook on the end, and pushed it into a metal link of the head collar. Now they pulled the horse's head up from above and Lewis pushed on the pole from below, and when they got it high enough the bottle was forced into the horse's mouth and upended. It swallowed most of it but some was splashed over them.

"Right, Lewis, throw a rug over him, don't let him get down and let's get him outside."

The horse was led out and for half an hour walked around the yard, and then brought inside and re-examined.

"Richard, get a bucket of water and let's try him."

The horse drank some water and then stopped and looked towards its flank. There was a rumbling noise and it passed wind.

"Well, Lewis, I think it's passing off, so we will go now, but walk him for another half hour and then try him again with water and a little hay. If he eats and drinks you can leave him."

"Yes, I'll do that, Sir, but before you go, will you give me four bottles of pink medicine, and can you come tomorrow morning and rasp two horses' teeth, they are quidding."

"Yes, I'll do that, and see you in the morning."

"Goodnight Sir," said Lewis and closed the gate behind them. As they drove back to the surgery Mr McAllister commented that he had had enough work for one day and hoped there were no more visits that night. Richard was pleased when there were none, because he had to catch the 7.40 a.m. train to Liverpool in the morning.

That summer he passed his first professional examination, a fitting reward for studying all through the Easter vacation, though he did make time to go to Westend to see Mollie and Lofty before they were sold. Later his father told him that Ezra and Martha had had a good sale and were staying with the Healds temporarily until they found a smallholding not too far from Droughton. So Richard with his two college friends Norman Robinson and Evan David Jones would in three months time begin their second year studying veterinary anatomy and physiology.

Richard went to Mr McAllister's at the beginning of the long vacation, and there found another change taking place. The vet was retiring because his health was deteriorating, but he sent Richard to see Colonel McGregor who had the biggest horse practice in the town and premises half a mile away. The Colonel saw him in the office in his surgery, and agreed at once to let him see practice with him and would not charge Richard a premium, provided he would work and help in the practice. Richard agreed at once to these terms and on the following Monday was at the surgery at 9 a.m. It was on the left side of a large square yard, at the bottom of which were six loose boxes, and on the right a shoeing forge. Outside this two horses were waiting while the ringing sound of the smith's hammers on the anvil echoed across the yard. It was altogether a more business-like set-up than Mr McAllister's had been. Richard was very impressed by it all and was a little in awe of the highly regarded Colonel. The office was a well-lit room with two large windows and the carpet was large and of Persian make. A large roll-top desk stood by the window and near it a Chippendale chair. The large mahogany bookcase was crammed with books and on top of it stacks of the *Veterinary Record*. In the centre of the wall crossed lances were fixed; to the left of them hung the Colonel's Diploma of Membership of the Royal College of Veterinary Surgeons, and to the right his Diploma of Fellowship.

When Richard entered the office the Colonel came into the room by another door and said, "Good morning, Mr Holden, would you like to come through into the works department."

Richard followed him into a rectangular room in the centre of which was a large table. Here a grey-haired bespectacled man was standing mixing some powder in a mortar with a pestle.

"Mr Wilkinson, this is Mr Holden, a student who will be here all the holiday, and he will be helping you when he is not with me."

"Good morning, Sir," said Wilkinson, and they shook hands.

"Mr Holden, stay with Bob while I get on," and the Colonel was gone, leaving a cloud of cigarette smoke behind him.

"Now, Mr Holden, when the Colonel's not around we use Christian names. Mine is Bob, what is yours?"

"Richard," he replied.

"Good; now on Mondays we dispense. Usually Tommy is here, but at the moment he is in one of the boxes getting it ready for an operation," said Bob.

Richard asked what Bob was making.

"Tonic powders for horses," was the reply. "This is the recipe book for all the medicines and powders and the drinks you can see on the shelves, and one look round tells you what has been used and so you dispense some more," said Bob.

"And what is this powder, Bob?" asked Richard.

"It's the top one on that page in the book," said Bob. Richard read *Pulv Gentian; Pulv ferri Sulph; Pulv Sodii Bic; Pulv glycyrrhizae*; all followed by Apothecaries' Script; it was all Greek to him; but soon under Bob's guidance he was putting a large spoonful of the powder on to a square of white paper and learning how to fold it correctly and make up the bundles of six powders and label them. They made up powders steadily until the Colonel came in and told Richard to go with him.

They went across the yard and into a box which was thickly bedded with straw, and there they found Tommy and a handsome young man with dark curly hair who gave the impression of being very self-assured and very smartly dressed, wearing a hacking jacket and buff-coloured breeches. He greeted the Colonel who turned to Richard and said:

"Do you know Mr Harrison? He's a final year student at the Royal Dick Veterinary College in Edinburgh."

They shook hands and Tommy brought in a half-bred colt, and put on its head the blinds, while the Colonel put on the twitch.

"Back him into a corner."

Harrison in the meantime had brought in a big sterilizer, which contained instruments, and then a portable wash basin and a leather case.

"Right, gentlemen," said the Colonel. "I am going to castrate this colt under local anaesthetic. Harrison, open the case, please, and take the lid off the sterilizer."

William Harrison knew the drill, and handed the Colonel a loaded syringe, the contents of which were injected into the colt's scrotum and testicles. While this was taking effect the Colonel scrubbed his hands and Harrison opened three wooden clamps. Selecting a scalpel, the Colonel quickly carried out the operation, and Harrison handed him the leather keepers and pliers.

"Right, Tommy, take the blinds off and the twitch and give his nose a rub."

Richard was surprised that there was so little blood, and that the operation had been done so quickly. The Colonel washed his hands and dried them; Harrison carried the instruments and the bag outside and Richard carried out the wash basin.

"Mr Holden, get a fork and take that bloody straw outside, and Tommy, let him have a drink of water and a small feed. Come along gentlemen," and soon they were in a bigger box where most of the floor was taken up by a casting bed—a very thick layer of straw covered by a tarpaulin which was secured to the floor. On this bed were laid out the casting hobbles, the spring D clip, the blinds and the twitch, and from the ceiling hung an electric fitment on which were four large bulbs. Along one wall was a large table and in the corner a white earthenware sink which was being filled with water from the hot and cold taps. Steam issued from the gas-heated sterilizer which was on the table with cloths and towels. The cupboard above was open, and full of bottles with various labels: Chloroform; Lysol–Poison; spiritus Meth; and jars labelled *Sapo. Mollis, Sapo. Hydrargyri Perchol* (Poison) and *Tinct Iodi.* Richard was fascinated but the Colonel soon had his attention.

"Now, gentlemen, the next is a three-year-old Shire colt. He is older than is usual because he was being kept for breeding but his conformation is not good enough, so we will cast and then anaesthetise him. Mr Holden and Tommy, you will keep his head up when he is down. Mr Harrison, will you bring Davies from the smithy, you will put in the spring D and give the usual dose of chloroform. Where is the mask?"

"Here it is, Sir."

"Right, turn the taps off, put some Lysol in the water and turn on the lights. Tommy, bring him in. When he is anaesthetised, Mr Harrison, scrub up and help me. Turn that sterilizer off, Mr Holden, put those gloves on and lift up the tray: don't touch the instruments."

In came Tommy with a 17-hands black Shire, Davies the smith following behind. The horse was a bit fresh but Davies held on to it and Tommy put on the blinds and then the twitch. Under the Colonel's directions the hobbles were applied and the horse cast. Davies and Harrison pulling the chain, the spring D clipped onto the chain, and Richard and Tommy struggled to keep the horse's head up while Harrison fitted the chloroform mask, opened the drawer at the bottom, and poured in the chloroform. Now the horse really struggled but they kept his head up and then suddenly he went quieter and was unconscious. The Colonel and Harrison washed their hands and arms.

"Davies, let the hobbles go, rope that top leg and pull it up and over."

Davies knew the drill and Harrison brought the tray of instruments. The horse was castrated and the Colonel called, "Catgut!" Harrison pulled out a long length and threaded a needle.

"Because the arteries will be large I am ligaturing them and then there should be no risk of haemorrhage."

The horse began to move slightly.

"Shall I give him more, Sir?"

"No, I've almost finished. Take the hobbles and the rope off him, Davies, and the mask—one each side of his head and don't let him get up."

Davies went out; the instruments were removed. The Colonel rose to his feet and said, "That went very well," and washed again. Later the horse was pushed into a sitting position, and finally rose, a little unsteadily, and after some more minutes Tommy led him out.

Richard noticed that the Colonel was standing by the table with his eyes closed, and was breathing a little quickly. He thought to himself that operating couldn't be as easy as it looked, and must be tiring as well. The Colonel went out and Harrison said to Richard:

"My name is Bill, what's yours?"

"Richard."

"Do you live in Droughton?"

Soon Richard knew a lot about the young student, and found out that Bill's father had been Mayor a few years before, that they lived in a big house not far from the Vicarage, and that he and the Vicar's son had been to a public school in the south of England.

After lunch at home, Richard spent the rest of the day with Bob Wilkinson, making up powders, lotions and dressings. The next day he watched while Harrison removed the clamps from the horse. Many operations followed: removal of tumours, docking, a poll evil and fistulous withers and many more minor ones. Quickly the weeks went by, but this enjoyable period ended tragically, when the Colonel collapsed and died suddenly one evening. Richard was upset and said to Bob that he had liked the Colonel and wondered where he would see practice now. Wilkinson told him to wait and see what happened because now two practices were for sale, but *locum tenens* would be found to run them in the meantime. So, after a year in which he had only seen Joan occasionally, he now went to Weston twice a week and they went for walks and twice he took her to the pictures; it was a firm friendship and very platonic.

Some weeks later Richard got a note from Wilkinson telling him to call at McAllister's surgery, where he learnt that a distant relative of the Colonel's had bought his practice and that Mr McAllister's had been sold to two young men, who were going to develop the cattle and small animal side of the practice. They said that Richard was welcome to come and see practice with them. Soon the late Colonel's practice was moved to new premises, two miles away on the south side of Droughton; the old yard and building were sold and later a new block was built with shops below and offices above.

The young partners did not buy Mr McAllister's house but one in a narrow road in the old part of town. The dispensary was in the cellar, the office and consulting room on the ground floor, and the operating room upstairs. Richard was surprised by this after the orderly way in which Mr McAllister's surgery had been arranged and the business-like arrangement of the Colonel's. One partner was a dour hard-working Scotsman, who was in charge of the cattle work; the other was a quiet man who was most unbusinesslike and always late for appointments. Richard went to the surgery for the last two weeks of that summer holiday and again at Christmas and Easter, but by then realised that he was learning very little because the Scotsman never asked Richard to go with him, and so he spent his time mainly with Bob Wilkinson in the gas-lit cellar making up medicines and powders. The consulting times were 9 a.m., 2 p.m. and 6 p.m., and though a steady trickle of people came, few operations were done, although many medicines were sold, and a lot of animals destroyed—dogs because they were suffering from distemper or stuttgart disease or the after-effects of distemper, and cats suffering from the flu. When he went to the surgery at the beginning of his second long vacation he found the Scotsman had left, Bob had retired and things were very chaotic, and so he told Mr Hendry that he would not be going again.

Richard was dispirited. He had failed in physiology in the second examination and so would have to re-sit that part, at Christmas. He was annoyed with himself because he had got second class honours in anatomy and passed in stable management and shoeing.

During the last year he had become friends with Bill Harrison and bought second-hand books from him, and a few times they had gone together to the local football match, Bill driving Richard there in his Frazer Nash sports car. At Christmas and Easter they had visited each other's homes and had dinner with their respective families.

So Richard was not prepared for the headlines in the local evening paper a few days later. "Sudden death of ex-Mayor's son." The report said that Mr William Harrison, MRCVS who had recently qualified at Edinburgh at the age of twenty-three and was the only child of Alderman William Harrison and Mrs Harrison, had been staying with relatives in Leicestershire. As a result of getting wet through while out cycling with his cousin, Mr Harrison had developed a very bad cold. Arriving home in Droughton his condition worstened and pneumonia had developed from which he died that previous evening. At the funeral the old Parish Church was full, the Mayor and Corporation were present, and Richard and his father sat behind the bereaved family. After the service they saw Tom Seed in the crowd and went to talk to him, and from him Richard got some very good advice.

"You go and see Major 'Johnny' Gillmour in Corchester and tell him I sent you, I know him very well. You could ring him up; here is the number: 696." Richard thanked him, but the information did little to raise his spirits from their low ebb. John, the Colonel and now Bill gone; he felt he wanted to get away and in the evening told his father so.

After dinner they went into the lounge and Ted closed the door and asked his son, "Now what is all this about wanting to get away?"

to be at the surgery in India Road, Corchester at 8.30 a.m. on the following Monday morning for an interview. Richard was pleased to get the letter so quickly after his father had made the initial approach, and thought how business-like—and remembered the Colonel with a pang of regret.

Richard came out of Corchester station at 8 a.m. into a square full of taxis and people; railway vans and horses; porters and trolleys. It was a hive of activity and he plunged straight in and walked up to the driver of a horse-drawn van and asked the way to India Road.

"Straight down the main road here for a quarter of a mile, then turn left and first right. Who do you want there? I know every works in this area, being Express Parcels."

"I don't want a works; I want Major Gillmour's the vet's," said Richard.

"You mean mad Johnny," said the driver, "It's a couple of hundred yards down on the right, you can't miss it."

Richard thanked him and strode along briskly and in twenty minutes was reading the highly polished brass plate outside the door of the two-storey stone-built building. The plate simply said, "J.C. Gillmour FRCVS, Veterinary Surgeon."

Below the bell in the door frame was a notice which said, "Please ring and enter". Richard did so and found himself in a square waiting room furnished with a table and stand chairs. At once another door opened and a lady wearing a smart white coat came in and asked, "Can I help you?"

"Yes," said Richard, "I have an appointment with Major Gillmour at half past eight."

"You are Mr Holden then?" the lady replied, "Please take a seat. The Major will see you soon."

Richard was looking at a copy of the *Tatler* when the lady returned and asked him to come through. He entered a consulting room and then turned left into an office. Behind the large flat-topped desk sat the Major who rose at once and said:

"Good morning Mr Holden, I am glad you are on time because I have a busy morning ahead of me. Now, as to seeing practice with me; you will come on a fortnight's approval, you will live in my house, St. Cuthberts; I propose you are here at 8.30 a.m. next Monday morning. You will need rubber boots, a warehouse coat, a mackintosh and a notebook and pencil for the practice and whatever further clothing you may require. So you have passed your second examination?"

"No," said Richard, "I was referred in physiology."

"Were you now? That's a pity—how did you do in anatomy?" asked the Major.

"I got a second class distinction," said Richard.

"Great," said the Major. "Now you can have a look round." He opened another door and bawled "Mr McDonald," and soon a fair-haired young man came in.

"William, this is Mr Holden, a veterinary student from Liverpool; Mr Holden, this is Mr McDonald." They shook hands.

"Show him round, William," said Johnny, and Richard followed the young man through a general office; dispensary; stock room; operating theatre; kennels; tack room; loose boxes; smithy; a very big yard, half of which was roofed over; and a garage for four cars. Upstairs were three rooms: a kitchen with a table and chairs for staff; a rest room with easy chairs; and a further stock room. He was very impressed by the buildings and their layout and with the general air of cleanliness and tidiness, and so arrived back in the Major's office for the second time. He thanked Mr McDonald, and then the Major.

"Right, Mr Holden, talk it over with your father and if you decide to come, be here at 8.30 a.m. sharp next Monday, but let me know by Thursday. You can phone me here. Goodbye." and with that Richard left, already certain that he would be happy in this practice.

With the consent of his parents he was there on time on the following Monday to be greeted with the order, "Good morning Mr Holden; go and help Brown load my car in the yard."

The vehicle was a Vauxhall with a canvas hood and side screens. Under Brown's direction he filled a suitcase with packets and powders and a crate with bottles of various liniments and medicines. Mr McDonald came in with two other men and Richard soon found out they were his assistant vets–Mr Edwards and Mr Wilson.

"Brown, how many staff are there here?" asked Richard.

"Ten," said Brown, "You'll soon get to know them. They are all nice except Mr Wilson, and Johnny's all right until he gets worked up."

At that moment the Major came into the yard, "Is my car ready, Brown?"

"Yes, Major," Brown replied.

"You've filled it with petrol, oil and water?" asked the Major.

"Yes, Major," Brown replied.

"Right, open the gates; come on man, jump to it." said the Major. Brown grinned and quickly opened the gates. "Mr Holden, go with Mr McDonald." With that he drove the car out of the yard.

Mr McDonald came out and said, "Put your stuff into my car, Richard," and soon they were in the Humber car driving out of the town into the countryside.

That first morning with Bill McDonald always remained fresh in Richard's memory. They visited farms and he watched cattle being examined; placentas removed; chaff taken out of cows' eyes; and angleberries removed from a heifer under local anaesthetic. The sun was shining, the countryside was lovely in July, and Richard's spirits rose quickly because Bill McDonald soon had Richard holding instruments and asking him questions about anatomy of the cow, and made him feel useful and part of a team. Before lunch they made a stop at the post office and Bill went in to ring the surgery to see if there were any messages. Quickly he came out, and off they went to a cow calving, and of course Richard was pulling on one calving rope while the farmer pulled on the other; the malpresentation corrected, the calf soon came–a heifer. They went back to Corchester in high spirits and Richard enjoyed his lunch with the Major, his wife Elizabeth and Bill for company. In the afternoon he watched Mr Wilson operate on two dogs and three cats in the theatre. By the end of the day Richard's misery was gone and he was certain he was going to enjoy being here, with all these new people in such a large practice. He soon learned that the Major was the one who dealt usually with horses, and the salaried partner Mr McDonald covered the practice to the south of the town while Mr Edwards looked after the north. Mr Wilson attended to the small animals and surgeries, having been a house surgeon at the Royal Veterinary College in London.

During the next two weeks he accompanied all the vets on their visits to farms and stables. He made himself useful whenever he could, and began to write up cases he had seen in his case book. At lunch a few days later the Major looked at Mr McDonald and asked:

"Well, Mac, do you think we should let Mr Holden continue seeing practice with us?" For a moment or two Richard was worried as to what the reply would be, because he was so happy here, but he need not have worried.

"Yes," said Mac, "He shows a lot of initiative and is beginning to be a help to me."

"Well, Mr Holden," said the Major, "It seems two great minds think alike, so we will be pleased to have you as a *bona fide* student. That means that you will be shown how to examine animals, and carry out work under our supervision, also the recipe book will be available to you. Can you drive a car?"

"No," said Richard.

"Well, in that case you will have to learn. You must also sign a student's agreement. Mr McDonald and I have decided not to charge you a premium provided your work here is satisfactory," said the Major.

"Thank you very much, Sir," said Richard.

"Oh, you can drop the 'Sir'," said the Major with a smile. "Now let's be doing, we can't sit here all day," and with that he rose and left the room.

"Come on, Holden," said Mac and so a friendship was formed which lasted for years.

They went back to the surgery, where the smith Walter Worthington was waiting for them and they all went to the Brewery where one of the dray horses was lame. Mac said, "I saw it this morning, Walter, and it must be pus in the foot, so I want you to take off the shoe and search it."

"Aye," said Walter and soon they were in a loose box in the Brewery yard. The horse was very lame, near fore, and the foreman backed it to the door. Mac made Richard tap the wall of the hoof with a hammer but the horse didn't flinch too much.

"Pick the foot up, Mr Holden," said Mac, "and hang on." Richard did so and lightly tapped the sole. The horse tried to snatch the leg away, but Richard hung on.

"Righto, drop it," said Mac, "Now put a twitch on him." Walter put on his leather apron, picked up the hoof and knocked off the clenches, hitting the buffer with the hammer, and then levering the shoe off with the pincers. The horse didn't object much to this, but when he thinned the sole with the drawing knife, it began to struggle. He tapped the pared-down sole until he found the most tender spot.

"Shake that twitch up now," said Walter, and with a very sharp searcher he deftly cut a small hole in the sole. Pus flowed out quickly. Walter put the foot down and said, "If you have to do this, Mr Holden, keep your face away when you cut through the sole, because if the pus squirts out and hits you in the eye it can give you a really bad eye or even blind you."

They now soaked the foot in a bucket of water to which lysol had been added. Walter then dried the foot and a piece of carbolised tow was put on the sole covered with a piece of thin tin sheet. Then the shoe was nailed on again, thus keeping the dressing in place, and the protruding bits of the tin sheet were trimmed off.

"Take the twitch off now, Mr Holden."

Richard did so and rubbed the big Shire's nose, while Mac gave the horse an anti-tetanus injection. When the foreman led the horse forward, Richard was surprised to see how much easier it moved already.

"We'll come and see him in a couple of days time. Stop his oats ration, for the moment; but get him exercised round the yard three times a day," said Mac, and with that they returned to the surgery, and Mac told Richard to go and help with the dispensing.

The room was like the one at the Colonel's with a big table, weighing scales, huge earthenware containers of drugs and small barrels containing oils, shampoos and disinfectants. Miss Neeve, the Major's cousin, was in charge, helped by Miss Davies, a blond sixteen-year-old, and Miss Horner, a brunette about twenty years old, who had a great sense of fun. The two girls were packing up powders. Miss Neeve was making worm powders for horses, and said:

"Mr Holden, get the small scales and weigh out 5 grains of arsenic for each powder, put it on the powder and gently mix it in with a spoon. I will fold them up. I need not tell you that arsenic is poisonous so don't lick your fingers."

It was a slow job and the afternoon was over when they had bundled up the last of the twenty-six packets of the powders and stuck on labels giving the instructions for use and a red POISON label. It had been a pleasant afternoon, and Richard now knew the girls' names and that they were in charge of the kennels supervised by Mr Wilson, and had also found out that Miss Horner helped as the theatre nurse at small animal operations.

Each evening he settled down to study after dinner, and had worked through his physiology notes, and begun to read the textbooks again especially, Halliburton's *Physiology*. Mac was proving invaluable because he helped Richard two nights a week, asking him questions and explaining things which Richard had not properly understood—he realised that he had not known enough about the subject at the last examination, but now he knew all about the essential amino-acids, the physiology of the heart and blood chemistry. Here Wilson helped him because it was his subject in which he had done a little research, because he was interested in anaesthesia in animals, and wanted to go back to the Royal Veterinary College in London and become a lecturer in the subject. Towards the end of the holiday Richard realised that he had become completely absorbed with the work of the practice and veterinary matters, so much that he had only been home twice in eight weeks and seen Joan once.

He passed the half of the second examination at Christmas, and spent ten days in Corchester, most of the time with Mac. One rainy, very dark night they went to see a horse with colic in the Canal stables. They were met in the yard near the canal basin by the man who looked after the twelve horses, and they followed him into the stable, their way lit by the light from an oil lamp he was carrying. The stable was long and narrow, and steel bins containing crushed oats were against the wall behind the horses, leaving a three feet wide passage to walk along.

"It's the sixth up, Mr McDonald," said the stable man. "And watch for the fourth one; it kicks,"

Mac had just walked past it and Richard was coming up to it, when it lashed out without warning; at the noise of the steel shoe hitting the steel bin they both jumped away but the bin was badly dented.

"Good God," said Mac. "That devil could have smashed my leg or Richard's. Why the hell don't you put it at the top of the stable?"

"Because this is the widest stall and it's easier to get up to his head because he tries to crush you if he can," said the stable man.

Richard walked briskly pass the horse and Mac began to examine number six.

"He didn't drink tonight, did he?" asked Mac. "No, OK, we will have to get some fluids into him, but first tie that kicker outside."

The horse was removed and Mac returned with a packet of powder, a long tube and a pump.

"Richard, fill that bucket with water and mix this powder in it, and turn the horse round please." It was brought out and backed into the stable again. The stable man held its head and Mac held its nose and quickly passed the stomach tube.

"Now, Richard, put the end of the tube onto that tube on the side of the pump; stick it into the bucket and start pumping."

The two gallon bucket quickly emptied and Mac withdrew the tube, and gave instructions to the stable man. Driving home Richard told Mac how John had been killed, and they talked about the dangers of dealing with animals. Mac promised to teach Richard to pass the stomach tube. By the end of that week he had passed it twice, and was very pleased with himself.

Arriving home he found great excitement—his father had bought a dark blue Morris saloon car. Having learnt to drive in the Army he used the car to go to work in a town ten miles away. He had been promoted and was now manager of the exchange. After Christmas they went to spend the day with Dick and Alice at Higher Hindshead, and Richard sat besides his father watching the movements necessary to drive a car. Some days later he went to the police station in Droughton, paid a shilling and was given a red-backed licence. That evening he tried to drive for the first time and narrowly missed a lamp-post, but by the time he went back to Liverpool, he had driven two miles without difficulty.

He worked really hard back at college studying pathology, Materia Medica, hygiene and dietetics, so much so that he began to get headache and eye strain. Easter was a pleasant break from study, and now that he was studying Materia Medica, dispensing was more interesting, but so varied—he spent one morning using white open-wove bandages and the plaster of paris used by dentists to make plaster of paris bandages, all stored in an air-tight tin box. Wilson one day let him watch the reduction of a fracture of the fore leg of a small dog. A cast of bandages was then applied and brown glue painted on each layer of bandages. It was put in the kennel to recover from the anaesthetic and with Mr Wilson they looked at all the inmates. On the Major's strict orders, all animals coming into the kennels either before operations or as boarders had to be examined and their temperatures taken, and Miss Davies and Miss Horner had to report to Mr Wilson twice daily after looking at all the animals. The cat pens were empty; all the cats had been sent home because one had become ill with a catarrhal cold, and Brown was scrubbing the cages with a solution of formaldehyde and caustic soda in hot water. The Major was annoyed and had told Mr Wilson in no uncertain terms to be more careful when examining cats and dogs. It was obvious that the two men were at daggers drawn. Wilson thought that the criticism was unfair, and was also fed up with the little free time both he and Mr Edwards had. They had four days, Christmas Day, Easter, Whit Sunday and August

Bank holiday free, and one week's holiday a year.

In July he passed his third professional examination with flying colours, and with Norman and Evan went on holiday to the seaside for two weeks. Using the car they explored the countryside as well. The little town was a fishing port and also very beautifully situated on a bay which had a long sandy beach. Many wealthy people lived there, others retired there, having lovely houses built. The plain behind the town extended for ten miles inland to the hills, and the whole area was well stocked with horses, cattle and sheep, and well-kept farms were numerous. Richard was now beginning to think about what he would do when he qualified in a year's time, and considered that this would be a pleasant area in which to practise. Back in Corchester he looked up the practice in the Register of Veterinary Surgeons, discovered that there were three practices in the area and so dismissed it from his mind.

The Major now began to take greater interest in Richard and he became the driver of the new big Austin car. He drove carefully and slowly at first, but the Major was always in a hurry, and used to say, "Come on, Mr Holden, drive faster; we have a lot of work to do." When Richard speeded up to 60 miles an hour, the Major would shout, "Slow down, you idiot, do you want to kill us both?" In spite of his temper Richard admired the Major and they were becoming friends as he made Richard do more veterinary work and so increased his confidence. They arrived at a farm one morning and after the Major had introduced Richard to the farmer he said, "Now, Mr Holden, I want you to blister this horse's shoulder with Red Blister. Clip the hair short with the hand clippers and rub it in for fifteen minutes. I'll be back in about half an hour."

Richard did as he had been instructed, and when the Major returned he said, "You've done a good job there, get the neck cradle from the car." This was fastened around the horse's neck so that he could not get round to lick the blistered area.

"Tie him on pillar reins for a couple of days and feed him from a nose bag."

They called there two days later and found the area scabby and tender and the Major remarked that the blister was just about right. Richard was pleased to learn afterwards that the horse became sound in two months.

It was in the surgical field that the Major excelled. Richard was his assistant, and having watched the late Colonel operate he was quite confident that he would prove his worth. The opportunity to do so came sooner than expected. The case was one of fistulous withers in a seventeen and a half hand Shire gelding which had been in a loose box in the yard overnight and starved. Brown led him out onto the tarpaulin which covered the thick bed of straw. This was under the roofed area, and so the lights were on. The twitch was applied and the hobbles, and Wilson and Richard easily pulled him over. The mask was fitted and Wilson gave the chloroform anaesthetic. Then the Major and Richard scrubbed up, and as the operating area had been prepared and disinfected the Major said, "Scalpel," and immediately made a foot-long incision from front to back of the swelling. Rapidly he cut out pieces of diseased tissue, with Richard holding the wound open with tissue forceps and occasionally getting sprayed with blood; while the Major shouted for forceps, and Richard clamped off the squirting artery. Now with a curette he scraped away the diseased bone. Richard kept swabbing away the blood until the Major was satisfied that all the diseased tissue had been excised.

"Now, pour in that antiseptic solution. Swab it dry, Mr Holden. How's the horse, Mr Wilson?" asked the Major.

"It's breathing nicely," said Mr Wilson.

"Good; now that roll of cotton wool, come on!" shouted the Major. Richard gave it to him and then poured in a pint of cod liver oil. "Suture and needle!" ordered the Major and, on getting them, started rapidly to sew up the wound.

"Take off the mask, Mr Wilson. Brown, keep hold of that head collar." Quickly the blood was washed off the horse's chest and the Major got to his feet. He looked at Richard and said with a twinkle in his eye, "Well, we are a couple of bloody men."

They took off the blood-caked rubber aprons and threw them into a big tin bath which was full of antiseptic solution. The horse was rapidly becoming conscious and when he finally decided to rise he did in spite of Wilson and Brown trying to hold him down. They managed to steer him unsteadily into the box.

"Give him a drink of water, Brown, and stay with him for half an hour, then give him a feed," said the Major. Brown, having done it so often before, just grinned.

"I like you helping me, Mr Holden, because you don't get in the way, and you anticipate which instrument I will need next," said the Major.

"Thank you, Major," said Richard in reply. "I really enjoy surgery and it is good experience for my final year."

At that moment Miss Neeve came running across the yard. "Major, Mr Loxham is on the phone. One of his prize cows has put its calf bed out."

"Right, tell him I'll be there in twenty minutes, and to wrap it in a clean sheet and keep pouring warm water on it. We'll want some men to help. Come on, Mr Holden; Brown, get the gates open quick."

The Major was in the car with the engine running as Richard jumped in.

"Are the strappings in, Brown?" asked the Major.

"Yes," was the reply. The Major drove out of the yard onto the road north and soon was doing 60 m.p.h., grumbling as he drove. "Come on, out of the way, you daft devils," as they roared past car after car. After ten miles they drove up the road to the farm and as the car stopped the Major was out, grabbing his apron and shouting, "Bucket of water and soap and a towel! Mr Holden, bring the strappings!"

When Richard entered the shippon the Major had already told a man to bring a big bale of straw and a rope, while two men were standing behind the cow holding the prolapsed uterus in a blood-stained sheet.

The Major issued a string of orders to the farmer. "John, get that rope round her forelegs and the bale under her belly, that's it; one man hold her nose; right, pull her legs from under her." The front end of the cow sank to the ground while the hind quarters were supported by the bale.

"Right, let me have a look."

The sheet was removed and Richard and the Major between them took the weight of the prolapse. It was the diameter of a bucket and about two feet long.

"Keep pouring that disinfectant over it," he said to one of the men, and then they began to squeeze and massage the prolapse up towards the cow's passage. They had returned half of it when she strained very hard, trying to expel it again.

"Bang her on the back, John. That's it! We are winning!"

Steadily the mass was getting smaller.

"Out of the way, Mr Holden, I've got it," and with that the Major pushed the rest of the mass into the passage.

"Give me that bottle; wash it first."

Richard did so and the Major pushed it into the passage, his arm following up to the shoulder. "I always do this to make certain both horns are back in place! Yes that's it." Out came the bottle and two pessaries were inserted. "Let her up, pull the bale out." He smacked her on the rump and she rose to her feet. "Put the strappings on, Mr Holden."

Richard did so and John Loxham said, "That was a good do, Major; she's that cow that won the first prize at the County Show."

"Yes I thought it was her," said the Major, looking at the dark red Shorthorn cow.

"Come along and have a proper wash," said John, and they went to the house. Richard was glad to wash the perspiration off his face and later gladly accepted a cup of tea, after refusing a whisky. The Major drank a large one and then said, "Mr Holden, you are the driver. We will see you again tomorrow, John; off we go." Richard thought to himself that the man beside him was a bundle of energy.

After lunch Richard wrote up the case of the uterine prolapse in the cow in his case book. He was entering only the more unusual cases now, having already entered the routine ones. The next day the roll of cotton wool was withdrawn from the wound in the gelding's withers, antiseptic oil was poured into it, and then a weighted cloth was spread over it. It took six weeks for it to heal completely and the horse went back to work on the streets of Corchester after three months.

Another unusual case happened some weeks later. Mac at breakfast asked the Major to see a cow for him at Mr Ball's, White Carr Farm; so later Richard drove the Major there. John Ball soon told the history of the case, how the cow had stopped milking and passing dung and then almost stopped eating, and that Mr McDonald had seen her the day before. The Major examined her, and found her temperature raised. Mr Ball said she had just stood quietly, not making a sound. The examination included pressing hard over the rumen, a rectal examination, and pinching and pressing down on her back. Finally the Major said, "I suppose Mr McDonald did all this yesterday?"

"Yes, that's right, and nothing happened," said John.

"Then bring me a strong fencing post."

When John returned with it, it was passed under the cow, John holding one end and Richard the other. The Major placed the stethoscope on the cow's chest.

"Lift now, bring it a bit further forward and lift again." The cow gave a little grunt and was uneasy. "I am certain, John, she has got a wire in her and it is probably just pushing through the stomach wall, so we will have to put her on a board."

Barrow-loads of manure were brought into an empty stall and tipped at the front; an empty corn bin was carried in and laid on its side making a side wall to keep the manure in position and a door was brought in and laid on top of it, so the door was two and a half feet high at the front, and sloped back to floor level at the back of the stall. It was tied firmly into position and strips of wood nailed across it.

They now led the cow into the stall, drove her up the door and tied her with a halter, leaving her enough rope so that she could lie down.

"If she doesn't pass dung tomorrow, let me know, John. For the moment just water her with a bucket and give her nothing to eat. If she passes dung, give her some new mown grass and nothing else," said the Major.

"I'll do that, Major," replied John. The next day she passed dung and was brighter, and after ten days she was put back in her own stall and was eating and milking well. Richard asked what would happen to the piece of wire.

"Two things," said Mac, "Either become encapsulated in a dense fibrous mass in the wall of the reticulum, or be passed on and degenerate in the gastric juices; the fibrous mass may join the second stomach to the diaphragm—you may see one when you are doing meat inspection." Some months after in the abattoir, a slaughterman drew his attention to the very thing—he had to cut the reticulum away from the diaphragm before he could finish eviscerating a cow's carcase.

While at the surgery one afternoon Richard saw Bob Whiteside come walking in. He went to talk to him, and found out that he had left Droughton because the Town Council had decided to build council houses very near the premises, so he had sold them and moved to Southall. This was a village halfway between Corchester and Droughton, and the Old Mill that Bob had bought was a half a mile away from the village. Richard asked Bob if he could go to his premises occasionally to look at carcases for pathological changes. Early one afternoon Mac left him there. As he reached the high wooden fence he smelt cooking meat and on going through the gate saw a long building half of which was two storeys high, the other half one storey; through the roof of the latter a metal chimney protruded pouring smoke across the river behind, and steam was coming out of the double doors. Bob met him and explained that they were boiling meat in a six foot tall steel container, using steam from the tall, upright boiler. From an overhead rail hung large pieces of meat from a previous boiling which were cooling. When cold they were put in clean hessian sacks and labels attached, and Bob told Richard that five nights a week they were taken to the station in Droughton for carriage to Belgium where the meat was sold for human consumption.

Richard's sense of rightness was offended by the thought that meat from diseased and worn-out animals was being used to feed poor people abroad, and said so to Bob who replied that if they didn't send it, he doubted that the people would ever eat any meat. He went into the other half of the building where there were two men cutting up carcases. The older one was introduced as Bob's uncle of the same name, so he was known as "Owd Bob" and his nephew who was named after him, "Young Bob". They were remarkably alike until the older man took off his cap when Richard saw that he was completely bald. The other man, Tommy, was young and fair-haired; like the others he wore clogs and chain-smoked cigarettes. Richard was not surprised because the smell was very bad, and though much of the raw meat, bones and carcases were covered with old tarpaulins, flies were everywhere, especially bluebottles. Both men wore round their waists leather belts on which were scabbards containing knives and from which steels hung, on which they continually sharpened their knives. It was fascinating to Richard to see how deftly but carefully they flayed a carcase, spreading out the skin on a heap of hides and throwing all fat into bins. Bob explained how nothing was wasted. The horns and hooves and bones were all collected by the manufacturer of glues and bone meal, and the fat went to an oil refinery for use in soap making and lubrication of machinery.

Richard's interest was focused on the pathological conditions he recognised—tuberculosis, peritonitis, pneumonia, mastitis, intestinal haemorrhage from lacerations at calving and many more. When Mac came to collect him at five o'clock he promised Bob to call at Christmas and spend a little more time there, and congratulated him on doing so well over the last few years.

"Well, I try to provide a good service. I never refuse a call and I pay for every animal I collect though often it is very little, a few shillings."

Richard thanked him, and during the rest of the holiday often noticed the Morris lorry with "R. Whiteside Horse Slaughterer" painted along its side, on the country roads.

In the last week of the vacation, he drove the Major to see a hunter described as "off colour". They followed the driveway round the mansion and behind found a stable block, in immaculate condition. A groom told them he was going to inform Sir Rodney of their arrival, and returned with a tall gentleman who was wearing an expensive suit. After shaking hands with the Major he led them into the stable and showed them a dark bay hunter mare, and then explained that she had fallen at a hedge two weeks before while being hunted. Since then she had become very stiff in her movements and was off her food. The groom picked up a fore leg while the mare's temperature was taken, which was normal, and the Major then noticed healed long scratches at the base of her neck.

"Was there wire in that hedge which caused these lacerations?" he inquired.

Sir Rodney said there was and grumbled about farmers putting barbed wire fences around their land and said how dangerous it was when hunting.

There were other old scars at the top of one of the fore legs. The Major took the head collar from the groom and then suddenly waved his hand at the mare's eye as though he were going to hit her. She jerked away and all her body stiffened for a moment.

"Sir Rodney," said the Major, "I am sorry, but your mare is developing lockjaw, which is sometimes called tetanus. Her eye has given the diagnostic sign, so now there is a lot to be done if I am going to save her."

Soon she was in a loose box thickly bedded with peat, the windows were covered with sacking and everything movable was taken away.

"I want her to be kept very quiet, no sudden noises; wrap sacking around the bucket handle; and oil that squeaking door hinge. Will you bring her some water now." The groom did so and on being offered it the mare drank some. "No hay now, give her sloppy oatmeal three times a day and try her with water each time. I'll give her some anti-serum now. Bathe those wounds until they are raw and squeeze out any matter. I'll be back tomorrow."

The next morning Brown put the horse slings in the car and their first visit was to the mare. The Major decided that her condition was worse and that she should be put in slings. A movable stall partition was turned out from the wall and bolted to the floor thus making a single stall, the mare was fastened to the manger and very quietly the slings were fitted. The Major cursed

Brown under his breath for putting so much grease on the pulley block chain, which was tied up out of the way once the slings were just taking the mare's weight. As she was still drinking, the groom was given liquorice powder to put in her gruel, and told to mash up apples into a pulp for her. Sir Rodney wanted to know how long she would be ill. The Major informed him that it would last at least ten days, and if she survived that length of time she would recover. He added that the fact that the groom had got a lot of pus out of the two deep wounds may have helped. All the wounds were covered with antiseptic oil and another serum injection given.

It was about a week later when they were hopeful that she would recover that disaster struck. The 7 a.m. phone call saying that the mare was very ill caused them to be on their way to her in ten minutes. She was lying half on her side in the slings, her legs out straight; she was quivering all over and sweating. Sir Rodney, wearing a dressing gown, came in.

"Don't you think she should be shot, Major?" he asked.

"I'm considering it—what was she like yesterday?" The groom replied that she appeared to be steadily getting better and had drunk everything given to her.

"Well something must have startled her for her to get like this," said the Major.

"I think I know what it was—one of our cats dashed out as I opened the box door," said the groom.

"Blast it," said the Major, "But we will have a try at straightening her up because every time her feet touch the stall division she has a spasm."

The division was quietly removed out of the way and the groom held her head. Slowly the slings were lowered until it was decided that they were at the right height, if she could stand on her feet again; ropes were put round her legs and the groom was told to pull her head round while they pulled on the ropes to try to get the mare straight. Two more men came in and when the Major said, "Heave," they all pulled, but as her hind legs touched the floor she had a violent spasm and her legs pushed her forwards. The breast piece broke under the strain; the mare slumped forwards and out of the slings, and lay on her side in a violent spasm.

"I'm sorry, Sir Rodney, it's no damn good. I'll have to shoot her."

"Please do," he replied and quickly walked away. Returning from the car the Major ordered everybody out and the pistol shot soon followed. The groom walked away vowing to kill "that bloody cat", and the Major and Richard followed Sir Rodney to the house. Over coffee Sir Rodney explained that he was grateful for all they had done, but was disappointed that she had had to be shot because she had been covered by a St. Leger winner in June and was four months in foal. "And I bet it would have been a winner," said Sir Rodney.

"It would have had better chances than evens to be that," said the Major.

This first case of tetanus he had seen stayed in his memory for a long time, and a few days later, back in the digs in Liverpool, he told the story to Norman and Evan, his two close friends. Norman was the son of a partner in a very big horse practice in a Midland city, and Evan's father ran an agricultural practice in Wales; so many stories were told of what they had seen and their experiences during the last three months.

Evan said it would be nice to see a horse for a change; he had seen nothing but cattle and the odd ewe throughout the holiday, in reply to which Norman said that he would be glad to change places with him, because in the city he had seen nothing but working horses. It was arranged therefore that at Christmas, Norman went to Wales and Evan to the city, with great benefit to both, because the subjects for the final examinations were extensive– veterinary medicine; meat inspection; surgery and obstetrics; including examinations as to soundness.

There was so much to read and watch, that Richard decided to resign from the OTC, even though he had passed both examinations A and B, but he was really sorry to have to forego his football on Wednesday and Saturday. The optician found that so much reading over the years was affecting his sight and so now he wore horn-rimmed spectacles, which Norman said made him look like an absentminded vicar! Too soon it was Christmas, when he spent a week in the Corchester practice, and one day went to see Ezra and Martha who were living five miles north of Droughton.

They had bought a ten-acre smallholding and had a new house built, the original one on the site being used as a store garage; there was a warm house for raising seedlings, and an office. Ezra was busy because he still had a lot of poultry to look after and a few store cattle, while Martha was enjoying herself growing roses.

By bus he went on to Bob Whiteside's as he had promised. He noticed two Morris trucks in the yard; each had been fitted with a hand-operated winch to make the loading of the carcases easier. At 6 o'clock they all went in the trucks to the XL Pub on the main road, and as it was Christmas the landlord gave you a meat pie if you bought a pint of beer which cost sixpence. Soon the locals, mainly farm workers and slaughter men, were joking and telling yarns and a sing-song developed when Charlie the local rat catcher began to play the piano. When Bob took him home at 7.30 that evening he was a bit tipsy and Richard realised that his mother did not like a knacker's lorry at her front door, but he made amends by going with her to socials and to church and to see their relatives.

Easter Monday, 23 April that year, found Richard driving the Major to Newport, which was thirty-nine miles from Corchester. They arrived at a well known stud farm and were met by a stable lad at the gate who directed them to the riding school. A tall, smartly-dressed man greeted them there.

"How nice to see you again, John, and who is this you have with you?"

"It's great to see you again, Sir," replied the Major. "And this is a final year student, Mr Richard Holden."

They shook hands, and turned to look at a mare which was being held by a groom.

"So this is 'Lucky Hand' and you want a Certificate of Soundness for her." Richard was at once all attention for this was one of the subjects in the final examination, but was unprepared for the Major's brusque command.

"Mr Holden, write down a description of this mare for me."

Richard examined the mare's teeth, measured her height and walked round looking at her carefully and then wrote:

A five year old bay mare. 16-1 hands. Star and stripe conjoined, finishing two inches above the upper opening of the nostrils; white to fetlock near hind.

The Major now conducted his examination, and when he had finished he had the mare trotted. The groom now mounted and the mare was cantered and then galloped in a figure of eight. The Major stood in the centre of the school, watching the mare's performance and listening to her breathing as she went past. Finally the gallop was stopped and the Major using a stethoscope listened to the mare's heartbeat, and then read Richard's description.

"Mr Holden, I wouldn't pass you in your final examination. We will now check a few things. The corner incisors are not meeting so the mare is coming five years. Get the measuring stick and we will measure her outside on level ground." They did so and the measurement was 16 hands. Richard, feeling a bit of a fool, waited for more criticism and it came.

"Hasn't the mare got black points?" asked the Major.

"Yes," he replied.

"Well, why didn't you put it in? And the mare has got a name, and look on the inner side of the off thigh."

When Richard looked he saw a white patch.

"Now we will rewrite it. 'Lucky Hand', a bay mare with black points, 16 hands, coming five years, star and stripe conjoined finishing two inches above the upper opening of the nostrils; white fetlock near hind; a roughly circular white patch about six inches in diameter on the inner aspect of the off thigh." The Major turned to his friend Brigadier Robert Page and said, "With this correct description I will send you a Certificate of Soundness for her by post tonight. Come on, Mr Holden, I hope you have learnt something today."

"Thank you very much. I have, and it will make a big difference when I next examine a horse for soundness."

"I'm glad you've taken it that way," said the Major. "You can't be too careful doing examinations for soundness. If anything is wrong there is a real dust-up and you may be sued and appear in Court and that's no good for a vet's reputation. So swat up dentition and colours and markings."

Back at the surgery Richard wrote up the details of the Examination for Soundness and then began to make up some cough electuary in the dispensary. Suddenly the door was flung open and the Major yelled, "Quick, Mr Holden, bring me some tannic acid, carron oil, oil of eucalyptus and some bottles of sedative! There's a horse on fire!"

"A what?" asked Richard.

"A horse, I said, you damn fool, come on."

Richard grabbed everything, put them in a cardboard box and ran out to the car. He put them in the back and had hardly got the door shut before the Major drove out of the yard into the traffic sounding his horn all the time, until they were going at 70 m.p.h. Richard was glad they were in the Austin saloon—the old Vauxhall would have been very draughty! Before they reached the farm they saw some men looking over a hedge. The Major lowered the window and shouted, "Where's the horse?"

One man said, "In this field. They can't catch her, Major," and in the distance they could see a heavy horse slowly trotting round the field with wisps of smoke blowing away from its back. Two men who had been chasing it finally caught the trailing halter rope.

They drove into the farmyard and the Major immediately walked across to a knot of people who were standing at the gate watching what was happening.

"Good morning, Mrs Isles," he said to a lady, obviously the farmer's wife. This is a bad accident, what happened?"

"I don't know really, except they were using paraffin."

"Well, would you please get me a clean bed sheet. I will want one soon," asked the Major.

"Yes," she replied and hurried away. By now the mare had been led to the gate and Richard could see that all the hair on the near side was burnt and along her back, and the smell of burnt hair and flesh was repulsive.

"The poor devil," said the Major, "She must be in agony, get me a quart jug of cold water somebody, and Mr Holden, bring me a sedative, the funnel and the stomach tube." The Major quickly passed the stomach tube and Richard mixed the sedative in the jug, put the funnel in the end of the stomach tube and standing on a bale, slowly poured the mixture into it. After a few minutes the Major touched the mare's back and she struggled, trying to bite.

"Obviously I am not going to be able to cut away that burnt hair, so her back and sides will have to be covered. Mr Holden, get a two-gallon bucket of warm water, dissolve that tannic acid in it and then soak the sheet in the solution." After giving these orders the Major turned to the farmer, asked for four bean poles and the help of two men, and told him to go and help hold the mare's head.

By now the mare appeared a little drowsy, so the Major, Richard and the two men supported the dripping sheet at each corner with a bean pole. They approached from behind her and then gently lowered the sheet onto her back. She did not struggle too much, even when Richard began to pour jugs full of the solution onto the sheet from the withers to her tail. "That will do now, let's have her in the stable. Now George, what happened?"the Major asked.

"Well, it was like this. She had a lot of old winter coat, so I brought her in and began clipping it off. Then I saw she was lousy, so I began cleaning her and rubbing her with a paraffin rag. Then father comes in and you know he always smokes a pipe–well he mainly seems to smoke nothing but matches, and though he is as deaf as a post, he can see a threepeny bit a mile off. I'd just finished her near side and was rubbing the paraffin in when he pointed with a lighted match in his hand and said, "Tha's missed some there," and he must have touched her because the hair blazed at once. She just neighed and plunged straight through the door smashing it open and went across the yard and into the field, so our Fred dashed to Robinson's to telephone you. Is she badly burnt?"

"I can't tell you, but we will come tomorrow and see how she is doing. I'll leave this solution and in the morning pour it over the sheet just like Mr Holden did."

The next day the wet sheet was gently rolled back and taken off. Lumps of hair and burnt skin were stuck to it, and large areas of the mare's back and near side were raw and oozing yellow fluid. The whole area was soaked in carron oil, a clean sheet tied in position and instructions left for the oil to be poured on twice daily. When they visited her two days later the mare was eating and brighter and parts of the raw areas were covered with large scabs. After George and the Major had been talking the latter said, "Come on, Mr Holden," and strode out of the stable. They drove out of the yard without saying any of the usual goodbyes.

"What's the matter?" asked Richard,

The Major replied, "The man's a fool, he does not want us to visit her any more, he says he cannot afford it, and they will carry on treating her–it's a pity as she's a good pedigree and has bred some very good foals."

It was over a week later that they were summoned to the farm again, where they found the mare in a terrible state. Obviously the sheet had not been taken off, nor the oil applied, so it was with great difficulty they got if off. The mare was sweating and breathing fast, her temperature was 105 degrees; pus was oozing out all over the scabby area, and smelt foul.

The Major stormed, "You know, George, you haven't looked after the mare, and all the matter has got into her system and she has developed septicaemia."

"Can't you do anything?" asked George.

"Good God no, man, can't you see she is dying? She should have been treated all last week but you told me not to come and now you are going to lose your mare and the foal she's carrying."

"Well in that case, you had better go," said George.

They did, and later learnt that the mare had died that afternoon. Even the account for treatment was never paid. "That's the sort that goes to the wall," said John and sure enough, in twelve months George went bankrupt.

It was a few days later that they met up with an old client. They were driving along the road which linked two villages, when they were stopped by a man who was a drayman and asked for a lift.

"What are you doing here?" asked the Major, "Get in." The man climbed into the back of the car and said that he had delivered two barrels of beer to the Kings Head and was in the pub getting the delivery signed and then having a drink. When he came out, the dray and the two horses were gone.

"You must have been a long time having your drink, then."

"Well, you know how it is. We got chatting and I'm not to five minutes because at the next stop, The Railway, I have my dinner and the horses their feed. Because I do this round every Tuesday the horses know all the pubs." So they speeded along the road and had almost reached the next village when sure enough they found the dray being pulled along steadily by the horses with no driver.

"Well, they are almost there," said the Major, "We will just follow them." Richard was surprised to see the horses cross over to the right side of the road and taking a wide sweep go through the narrow entrance into the pub yard without touching either side.

"Well I'll be damned," said the Major, "I would not have believed that if I had not seen it." The drayman got out and ran into the yard to find the landlord standing there.

"So that's the game now, you let the horses do the work while you drive about in a motor car."

"Oh, stop your noise," said the driver, "And help me roll off those barrels." Richard recognised the Shire with a white patch around the eye, as the horse which had had pus in the foot, which Walter had opened up and drained in the surgery yard.

The next morning Brown was busy putting the hobbles, the blinds, the mask and the chloroform into the car together with everything else necessary for gelding horses. Richard and the Major were ready to be away at eight thirty, because they had a busy morning. All the Shire colts in an area were brought to one farm on one morning for castration. This was done because it was cheaper and a plentiful supply of labour was always available—men who could handle Shires; also the operation had to be done before flies appeared in the late spring.

On arriving at the farm the Major soon had everything organised. The searing irons were put into a fire, with instructions only to allow them to get red hot and when he shouted "Irons!" to put them in a dry bucket and bring them as quickly as possible. Everything went smoothly and four colts were castrated, then there was a break for a cup of tea. The operation on number five was half over and the Major shouted, "Irons!" There was no immediate response so he bawled at the top of his voice "Irons!" and as the flustered youth came running up he pulled the iron out of the bucket and thrust the red end at the Major who without looking up grasped it. With a howl of pain he jumped to his feet shouting, "You bloody fool!" and plunged his hand into the bucket of disinfectant.

"Mr Holden, finish it while I attend to my hand." Fortunately the spring clamp had remained in position and Richard seared the stump and then operated on the other testicle. He at once went to look at the Major's right hand, and there was a swelling the size of half a hen's egg. Richard poured eucalyptus oil over it and bandaged it tightly as directed by the Major and then proceeded to operate on the other two colts. He was pleased when they were driving back to the surgery to be told,

"Richard, I could not have cut those last two colts any better myself."

Richard took a break from his studies on the Whitsun weekend, and spent a day at home, and then went on to Corchester and arrived just in time to accompany the Major to a mare which was having difficulty foaling. The big sterilizer which contained the embryotomy instruments was put in the car, together with the chloroform and mask. It was a warm, sunny morning. The Major drove rapidly the seventeen miles to the farm and in his usual manner grabbed his apron and rushed into the box shouting orders. So two buckets of hot water were brought and two bales of straw placed behind the mare. After putting on his apron and scrubbing his hands and arms he ordered, "Right, pick up her foreleg." He then stood on the bale and having washed the mare's vulva, began to examine her and then said:

"This is a bad one, it's wry neck and the foal is dead, there is no movement at all. Mr Holden, give me two sharp hooks on the long ropes."

Richard got them out of the sterilizer and the Major passed them inside the mare, but only managed to get one to hold. "Right, pull, Mr Holden!" Richard pulled and the mare strained and the Major struggled to try and pull the foal's head towards him but it would not move. He finally got down off the bale and told the farmer that the mare would have to be given chloroform, and that this could be dangerous, but there was no other way of stopping the mare straining and bringing the foal's head into the correct position. The farmer agreed that this should be done, and said that he was sure the Major would foal the mare. So after more straw had been laid on the floor, the mare was anaesthetised and Richard gave the Major the embryotomy knife and pulled the rope tight. The major on his knees worked away and sweated and cursed, until he asked for another hook. Once this was fixed in the foal's skull he told Richard to pull gently.

"Great," said the Major, "Now hard."

On doing this, out came the foal's amputated head. He rose to his feet and looked at the mare and said, "Open the tray in the mask, she won't want much more. Mr Holden, rope the fore legs because I must sit down," and he slumped onto a bale.

"Are you all right Mr Gillmour?"

"Yes, but my heart plays up. You pull on those ropes now and Richard, keep your hand on the stump of the neck." Willing hands seized the ropes; soon the foal was delivered and the placenta came with it.

"Take the mask off quick and put some pessaries in her. Is she all right inside?"

Richard examined her carefully and then said that she was, so the farmer and his men pulled her head round, pushed her into a sitting position and held her there. After washing Richard put all the equipment back into the car and the farmer asked them into the house.

"Not yet," said the Major, "I want to see her on her feet first."

He got to his feet, washed and put on his jacket and then examined the mare. Telling the two men who were holding her head to hang on, he gave her a slap on the rump and she got to her feet.

"Well done, Sir, that's a good do, come on into the house now."

They followed him and were glad of the cake and tea his wife provided.

Driving home Richard asked how long the Major had had a bad heart.

"I haven't got a bad heart, but extreme exertion makes my heart beat very quickly and I become a bit dizzy—I am glad you were with me to finish the job in fine style."

Richard said that he had been grateful for the opportunity of foaling his first mare, and was glad that everything had gone well in this case. The Major said that they had been lucky, because already that year he had had to shoot five mares because he could not deliver the horribly deformed foals which one stallion was leaving behind. They had driven a few miles when he suddenly exclaimed, "Well I'll be damned, talk of the devil, here is the stallion in question." Ahead was a great Shire stallion being led by a small man who travelled the stallion for the Buckton Society. "He's called George Fletcher. He takes the stallion to a pub yard and the mares are brought there to be covered. He stays in the pub at night and they do say he's as active as the stallion but he has only three children that I know of." Richard thought that more happened in the countryside than one might expect and that he was learning all the time and not only about veterinary matters!

After lunch he went with Mac to dock seven foals, the last for this season; most of them were well grown and about nine months old. There was quite a crowd of farmers and helpers present when they drove into the farm yard and the docking irons were put in the brazier to get red hot. The first foal was backed up inside the box until it was touching the close door. The tail was lifted over and strong twine tied tightly round its root. Mac injected the local anaesthetic, and after a few minutes the docking knife was brought, the farmer indicated the length he wanted left and the tail was cut off. "Irons," said Mac and quickly seared the stump; Richard shook the powdered resin over it and Mac melted the resin until a good seal had formed. After telling the farmer to inspect it a few times to see it was satisfactory the foal was led out and another took its place. During the afternoon Richard did two and Mac the rest and everything went off quickly and smoothly.

At seven the next morning he was on the train going to Liverpool and thinking about the final examinations he would have to sit in six weeks time, and about Joan who had got her Diploma and after a temporary post had applied for a post with a big catering firm in London called Lyons. With a feeling of guilt he realised that he had neglected her these last twelve months and wondered if this would be a parting of the ways, something he did not want to happen; but she would have to wait until July. When in that month the examinations ended the fourteen students waited anxiously, Richard with Norman and Evan his friends, for the results to be announced. Three had failed and Norman was one of them, much to his friends' consternation. Evan had got a Second Class Honours in Medicine and Richard had achieved this in all the examinations. He could hardly believe it, but was intensely happy and relieved when he told his mother the news on the telephone.

It was a busy afternoon. He paid his fee as a member of the Royal College of Veterinary Surgeons, took the oath, and signed the declaration to obey all the Act Charters and Bye Laws of the college. He had a short interview with the Secretary to the Board who wanted to know what he was going to do and then told him to keep in touch. Back in the digs he packed all his books and belongings into two suitcases, and found he could hardly lift them. Then came the final break; as he said goodbye to Norman and Evan he felt a curious mixture of sadness and happiness and was almost in tears when he put his two cases in the taxi which took him to the station.

His father met him at Droughton, congratulated him and drove him home, but Richard was surprised that a celebration party had been arranged so quickly. Ezra and Martha, and the Healds were there; they congratulated him and then went into dinner during which Ezra proposed his health. It was however only a lot later when he was going to sleep that the sentence, "I'm a vet," kept chasing round in his brain. The next morning he spent in his study; books were arranged in the bookcase; old papers and revision notes and magazines were all thrown into the waste paper bin. The house was quiet because his sister was in London taking her professional examinations, so he got his bike out of the shed, oiled it and went out on it to the Westminster Bank and arranged for his account to be transferred from Liverpool.

Arriving home, he telephoned Joan and was disappointed that there was no reply; so he got the service book from the car and spent the rest of the day in the garage learning how to grease the car and change a wheel and getting to know how it worked. When he talked to Joan on the telephone next morning, they arranged to go for a trip to the seaside in the afternoon, and she later arrived in a new Morris saloon. Richard felt a little like her poor relation; he hadn't much money and his university blazer and slacks were old, but Joan looked marvellous and was wearing an expensive blue costume. It was a pleasant break and he managed to kiss her just before she drove off home so he was in high spirits because she had invited him to go to their house in Weston on the Sunday. During that afternoon they played tennis on the courts at the back of the house, but stopped when it began to rain. They went into the house into the lounge, and she put on the gramophone the Gershwin song "The man I love", and soon he was sitting on the settee holding her in his arms. Her mother however persisted in interrupting Richard's courting and finally a maid brought in afternoon tea on a tray. When they had eaten, Joan suggested that he left, because she had to go out with her mother that evening. When he left he felt very frustrated because he never seemed to make much progress in his courtship of Joan, and he knew that, though he had occasionally been out with other girls, he loved Joan intensely.

Finally he went to his Uncle Dick's farm for a working holiday, and was soon hard at it helping with the clip and shepherding on the hill. At night he and Dick talked for hours about new treatments for sheep diseases, and new management methods, and the days passed quickly until the morning a telegram arrived which read, "Temporary post at Corchester". Arriving home he was pleased to see that his father had had his Diploma framed and that it was hanging in his study. He learnt that Mr Wilson had left and that his replacement would not arrive for some time so the Major wanted Richard's help. On the telephone he asked him to commence work the next Monday morning, which he did. As he walked down the hill from Corchester Station he was determined to make a name for himself as a vet.

III

"Good morning Richard," said the Major, "and how did you do in the final?"

"I got 2nd class honours in all the examinations."

"Congratulations. You did do well. Are you thinking of doing research or teaching?"

"No, I still want to be a practitioner," replied Richard, and so he was offered the temporary post of assistant. The terms were three guineas a week, live in at St. Cuthbert's, and the usual holidays. Mr Wilson had gone back to London College to teach and do research work, and his replacement Mr Allen would not arrive until October. Richard was given the Austin 7 to drive and was told that he would help Mr Edwards in the country to the north of the practice and also do small animal work, which he found the Major shared with him. But today was Monday, and he found that he had to help with the dispensing all morning, just as he had done when he was a student, and in the afternoon had to help Miss Horner and Miss Davies.

A farmer who was a poultry breeder, some years previously had bought two Old English sheep dogs to guard his flock, and as they were a male and a female he had bred from them and so now had five. They were loose from dusk to dawn and had stopped the stealing of poultry which had occurred previously. They were all muzzled when they arrived and were covered in very thick coats of matted hair on which mud, chicken droppings and excrement had dried. While Richard held them the two girls set to, using the Cooper Stewart electric clippers. When the first dog was finished they had a veritable "door mat" of hair, and because he had fleas and ticks they dusted him with Cooper's anti-parasite powder, so he looked half the size and was almost snow white. While Richard struggled to hold the dogs, he enjoyed talking to the two girls and joking with them, having had very little contact with girls previously. He found he was attracted to the brunette Miss Horner, who was well dressed and had a good figure hidden under the white coat. The dogs were finished by 5.30 p.m. and Richard just had time to go to St. Cuthbert's and have some afternoon tea before he had to return to the surgery for 6 o'clock.

He treated all the cats and dogs presented and Miss Neeve showed him where various pills, lotions and small animal instruments were kept. She also collected the money and gave the receipts so it was 7.30 before they had finished. After saying goodnight to Brown they drove up to St. Cuthbert's and had dinner, a happy affair during which Richard had to stand quite a bit of teasing from the Major and Mac, the latter saying "Well we can throw our books away now, second class honours indeed, we only need to ask Richard for the answer to any difficulty," The Major answered the telephone when it rang, and returning said to Richard, "That's Tom Watts at Lonbarrow; he has a cow which can't calve, I told him you would not be long."

Richard delivered a live heifer calf and when he drove the car into the yard after a return trip of 32 miles at 10.45 he hoped that in future he would not have to work 17 hours every day.

Mac advised him to join the National Veterinary Medical Association, which he did at once and when he was not on duty he often spent his Sundays reading its paper *The Veterinary Record*. He went home for a party which was given for Mary who was now a Licentiate of the Royal Academy of Music. Richard had an HMV gramophone, a table top model which played records at 78 r.p.m. using a steel needle. During his university days he had bought quite a few records, some classical, some popular, of music which he enjoyed, so he was able to discuss the work of various composers with Mary's friends, all of whom were musicians of both sexes, young, enthusiastic and lively. So after a buffet supper he was not surprised when in turn they played various instruments and finally played some chamber music. It was an enjoyable evening which was the spur which drove him on to buy more records of works by Elgar—his favourite—Beethoven, Brahms and others. Such breaks helped him over the first few weeks, because he found he was given more important work to do; was also on duty one night in three and still doubted his own ability.

One evening he went miles to the Home Farm of the Teren estate, to a calving case which was an impacted breech. Though he tried very hard to get a leg back, he felt he could not without rupturing the uterine wall. He explained this to the farm bailiff, who allowed him to telephone the Major for assistance. This was readily forthcoming, and when the Major had examined the cow he mixed up Lux in warm water which was then pumped into the cow's uterus. Soon two feet were protruding and were roped and a very big live bull calf was delivered. At home later the Major told Richard that he was pleased that he had called for assistance, because if he had tried to calve the cow without more fluid, he would probably have killed the cow.

"As they are full pedigree Herefords, I think they would have sued me, and of course it would have damaged our reputation, so don't worry about it. If you are in difficulty, always call for either Mac or me." Richard thanked him and felt better, and next morning got a packet of Lux from the store room.

Some days later he visited a farm to see a cow "off colour". She was slavering and had a very swollen lower half of the neck. The farmer gave no history

of the case when Richard questioned him except that the cows had got into
the turnips. He immediately thought of choke, but the cow was not blown so
he dismissed that from his mind. The temperature was 104½°F and the pulse
110 per minute. He tried the cow with a bucket of water but she would not
drink. When he told the farmer that the cow was very ill with a septic swelling on her neck, he was asked what he was going to do about it. Annoyed
with himself for not being able to come to an accurate diagnosis; and with the
farmer for his hostile and unhelpful attitude, he told him he was going to find
Mr McDonald and come back with him. Mac listened to the story and said:
"I don't trust old Bob at Barn End, but come on, and we'll see what we can
make of his cow."

The welcome this time was different.

"Good afternoon, Mr McDonald. I'm glad you've come because this lad
doesn't seem to know much about the job."

Mac spun round. "Bob, let me tell you something–this lad, as you call
him, is Mr Holden and he's a far better qualified vet than I am, and as for
your bloody cow I would not touch it with a barge pole, because it's dying
and one of you has killed it."

"I don't know what you are talking about," said Bob.

"Oh yes, you do," and the accent was becoming stronger and the voice
louder as Mac went on, "That cow got a turnip stuck in its throat and you
pushed something down to shift it and you didn't, you've just torn her food
pipe open."

"Nay I didn't, it was Tom." Tom looked sheepish and Mac asked:

"Well, what did you use?"

"A walking stick," said Tom.

"Well, you were a damned fool; get on to Bob Whiteside; you will get a bit
more for her if he kills her."

With that they left, and next day at Bob's yard they found the oesophagus
torn and the turnip in a mass of blood and stinking fluid in the muscles of
the neck—the cow had died before Bob had got to the farm. A week later
when Richard went to the farm again to remove a retained placenta from a
cow, Bob and Tom acted as though nothing unpleasant had taken place previously.

That evening at dinner he kept rubbing his right arm, and Mac said that it
was obvious he had been cleansing a cow. Richard replied that he had, and
Mac told him to go and soak his arm in warm disinfectant solution and let it
dry on, and if he were doing any obstetrical work always to use the Major's
antiseptic soft soap—which was a very mild, soft soap he had specially made
at the soap works and to which he then added *Ac. Carbolici Glyc,* and *Ol.
Eucalypti.* There were tins of it in the surgery. Elizabeth, the Major's wife, a
very placid woman, often left them round the dinner table discussing technical things. One evening the verbal battle was prolonged because Mac wanted

to vaccinate his two Border terriers against distemper using the virus–serum method. The Major said that he was not having live distemper virus brought anywhere near the surgery under any conditions, but Mac stoutly defended its use saying that it was an attenuated virus.

"Fat lot of good that will be if the virus suddenly reverts to full virulence in my kennels. I would have to shut up shop."

In the end he ordered the vaccine and used it on his dogs during his annual holiday with no bad effects.

Now the battle began again.

"How do you know they are now immune?" asked Johnny.

"I don't," replied Mac, "but you will find out if we have another bad out-break of distemper; my dogs will not get it."

June proved Mac right and the Major immediately became enthusiastic for the use of the vaccine. It was on the morning of the first Friday in October that the Major called Richard into the office, closed the door and said, "Well, this is the parting of the ways, Richard. Mr Allen has telephoned and will be here on Monday, so thank you for all your help and here is your cheque up to date. Will you stay for lunch?" Though Richard knew the job had been temporary, to be suddenly dismissed like this hit him like a thunderbolt so he quietly said, "No, thanks, I'll go and collect my things," and having shaken hands walked out, a bit dazed by the suddeness of it all. He said his goodbyes to everybody and as he walked to the station he thought, what do I do now? I am unemployed.

Richard opened an account at the post office with the Major's cheque, so that he could always get some money if the banks were closed, and had been home three days when he had a surprise. He answered the telephone and a voice asked for Mr Richard Baden Holden. When Richard said he was speaking he was told to hold on, and the Secretary of the Board of Veterinary Studies suddenly spoke and told him that he had given Richard's name and telephone number to a practitioner at Fernhall in Shropshire who wanted a good assistant at once, and that this Mr Buxton would be in touch. Richard thanked the Secretary for his kindness, and later in the day gave Mr Buxton the Major's name as a reference. The reference must have been a good one because that evening Mr Buxton rang back and asked him to go to see him on Thursday with a view to starting work at once; so Richard went up to the bedroom and began filling the suitcase he had just unpacked.

After changing trains he arrived at the Halt on a little local train. He was the only passenger to alight, and was glad that Mr Buxton met him because he appeared to be miles away from anywhere. Mr Buxton told him that it was a mile and a half to the Halt and that the practice was one third in Shropshire and two thirds in South Cheshire. They finally turned into a drive which led up to a fine-looking black and white half-timbered house. Ivy Bank was an early seventeenth century house, with latticed windows and many rooms with uneven oak floors and massive oak doors, and Richard thought it was wonderful. At dinner the maid waited on Mr Buxton, Megan his unmarried sister and his mother, and they were all very friendly. Later Richard and Walter Buxton went into a room at the back of the house which was the practice office. Walter told Richard that his father had died suddenly ten days before after being head of the practice for nearly forty years, and that it was mainly a cattle practice. He offered four pounds a week, live in, and Richard would have a Morris Minor car to drive. There was a half day off weekly and ten days holiday a year. Richard accepted the post and signed a binding out agreement.

Next morning, after Walter had drawn a map showing where the four farms were situated, Richard set off with his confidence restored. Soon he drove up a potholed muddy lane into a very dirty farmyard, and went with the farmer into a shippon where Richard was shocked to find the cow muck shovelled up against the wall. It was at least a foot deep and he had to walk through puddles of urine. It was very humid and he noticed that sacking was stuffed into every hole, so that there was little ventilation. After dealing with the cow he was glad to get out of the foul conditions into the cold autumn air, but the next two farms were the same.

The dairy farm was clean and well run, the shippons had been swept and straw scattered behind the cows like the farmers did in the Corchester practice. At lunch Walter told him that many of the smaller farmers only cleaned out their shippons once a week, and that the hygiene of milk production was very poor. After a month Richard realised that the only animals he had treated were cows, and more cows, but he was enjoying it and could now understand the local dialect. He began to smoke more cigarettes and sometimes he and Walter would walk to the Eagle and Child at night and have a pint of beer, and so he got to know some of the local farmers and their sons, and the tradespeople in the village. The church was Norman to Perpendicular, with two Norman doors and a fine west window. Richard went to matins every second Sunday, and always felt refreshed and relaxed after the service. As the weeks went by he passed a probang to relieve choke; cast a cow and with three men rolled her until the vagina was untwisted and delivered a live calf; and found that the cow with suspect foot and mouth disease only had half a sardine tin jammed between the molars in her upper jaw.

Walter gave him a list of farms to visit one morning and told him to get to Halton Farm at twelve o'clock, when the farmer would be there. When at a quarter to twelve he arrived at the farm gate he saw the track went 300 yards across the field to the buildings, so after opening the gate he drove up to them. He walked into one shippon which was full of cows and then into the second which was about half full and there he saw a cow tied on its own. She was covered with sacks, and was not eating. He had taken her temperature and was listening with his stethoscope to her stomach movements, when he realised someone was behind him; he turned quickly and saw a big man with long matted hair and a thick beard which covered his face. His eyes were very dark and wild and his clothing was tied about him with string.

"Hello, I didn't hear you come in," said Richard. "I'm the vet from Mr Buxton's. Have I got the right cow?" The man nodded.

"I thought I had found the right one. You know she has been ill for a few days; she has got slow fever and I am going to give you some powders for her." As he walked towards the door the man tried to get behind Richard, who quickly side-stepped, and then kept his eye on him.

"These are the powders and I'll put the directions on them. Dissolve half a pound of black treacle in a pint of hot water and allow to cool, mix in one powder and drench the cow. Repeat twice daily and don't give her any cake–I'll come to see her in two days time." The man took the powders but never spoke and Richard slipped into the driving seat and drove away quickly. As he reached the gate he met a woman cycling towards him, who at once jumped off and came to the car.

"You are early, Mr Buxton said you would not be here till 12 o'clock."

"Oh, it's all right," said Richard, "I've seen the cow and given your man some powders for her. He's not very talkative, is he?"

The woman looked at him and said, "No, he isn't. When will you come again?"

"In two days time."

"Well, will you wait here until I come at 12 o'clock?"

Richard promised and was there at twelve and waited for fifteen minutes before he got fed up and drove up to the buildings. The cow was brighter and had passed some dung, and she was dragging bits of hay out of his hand when he was aware of the man's approach. As he turned, the man was holding a pitchfork in both his hands pointing towards him.

Richard said, "She is improving and I'll give you some more powders. When she has had them I think she will be better." The man never spoke and behaved as he had done two days earlier, so Richard drove off and was at the gate when the woman arrived wheeling the bike. She was out of breath and said, "I am sorry I am late but I had a puncture. Are you all right?"

Richard replied that he was and said that after more powders the cow should be better, and drove off. When he mentioned this to Walter, the latter said that he had heard that the woman's brother was a bit peculiar.

"I don't know about peculiar," said Richard, "I think he is mad." He was proved right, when six weeks later the brother killed a potato merchant with a pitchfork. It took three hefty policemen to overpower him and get him into the ambulance which took him to the asylum.

He spent the three days of the Christmas holiday at home, and on the first night saw Joan in Droughton and wished her all the best, but she said she was in a hurry, and walked away. Richard stared after her for a moment thinking how lovely she was, and how her beautiful grey eyes had sparkled. He was waiting at the tram stop when a car passed and Richard saw Joan sitting beside the driver who was the owner of a furrier's shop in Church Street. The man was wearing a dinner suit, so obviously they were going out to dinner. Richard's euphoria drained away, and some of the brightness of the Christmas Eve dimmed. He suddenly thought what a fool he had been; he should have got in touch with her earlier, and arranged to spend the Christmas days together; also, though he had sent her a card he had not bought her a present. She must think I am not interested, but it's all my own stupid fault. Here I am with plenty of money, well dressed, all on my own with no companion; and in a black mood he went home and spent the evening with his parents. Mary was not at home; she was at a party she was giving, helped by her friends, to old people in the Church Hall in Droughton. After attending the late Eucharist Richard lay in bed listening to the church bells ringing in Christmas Day, as he had done every Christmas since he was a little boy, and in his misery he fell asleep.

Towards the end of January on a bitter snowy morning he arrived at the dairy farm at 8 a.m. to see two cows which were "off colour". It was a herd of 90 pedigree cows from whose milk was made the creamy pink Cheshire cheese for which the farm was famous. Tom Baldwin met him, and took him into the big shippon saying, "I'm very worried, Mr Holden; since I telephoned another cow has become ill."

Not far from the door which Tom closed behind him were two cows which were breathing rapidly; their temperatures were high and pulses rapid. Chest examination revealed pneumonia present.

"Tom, were these cows well yesterday?"

"This one wasn't but the other was, I wish now I had never bought it, but it looked fit and milked very well the first two days, and it has a very good pedigree," replied Tom.

A good-looking girl called, "Dad, this one's not right."

"Good Lord, that's four now." Richard was already beside the cow which had not eaten and had a foul-smelling diarrhoea; and the fourth was showing the same symptoms.

Richard said to Tom," I am certain you have got a highly infectious condition here; can you isolate these cows?"

"No," said Tom, "With this bad weather everything is inside; all the boxes are full."

"Well then, we will have to treat them where they are," and Richard gave Tom the fever drinks, the powder to stop dysentery and instructions for wrapping the cows up, though the shippon was very warm and humid, and then promised to return at midday. Back at Ivy Bank, over a late breakfast, Richard gave Walter the story to date.

"I don't like the sound of it, he obviously bought trouble and whatever germ that new calved cow had in her system was activated by travelling all that way in a freezing cattle wagon. We have a lot to do but I'll meet you there at half past eleven."

They were met by a very worried Tom who said, "I'm glad you've come, Mr Buxton, because this job is going from bad to worse; there are seven of them now, some blowing and others scouring."

After examinations of all the cattle had been done, the three men went into the dairy and discussed the condition, ruling out castor bean poisoning or arsenic; nothing could have come from the hay, which was good, and the cattle cake had been fed for a fortnight. They discussed the causes of pneumonia and black scour and finally decided that it was a form of transit fever, brought by the newly purchased cow. Tom wanted to know how they were going to stop it spreading and they had to admit they did not know, but Walter said "I know the man who will know."

"Who is he?" said Tom, "Get him here as soon as you can."

"He's the Professor of Veterinary Pathology at Liverpool, I'll ring him up as soon as I get back. Meanwhile here are more powders and medicine." The two vets washed their rubber boots with Jeyes fluid and went to have lunch, over which they argued about the cause of the trouble. Walter thought it was a virus but Richard said it was a germ–a virulent bacterium. The Professor came next morning with his assistant. They were taken directly to the farm and saw two dead cows lying outside the shippon door. Tom thanked the Professor for coming and they all accompanied him as he inspected the fourteen sick animals. Twice he removed his spectacles and wiped the lenses, and watched his assistant taking various samples.

Finally he turned to them and said to Tom, "I think there are three causes. One is the very cold weather which affected the cow you bought which was carrying the germ, the second is the humidity and lack of ventilation in here, and the third is the cows' reduced resistance as the winter goes by. They have been in for almost five months now with no sun on their backs and no Johnny Green Grass."

"I can see that," said Tom, "but how are you going to stop it?"

The Professor looked at them all and said, "Open the shippon doors and turn the cows out."

"What!" yelled Tom, "It will kill them."

"I am certain," said the Professor, "that you will kill a lot more if you leave them in here. Wrap them up with sacks if you want, but feed them their hay outside, and as to the ill ones, treat them symptomatically, but leave them in here wrapped up in sacks with all the doors open. I want all the side and roof ventilators wide open as well, and in the meantime I will see if I can get a serum which may help.

Tom said, "Well, thank you, Professor. It sounds drastic, but if it stops it I will be really grateful."

Over lunch the Professor said that in his opinion the cause was the bacterium Pasteurella–a virulent strain which he hoped to recover from the samples he had taken. It was agreed that serum might help and so this was ordered at once by telephone. Richard collected it at 5 a.m. from the guard on the milk train when it stopped at the Halt. By now three more cows had died and two, very ill, would obviously not live long. He spent the morning injecting all the cattle and the herd was improving; no new cases had occurred. Doris, Tom's daughter, filled the syringes for Richard and one of the men held each cow's nose while it was being injected. The two very ill cows died that night, but next day Tom was pleased with the herd and the milk yield was rising, but the farm reeked of Jeyes fluid with which the men were scrubbing out the shippons and boxes.

As he was leaving, Richard on impulse asked Doris if she would like to go to the pictures in Newport on Saturday night, as with the thaw the roads were open and it was his night off. They enjoyed the film, and in the semi-darkness of the back row, held hands and kissed twice, then later sat in the car eating fish and chips out of newspaper. Driving back to the farm Richard appreciated how attractive Doris was–pretty, intelligent, and amusing. He did not however get a good night kiss because arriving at the farm Doris said cheerio, jumped out and was gone. Richard thought it was a good beginning though, and made a mental note to buy a box of chocolates next time.

The first time he went to Church Farm he had to operate on a newly calved cow which had a blocked teat. Carefully he disinfected the teat end and when the owner had her by the nose and the tail was pressed upwards by one of the men, he got a sterilized McLean's teat knife and cut the teat end once and then again at right angles to the first cut. The milk which flowed freely from the swollen quarter was caught in a bucket and given to the calf which was in front of the cow. He now showed the farmer how to dip the teat into the disinfectant solution and also the bougie, which was then pushed into the teat canal leaving the frayed end protruding, and to do this after milking for three days.

The man now went to the other end of the shippon and with another started loading bricks and dirt into a wheelbarrow. When Richard asked what they were doing the farmer told him that they were repairing the standings and cleaning and whitewashing the shippons to be ready for the new Milk Scheme. A week later, in response to an urgent message that a cow was down, he arrived at Church Farm again, to be met by the farmer who said, "I'm sorry Mr Holden, you're too late; she's just died."

"By Jove, that was quick," said Richard. "How long had she been ill?"

"Only since this morning, she didn't eat her cake and gave no milk, so I gave her a fever drink, but when we came out after breakfast she was down."

The cow lay opposite the door in the 7th standing and when Richard saw the bloody froth at her nostrils and the blood-splashed dung behind her, he was fairly certain she had died of anthrax. He told the owner, who would not believe it, but Richard made him take precautions at once. He blocked up the drain and strong disinfectant was poured over the dung and at the front of the cow. Richard told him that he would report it at the police station in the village. He called at the farm a few days later and the farmer said that the Inspector had diagnosed suspect anthrax and that the carcase had been burnt. On trying to find out where the germ had come from, the records of the Diseases of Animals Acts had been searched in the police station. They found an entry from eleven years before that a cow had died of anthrax in No 7 standing in the big shippon at Church Farm. In repairing the standing the farmer had brought the germ to the surface and as he fed cake on the floor the cow had eaten the germ in the soil which had stuck to the cake. What a quirk of fate, thought Richard; in trying to improve his lot, he has lost one of his best cows.

A few days later, his father telephoned to say that Aunt Martha had died, having been ill for six weeks, and that the funeral would be in three days time but Richard had to tell him that he could not go to the funeral. That evening he wrote to Ezra, a letter of sympathy, in which he promised to visit him during his next holiday.

It was one morning after Easter that Walter asked Richard if he would operate on a dog next morning. A gamekeeper left the dog, a big clumber spaniel, at the surgery next morning, and as there was no operating theatre, the two vets scrubbed a table with disinfectant, and boiled the instruments in a sterlizer. The dog appeared friendly when they lifted him onto the table and Walter held him as Richard moved forwards to tie a muzzle round his nose. Without warning the dog lunged forward and fastened his jaws on Richard's right hand, the canine tooth sinking into the knuckle joint of his first finger. Richard yelled and Walter tried with all his might to force the dog's mouth open, but it merely growled and bit harder. Richard shouted, "Walter, get him off! He's chewing my finger off!" and Walter picked up the heavy claw hammer they used for opening wooden drug cases. With one blow he killed the dog and Richard, crying with pain, withdrew his mangled hand from the dog's mouth. He plunged it into a basin containing disinfectant, and then Walter bandaged it. Richard, worried about the events of the last few minutes, said to Walter, "What are we going to tell the owner?"

"Oh, I'll just say it died under the chloroform, don't worry. Go through into the kitchen and ask Megan to make you a drink, you do look white; and I'll clean up here."

The tea revived him, but he realised that he couldn't work for a few days. That night his hand and arm became painful and it was a long time before he got to sleep.

After a late breakfast, he went through into the surgery to find Walter and to ask him what he should do. Walter in an offhand manner, said, "In a way the accident has forced my hand. You will have noticed how the practice has gone quiet now the cows have been turned out, and so there is not enough work for two of us. You will be unable to work for a bit with that hand, so I've decided to dispense with your services at once, because I will be able to manage on my own. I will go and write out your cheque now and I will give you a good reference because you have done very well since you came."

With that he left. Richard was stunned by the sudden change in his fortunes. He went to his bedroom and soon packed all his things into his suitcase, and then, sitting on the bed, put his head in his hands, and in despair thought, now what shall I do, I am sacked again. The atmosphere at lunch was rather strained, and later Walter ran Richard to the Halt to catch the train. When he changed trains at Crewe, he remembered that he had not let Doris know what had happened, and wondered what she would think of him for not informing her.

His spirits rose as the train drew into Droughton and soon he was on his way home in a taxi. After his mother had made him a cup of tea and listened to his story she sent for the Doctor who soon came and immediately took a serious view of the injury, and ordered hot kaolin poultices to be applied three times a day. Even with this treatment, by the end of the week vile-smelling yellow pus oozed from his wounds, his hand and forearm were swollen and he felt ill in himself and very tired with getting very little sleep. The next week his father took him to the Infirmary; there he was given an anaesthetic and the surgeon cut open the skin on the back of his hand and drew out a cigar-shaped core of necrotic material. When he came round from the anaesthetic he found his bandaged hand in a sling hanging from his neck, and his father's strong arm supported him for some time before he drove him home. It was another fortnight before his hand was healed and he began to go for walks to try and get fit again.

Each weekend Richard looked in the "Appointments Vacant" column in the *Veterinary Record* at the two or three posts advertised there. He never got a reply from the first one he wrote to, but he did from the second asking for more information, so he replied at once. One evening he telephoned Doris, and told her what had happened. She was sympathetic and told him that she was going to College to get a Diploma in Food Manufacture and as he was not coming back to work with Walter, it had been nice knowing him and cheerio and the best of luck and rang off. Some how he did not feel bitter towards her—he liked her too much for that—but that chapter was ended and so he must make a fresh start.

In reply to his second letter Richard was asked to attend an interview at 10.30 a.m. on the following Tuesday morning at an address in Lindley, a town fifty miles away. He walked up the hill from the station on that sunny June morning and was nervous when he rang the bell at the door of the large stone-built house, but he was quickly put at ease by the charm of the cheerful man who asked him inside, and introduced himself as David Lewis. He was a plump, short man, with thick, black hair and lively black eyes, and his voice betrayed his Welsh nationality. He soon explained that it was a mixed practice, mainly large animal, and was divided into three parts, a northern, a central, and south-western part and that the successful applicant for the post would be in charge of the south-western branch practice, where the surgery assistant lived with her husband in a flat over the practice premises, so no accommodation was provided. The partner in charge of the eastern part now arrived, a tall soft spoken Scotsman called Alistair Duncan. Now they both asked questions and then took Richard round the house; everything to the right of the front door was private, that to the left was the practice building. Two large terraced houses had been joined together and the entrance to the left one was at the left end; a discreet notice saying "Surgery, please ring", was beside the door. Internally there was communication between the left and right halves. It was well laid out, with a waiting room, consulting room, dispensary, office and operating theatre and kennels all on the ground floor. In the cellars were a stockroom and a general room where large animal instruments and equipment were stored. Upstairs were a small laboratory, library and staff room. After the tour they went through into the right half, a very lovely well-furnished house, and Richard was given coffee before Mr Duncan took him by car to Holme. On the way Richard learnt that the present assistant, who was really a salaried partner, had been given the sack and was leaving this weekend; the reason for his dismissal was the fact that the turnover of the practice was only £700 a year and this barely covered wages.

"Really, he is lazy," said Alistair, "His wife is the only child of a wealthy farmer and cattle dealer and they want for nothing, so he seems to have no incentive to work."

They stopped outside a large shop. The lower half of the plate glass window was painted and opaque and on opening the door a spring mounted bell rang noisily. A young man quickly put down a newspaper and got to his feet.

"What are you doing here?" asked Alistair.

"Oh, I had just called in to see if there were any messages, and to have a cup of tea, so Cheerio," and with that he walked out of the door. Richard thought that his spotless suit and shiny brown shoes did not show any evidence of having been in a stable or shippon that morning.

"That was Tony Green," said Alastair, "he is always rude," and with that they left the waiting room and went into the consultation room, behind which was the office. The day book on the table showed one visit for that day. On the left of the room steps led down to a cellar, the front of which could have been used as an operating room; the rear room was a dispensary and store. The door at the end of the office opened and a small, bespectacled, dark-haired woman came in.

"Good morning Mr Duncan," she said, "Mr Lewis rang to say you were coming."

"Good morning, Mrs Steel. We were just going, unless Mr Holden here wants to see anything else."

"No thank you," replied Richard. With that they left, and in two minutes they were at Holme Station. Alastair thanked Richard for coming and, after asking him if he had done much horse work, said that he and Mr Lewis would be in touch after they had seen two more applicants later in the week.

On the train home Richard considered the job: £6 a week live out, a car provided and the usual holidays. Also, if after three months he had proved satisfactory, a junior salaried partner's agreement would be offered, and the usual binding out agreement would have to be signed. He wondered why, though they were very clean, the premises looked neglected and thought the old bench and torn lino in the waiting room gave a bad impression; there was no comparison to the Colonel's or the Major's establishments.

On reflection he decided to accept the position if it were offered to him, because he felt he was putting on his mother and also his money was beginning to get less again.

He went to see Ezra as he had promised, and found him an old man—Martha's death appeared to have aged him ten years. He was being looked after by Martha's widowed sister, Mrs Lee, whom Richard had heard about but never met. The house was spotless and the home cooking delicious, but outside it was obvious Ezra was allowing the smallholding to go to seed; weeds were growing everywhere and only the poultry and the calves appeared well and cared for.

Nevertheless, he was interested in all Richard had done, and particularly wanted to know what ideas he had for the future. Richard said that in time he would like his own practice, and so was saving money until such time he would have enough to set up practice on his own account; to buy a practice was out of the question. Ezra walked with him to the bus stop, and made him promise to come again. Richard did so and waved to his uncle as the bus roared away. Somehow he knew he would never see him again.

At home he began to get everything put together that he would need in his new job, and to pack a suitcase. Suddenly he stopped and asked himself how he knew he had got the position. He began to wonder if he were beginning to take after his mother who could foretell the future, and was fey – she could always foretell death.

IV

The letter arrived on Friday, offering him the post, and asking him to telephone Mr Lewis if he could begin work on Monday. He could live at the house in Lindley until he could find suitable accommodation in Holme.

On Saturday morning, in the best jeweller's in Droughton, Richard bought his mother a solid silver cake stand, because she had not taken any money for his board all the weeks he had been at home, and he knew she wanted one. Just before tea on the Sunday he went into the kitchen and said, "Mother, put the cake on this." She was thrilled and flung her arms round him and kissed him, and a very happy meal followed. His father took him to the station, and his two suitcases and his boxes of books were put in the guard's van of the 6.50 a.m. train to Holme.

There a taxi took him to the surgery in High Street. Mrs Steel said she was pleased he was early for the morning surgery and gave him a cup of tea. There were only two patients between 9 and 10 a.m. and later he passed the time in arranging the pills, lotions and medicines in an orderly manner, and then by cleaning a Morris car which was very dirty both inside and out, as left by Mr Green in the yard at the back of the building. He had his lunch in a café across the road, and then telephoned Mr Lewis and received permission to go to Lindley to collect a stock of medicines and drugs to bring back to the Holme surgery. That evening he saw three patients between six and seven o'clock and at dinner with the Lewises asked if he could begin to improve the appearance of the Holme surgery while he had so little to do. David was enthusiastic and told him he could spend up to £5 without permission being required. After surgery the next morning he went to the police station and introduced himself to the station sergeant who immediately said he knew Mr Lewis and promised to get him the address of some good lodgings. He also advised him to have his lunch in the Sitting Goose Hotel because it was the best in the town. Holme was an industrial area set in a fertile valley which was intensely farmed and was walled in on the east by mountains and moors. Back in surgery he found a map of the area. Getting the names of the farms from the ledger he plotted them on the map, and was surprised at how few they were.

The telephone rang. Richard answered, "Lewis and Duncan, Veterinary Surgeons; Mr Holden speaking."

The voice said, "This is Jim Benson, Ravenswood, I want a vet quick. I have a horse with colic, will you come straight away?"

"I'll be there in fifteen minutes," replied Richard after consulting his map. The lane up to the farm was rutted and bumpy and followed the river bank, and a large herd was grazing in the fields.

"Hello, what did you say your name was again? I didn't catch it, on the 'phone."

"Holden, a very common name round here, where's the horse?"

The farmer took Richard to a loose box and he soon diagnosed a case of spasmodic colic in the big Shire. While one of the men held the horse, Richard passed a stomach tube and the two gallons of diluted medicine was soon pumped in by the farmer, after which the horse was taken for a walk.

"I've never seen that done before," said Mr Benson, "but I must say it's easier than using a drenching bottle. Thank you for coming so quickly, because I haven't had your firm for a year. I fell out with that Mr Green. I've been having Lonsdale's but there was no vet in when I rang them so that's how I came to ring you. While you are here would you look at two cows?"

The first was a cow with a bad "foul in the foot", which Richard cleaned up with antiseptic, then after applying iodoform ointment bandaged the foot firmly. The second case was a chaff in the eye. Richard poured in a little cocaine solution and then kept squirting warm water from a hypodermic syringe until finally he washed out the chaff. The horse, which had dried off a lot, was standing outside and looked easier and drank when led to the trough. Richard gave instructions for care of the horse and said he would visit the lame cow in three days time.

As he drove away, he thought to himself that that was the first bit of real work he had done since he arrived. As he drove up High Street, he could see Mrs Steel wearing her white coat standing outside the surgery and as he stopped she opened the car door and said, "Do come quick, there's a dog here bleeding to death."

The black and white collie had got loose and run into the hay field and the mowing machine had almost amputated the left hind leg above the hock, from which blood was dripping from a blood-soaked bandage.

"Get your hand right up inside the leg and with your fingers on the bone, squeeze hard."

Richard quickly cut away the string and bandage, cut off the thin strip of skin and let the torn lower leg fall on to the table, dipping the stump into antiseptic solution. He got a pair of Spencer Wells forceps from the sterilizer, said to the farmer, "Release your grip," and deftly shut off the squirting artery.

"That's better, now let's get a bandage round his nose. I don't want Mrs Steel bitten."

"He won't bite while I'm here. I'm Bob Mattinson. He's my best working collie and I want him saved if only as a stud dog."

"Right, I'm Mr Holden. I am now going to clean the stump, ligature the artery, inject local anaesthetic and then stitch the skin to try and cover it."

When it was finished and all bandaged up Mrs Steel brought in cups of tea. Bob said that he farmed High Halsteads, a big sheep farm. He bred his own sheep dogs and took part in dog trials, as a result of which he sold his dogs all over the north of England.

"By the way, I sold one to Dick Holden at Higher Hindhead a few weeks ago, are you any relation?"

"Yes, he's my uncle," Richard replied. "It is a small world. Anyway, get your wife to cut the foot out of an old sock, pull it up the leg over the bandage and tie it to a girth round his chest. I don't want him chewing that bandage off," and Richard gave the dog the rest of the sweetened milky tea in a dish. Bob brought the dog back three times that week and the stump healed very well. He was so pleased that at the last visit he brought Mrs Steel and Richard half a dozen eggs each.

The Sitting Goose was the best hotel in Holme, and run very well by the Misses Howarth; it had been in their family for eighty years. The dining room was almost full when Richard walked in.

"Just one?" enquired Miss Howarth. "Very well, you will have to share a table with Mr Lord the chemist, and your name is?"

"Richard Holden, I'm the vet from Lewis and Duncan's up the road."

"Yes I know; then sit here please. Mr Lord, this is Mr Holden."

Soon the two were talking about drugs, and Jim Lord told Richard that it was time that Lewis and Duncan got another vet to run the Holme practice, because he was always dispensing recipes for farmers and dog owners. Richard jokingly replied that it would be nice to put a stop to that. As the weeks went by they became good friends, even though he only had lunch on Saturdays and Sundays in the hotel, because he got good lodgings quite quickly, recommended by the police sergeant.

The three storey stone built house was in the area called Valley View. From his bedroom window, Richard could see right across the town, and the Town Hall Clock, the spire of St. Pauls Church and the square brick block of the Royal Infirmary appeared very near, though slightly obscured by the smoky haze even on a summer's morning. The other four young men who lodged there were a teacher; an assistant foundry manager; a curate, and a member of the Borough Treasurer's staff–a jolly bunch of young men, and Richard found he was the busiest of the lot. From going to calve a cow at 6 a.m. sometimes, his day did not end until 8 or 9 p.m., and he was glad that every second Sunday was his day off, when Mr Lewis covered for him.

The 8 a.m. visit to the local saleroom to a "mad dog" gave him later the opportunity to refurbish his surgery. It was obvious that the guard dog, which was loose at night in the building, had got the spring clip of his lead embedded in his foot, and had then got the lead caught under a heavy sideboard. Every time the dog moved it was in agony and was snapping at the steel chain lead, growling and slavering.

Richard told Mr Reed the owner to go and find some wire cutters, while he went out to his car and brought in his dog catcher. Richard slipped the loop of the catcher over the dog's head and pushed his head away, and Mr Reed cut the lead. The dog limped forward and grew calmer, a muzzle was applied and Richard hung on to the Alsatian while the clip was cut off. Maurice Reed was very grateful because he said he had thought first of shooting the dog because he could not get near it.

As a result, the surgery waiting room had the floor covered in red linoleum, and was furnished with eight stand chairs and a small table on which soon appeared copies of *Our Dogs* and old copies of *London Life*, the *Tatler* and *Answers*. The bench was taken to pieces and the long pieces of wood made good shelves when erected in the cellar, which Richard made into an operating theatre for small animals, because a sink with hot and cold water was already fitted and electric light was available. The ceiling and walls were "walpamured" white and a keytable and a cupboard made up the furnishings. He got a joiner to make a wooden box 14 inches long, 7 deep and 7 wide with a top of bevelled plate glass which was pushed into position along a groove let into the top of each side. At one end was a brass inlet nipple. He brought an anaesthetic apparatus back from Lindley; this was a glass container with a removable lid which had an inlet and outlet pipe. Ether was poured into the container, a Higginson syringe blew air through the inlet pipe and the ether and air mixture was blown into the box through a tube attached to the nipple. It was easy to see when a cat became unconscious; then it was lifted out and the anaesthesia was continued using a metal mask, which had a rubber rim. Soon, with Mrs Steel as anaesthetist, Richard was castrating two or three cats a week.

One Monday morning he went to the stable of the local coal merchant to treat a horse with a thick leg. In all his horse cases he used Major Gilmour's recipes. After examining the horse he mixed up the 1lb. powder in 2 gallons of water, passed the stomach tube and had it pumped in. The merchant watched him and then said "Well I'll be damned; I thought our Jim was pulling my leg." His wife was Jim Benson's sister, and had told Bill Bond how the new vet had pushed yards of hose pipe up his horse's nose and how quickly it got better.

"I use it because it is a better way of treating horses. This horse gets only water and sloppy bran and no bedding in his box–I'll be here tomorrow."

The treatment was repeated next day and by Wednesday the horse was almost better, so light diet and exercise were ordered.

One evening he had to go and help out at Lindley, because David was at a prolapse case, when a case of a cow bleeding badly came in. Richard soon reached the farm to find a cow had been hiked (horned) in her udder–there was a five-inch tear almost separating the hind quarters. Acting a bit like the Major he barked out orders, the cow was cast quickly, the hind leg held back, the wound washed with antiseptic, the artery found and ligated and then the skin sutured and fly-repellant antiseptic oil applied. He then went on to David's surgery and found that he had arrived home. Richard was invited to have some supper and soon they were talking technicalities about parturient apoplexy or milk fever. David still blew up the cow's udder with oxygen, but Richard wanted to try the new calcium treatment. In the end it was agreed that Richard could try it, but David advised him to join the National Veterinary Benevolent and Mutual Defence Society at once; the entrance fee was only a guinea.

Richard joined the Society and then got some back numbers of the *Veterinary Record*, and read up all he could about milk fever. Jim Lord supplied him with calcium chloride and distilled water and he boiled 1 ounce of the powder in 12 ounces of water, filtered the solution, and closed the bottle with a boiled rubber bung. He was determined to try this new treatment because only about two-thirds of cases got better and they often lost a quarter with mastitis. For advice he rang the Major because he was certain that he would have tried it.

"Yes, it works very well, Richard. How nice to hear from you. So you are in Holme, plenty of cattle round there. Use a long needle, a flexible connection and a twenty mil. syringe. I get the jugular vein up by pulling a calving rope tight round the neck, but you can use the mammary vein. But whatever you do be certain the solution goes into the vein because if any gets outside you get a big swelling and then a slough. Glad to be of help, all the best and Cheerio."

As autumn came the weather turned showery and Jim Benson asked Richard to go and look at some lame cows. The potholes in the lane were filled with water and mud was everywhere.

"Mr Holden, I want something doing about these lame cows, I'm getting too many of them. I've nine lame this morning; it's far too many out of a hundred cows."

So Richard examined them, finding that some had foul and some ulcerated soles, and they all resented treatment—it was a sweaty dirty job, dealing with them. Then they went and walked to the field gate. The gateway was very muddy and clinker had been spread.

"Well, Jim, the first thing I want you to do is stop using this gateway. This wet clay land is making your cows' feet soft and the clinker is causing trouble, it's so rough. I think the best thing is to make two new gateways on that higher ground opening on to the old lane and use them alternately."

"Aye, but Mr Holden, it's quarter of a mile further that way," said Jim.

"I know that, but it's a tarred road all the way and the cows' feet will be drier. I also want you to dig out the ground just outside the top door of the shippon, line it with a tarpaulin and make up this solution in water according to the direction on the bottle. Do that for two days, empty it and refill it with this antiseptic solution, change over every two days and I think we will get things to mend."

Soon there were only two lame cows; one took a long time to get right, and the other went to the butcher.

So Richard could not understand the message one morning a little later which said more cows were ill. It was not the cows however which were affected but the calves and heifers. They walked to the far field to inspect them and found many were coughing.

"They've got husk, Jim."

"Are you sure? I've never had it before," he replied.

"Yes, I am sure," said Richard, and they walked on and found a heifer dead. "I'll examine a blood smear for anthrax and if it's negative I'll ring Berry the horse slaughterer and ask him to open it here. I'll let you know the time."

The smear test was negative, so he asked Berry to get the lungs out of the carcase. When he opened the trachea and used a magnifying glass, fine worms could be seen in the froth. Jim was astounded, but immediately sent his men to bring in all the affected animals and give them dry food. Jim collected a large bottle of husk medicine from the surgery and went back to dose them all. Next morning Richard went to inject them all intratracheally, finding that one had died during the night, and that out of the 33 remaining four only were healthy.

"Jim, these four—did you breed them?" asked Richard.

"No, I bought them at a dispersal sale in spring," said Jim.

Richard explained that these animals had probably recovered from the disease, but were carriers and had brought the disease with them. Another died but the others slowly recovered and the pasture was ploughed up.

The three months had passed and David asked Richard to Lindley one night for dinner. He and Alastair Duncan arrived together and soon the promised agreement was being discussed. It was agreed that Richard's position was permanent, and his salary was confirmed at £8 a week live out, this to be reviewed in 12 months, and eleven days holiday a year.

Richard would be in sole charge of the Holme practice, which would be self-supporting, except for the motor car, which David and Alastair would replace soon. Apart from the chairs, tables and cupboards, which had been recently purchased, there were no tangible assets at Holme. The practice premises were rented on a long term lease. This surprised Richard, who made up his mind to buy them. So the assets were current debtors and cash at the bank, and the outlook was good, for the accountant's figures for the first three months showed that the turnover had been £280.

It was agreed that a profit-sharing scheme should form the basis of a salaried partner's agreement, Mr Lewis receiving 3/7 and Mr Duncan and Richard 2/7 each. The usual clauses about obedience to the senior partner's orders, efficiency, punctuality and binding out would be included. This was the substance of the agreement they all signed at Mr Lewis's solicitors some days later. Richard, believing in the word of the partners, never questioned anything, not even why Mr Duncan should have 2/7 of the profits, and did not consult a solicitor; he was so busy he never thought of it. But he did realise that having thrown himself heart and soul into his work he had neglected everything else including himself. He wrote to Joan a long letter telling her all that had happened, then rang Uncle Dick and had a nice talk to him and Alice, who invited him to go and see them one Sunday.

Fishers, the tailors in the High Street, never had a window display. Usually there was one roll of expensive material on a stand and nothing else. Inside it was a shop, with many fitting rooms, a large display department, a busy workroom with many tailors; it was a centre of gossip and interest for all of the area's prominent business men, landlords, and professional men, Richard was lucky in that he was welcomed by Mr Fisher senior when he entered the shop, and soon had all his measurements entered in the clients' ledger for the making of a hacking jacket in russet cavalry twill and a pair of fawn trousers in the same woollen material. While this was going on Mr Fisher extracted a lot of information as to Richard's profession and background and entered this at the bottom of the page in the ledger.

In the practice he noticed new names appearing in the day book, one of which was that of Whittaker, Buck House Farm who had a cow down after calving. Richard found a cow with milk fever lying in the standing and immediately decided to try the new treatment. By the time he had injected the whole bottle the cow had lifted her head and was looking round.

"Mr Holden, that's quick," said Lawrence.

"Yes, it's a new treatment that so far appears to be a lot better than the old one because you don't touch the cow's bag," said Richard. "Just let's have a bit of soil and straw scattered round her and we'll see if she will get up." She did, Lawrence was delighted and after being told to milk her lightly for two days thanked Richard and said it was a "ruddy miracle". Over the next few weeks so did other farmers, including Alwyn, Lawrence's brother who farmed fifteen miles away, at Barn End, Thursby.

Richard was now a good driver of a car and always went quickly, so much so that the new Austin car was quickly christened "the Flying Bedstead" by some of the farmers, especially those who saw Richard driving very fast along the main west road. It was strange, but the accident happened when he was going very slowly up Crossings Brow on a very wet Tuesday morning. He had to stop at the level crossing and after the gates were opened set off, up the steep hill, staring ahead through the blindingly heavy rain. Avondale Road ran diagonally across the Brow from above to below and just as Richard was driving across the junction in second gear a heavy lorry coming from the higher part of Avondale Road crashed into his car and pushed it onto its near side. As the car turned onto its side, he felt an intense pain in his left hand, medicine bottles crashed about him and he found himself up against the passenger door, while the scream of metal on stone was deafening for a few moments. Then it stopped and there was another crash as the lorry plunged through a garden wall.

The butcher in the corner shop told his assistant to ring for an ambulance and ran out to the car, to be joined by the grocer and people from the post office. Richard rubbed his hands over his face and quickly came to his senses. Helped by the grocer and butcher he got out of the wrecked car, and was taken into the shop and given a stool to sit on and then a mug of tea. A policeman arrived on his cycle and then three men appeared carrying the lorry driver who was semi-conscious and bleeding from his head, and laid him on a table at the back of the shop. Richard had rubbed his bleeding left hand over his face and looked a gory spectacle, so much so that the ambulance men were going to put him on a stretcher until he protested that he was not hurt. Then they saw the lorry driver and he was carried out.

After giving a statement to an inspector of police, Richard got a taxi back to the surgery and cleaned himself up, and bandaged his hand which had been torn by the ignition key. He then rang David who at first was very annoyed, but calmed down when Richard explained that it was not his fault. After this he walked to Howarth and Brown's garage at the end of the road, told them where the wrecked car was for them to recover, and hired another car. He felt upset and tired for the rest of the day but finished all his work, though he was very disappointed that one of the partners had not offered to help him. When the case came up in Court, Richard was exonerated from any blame, because the brakes of the lorry had failed; it was carrying three tons of coal more than it was authorised to carry. It had no horn, an inefficient silencer, and the rear number plate was missing. The practice was awarded damages and expenses, so finally Richard had a brand new Austin car which did a lot for his morale.

Events often occur in threes, and after his first court appearance, he soon appeared there again. The message on the Monday was to visit a horse with a thick leg at Gardners, but when Richard got there and examined the horse he realised it was not the usual type of thick leg. The horse was sweating, had a temperature of 105 °F and a rapid pulse. The off hind leg was swollen from haunch to foot, he could feel gas under the skin, and a bloody serous fluid was dripping off the hair in various places. With a pair of curved scissors he cut the hair away at one place and saw a small round hole from which the fluid was oozing. Every wet patch proved to be the same. He looked at John Gardner and said:

"You know, this is not an ordinary thick leg. In my opinion these holes have been made by a sharp instrument like a bradawl, and this horse is dying."

"It's strange you should say that," said John "because when I came in on Saturday night there was a pitchfork just inside the door on the ground and they are never left there usually, they are up in the hay loft."

"Will you bring it, John," said Richard and when they measured the distance between the holes it was exactly the same as the distance between the tines of the pitch fork, on which they could see hairs and dried blood.

"John, this is a job for the police. You go and bring them; I'll wait here,"

John came back with the sergeant in about half an hour; he listened to the history, saw the holes, and then asked:

"Mr Gardner, have you fallen out with anybody lately?"

He pondered for a moment and then said, "No."

"Are you certain? Think hard."

"Well, I don't like to blame anybody but I did sack Jack Hall last month for pinching hen food," replied John.

"Thank you," said the sergeant, "I'll be off now and continue my enquiries and let you know." The horse was breathing very rapidly and swaying on his feet, and John asked if he should have it shot.

"That's up to you, Mr Gardner, but I want to be at the post mortem so let me know, won't you?"

There was no need to; the horse died shortly afterwards, and the post mortem showed how deeply the tines of the fork had been driven into the horse's leg. When Jack Hall was visited by two policemen he at first denied all knowledge of the case, but two witnesses identified him as the drunken man staggering away from Gardner's on the Saturday evening. Then he broke down and confessed that he did it to get even with John Gardner for sacking him. In court Richard as the professional witness gave his evidence clearly and efficiently. Jack Hall was sent to prison where he was safe from the anger of the local people.

"Jem" Braithwaite was a well known local character who farmed High End with the help of two men; there he had fifty milking cattle which enabled him to supply a large area in Holme with milk. People could rely on him, he never missed a delivery and was never late. He left the farm at 5.30 a.m. every day to begin delivering milk from his beautifully varnished cart which was drawn by a heavy horse. One morning a policeman saw that the horse was lame and stopped Jem and told him he could not work the horse. Now Jem was very deaf and pretended not to understand, and as soon as the policeman walked away, got back in the cart and continued delivering milk.

The policeman stopped him again, made him take the horse out of the shafts and impounded it, taking it to the police station.

Richard had to go and examine it and found it lame off fore. As a result Jem was summoned to appear before the Court two days later at 10 a.m. Richard was amused to find the court room packed with men, a lot of them Jem's farming friends, and he stood in the dock shouting greetings to them. Silence reigned when the magistrates entered, and soon the clerk read out the charge. Jem was waving to a friend he had just noticed. The policeman standing besides him touched him on the arm and said:

"Pay attention to the Clerk."

"What?" shouted Jem.

The officer shouted back, "Pay attention to the Clerk!"

"Why?"

"Because he is reading the charge."

"What for?"

"Because you worked a lame horse."

"Where is the Clerk?"

"Over there."

By now people were beginning to be amused by the farcical proceedings. The clerk started again. Jem bawled, "I can't hear thee!" The magistrate intervened and told the policeman to repeat each sentence in a loud voice to Jem.

"That you did at 7.40 a.m." repeated the policeman.

"If Mrs Harris had come out quicker with her jug I'd have been round the corner and I wouldn't have been spotted."

"Don't interrupt."

"Well I'm going to tell my side of the story, it's too one-sided."

Richard's evidence was conclusive, and so Jem was fined, though his friends said it was the best free show they had witnessed in years. Jem changed his route so that in future he did not go along that road at 7.40 a.m., and he still employed Richard as his vet.

The day book was now showing anything from 4 to 7 or 8 visits a day and the number of people coming to the evening surgery increased. Richard began to inject dogs with virus serum against distemper, including the two dachshunds from the Sitting Goose. He was just finishing his lunch in the hotel on the Saturday morning when Miss Ruth Howarth told him he was wanted in the surgery at once. Mrs Steel told him that his father wanted him to telephone home as soon as possible. Before he picked up the phone a voice inside him said "Ezra" and he shivered momentarily. His father told him that Ezra had had a severe stroke on Friday morning and had died in the early afternoon, and that the funeral would be at 11 a.m. on the coming Wednesday. Mr Lewis gave him the day off. Richard arrived home, and was in tears as he looked at the white face of his dead uncle lying in his satin upholstered coffin, and his father led him away as the undertaker screwed on the coffin lid. All his uncles and their families were present at the graveside to watch the coffin lowered into Martha's grave, but Richard had to leave them all in the early afternoon to get back to Holme. Some weeks later the solicitor's letter informed him that he was one of the beneficiaries under the will. Ezra had left him £500, and his sister £250.

Spring was late and mild and the practice was busy with all the spring calvings. Richard castrated two shire colts, and docked some foals. When Alastair Duncan asked him if he would do some horse work for him, Richard's morale was given a big boost. It was arranged that he would operate on two colts, which meant that he left Holme at 6 a.m. and after successfully operating arrived back at his surgery at a quarter past nine, to find a full waiting room and some visits waiting. Mrs Steel gave him a cup of tea and he worked on, and then bought a meat pie and ate it on the way to his first farm visit.

"You've taken your time to get here," said Tom Carr.

"Yes, I'm sorry, but I had to go to Refton."

"Refton," said Tom, "that's a hell of a way to go."

"Yes, I know," replied Richard, "but I was operating on two colts for Mr Duncan."

"Tha sees he pays you," said Tom. "Come on, cow's in here." Richard was relieved that the heifer calf was alive, and soon delivered it. He was on his way to his car when Tom said, "Don't be in such a hurry–there's another one yet." This was a beast with wooden tongue, so he lanced the tongue, rubbed in some iodine crystals and gave Tom a bottle of medicine with which to continue the treatment.

It was a long day which only ended after he had treated a horse with founder at the LMS Railway stables at 9 o'clock that night. He arrived at the digs just in time to go with George, Alec and Robin to the Rose and Crown to celebrate George's birthday. When the landlady joined them they almost got her tight, and Richard felt a new man at closing time—it had been a jolly evening which had been more enjoyable because it had been unexpected.

During the next few weeks he made five visits to the Refton area. As a result he found himself operating on dogs and cats after evening surgery, dispensing on a Saturday evening, and his car was very dirty. When he asked David and Alastair if he could have some assistance, it was politely refused, even though David now had an assistant, Mr White, to help him and Alastair. Richard, faintly annoyed, said that he would try and get someone part-time who could come in perhaps two half days a week and they agreed to this.

The Siamese cat was miserable, and resented Richard examining the matted fur round his neck, but the big white-haired old man held him firmly while the hair was parted and the skin washed with antiseptic, revealing pus oozing from a few places round the neck. It had been like this for almost three weeks and had come on quite suddenly after it had been at his sister's for a few days.

"I am certain there is something buried under the skin, Mr Wilcock. You will have to leave him and I'll give him an anaesthetic and see if I can find out what it is."

Mr Wilcock looked at Richard and said, "He means a lot to me, and though I haven't much money I'll pay anything to get him right."

"We will see about that later. He's not been fed, has he?"

"No, he's only had a drop of milk today." So the cat was anaesthetised and the forceps drew out a bit of rubber. Richard clamped it and then cut it. "I think it's a rubber band, Mrs Steel." He carefully pulled on the clamp and out came the rest of a rubber band. He syringed Eusol into the holes, and put the cat back in his basket to recover.

Mr Wilcock was first for evening surgery and soon explained that he thought the rubber band had been put on the cat's neck by two mischievous grandchildren who stayed at his sister's during the day so that their mother could go out to work. He was profuse in his thanks because he explained it was his late wife's cat and his sole companion. He counted out the seven shillings and six pence on the table and said, "I can't thank you enough. If you ever want any help, do let me know. I am a retired dispenser but I would do anything."

Richard could hardly believe his ears and said, "Where do you live?"

"Station Row, it's not far," said Mr Wilcock.

"O.K., you come back at half past seven."

Mr Wilcock proved invaluable; medicine bottles were beautifully wrapped in white glazed paper and the ends closed with red sealing wax; on Wednesday afternoons he and Mrs Steel did all the dispensing, referring to Richard's recipe book or Hoare's *Materia Medica*. On Saturdays the car was cleaned, rubber boots washed, calving ropes boiled, and the car boxes filled with powders and medicines. He was a godsend to Richard and all for eight shillings for two half days. Everybody called him Willie, but there was one snag—he smoked the foulest smelling twist in his pipe. Richard later found out that he also helped at Lord's the chemists, and on Saturday night at 9 o'clock scrubbed out a butcher's shop.

By summer that year it was apparent that more accommodation was necessary; the back cellar was crammed full of tea chests and wicker baskets which were used to transport bulk drugs. There were also cat baskets and harness and hobbles, and large animal instruments hanging on nails driven into the walls. It was always cold because there was only a one bar electric fire to heat it; Richard would not allow an open fire with so much inflammable material about. Across the back from the yard, was a small stable in good repair, which had been empty for some time. Willie Wilcock soon found out that Mr Seed from the saleroom owned it, so Richard went to see him one lunch time, and they made arrangements to meet at the stable that evening.

David Lewis agreed with the idea of using it as a storeroom, kennels, and garage, so Richard and Mr Seed met that evening and it was agreed that one stall partition be removed and the double stall made into a loose box; the door would be widened and with the removal of another partition a stock and storeroom could be made and at the end a kennels and cattery.

The weekly rent was very little, and Mr Seed soon found second-hand shelving, doors, and two trestle tables to put the cat cages on. Willie helped the joiner to carry out the conversion, and then worked three half days a week; among other jobs he whitewashed it all through. The loft was left untouched, but the idea was to use it later. George, the foundry under-manager who lived in the digs, soon fabricated six steel cat cages which Willie painted white, and soon they were very rarely empty. Richard never told the partners that he paid Willie to help Mr and Mrs Steel decorate the flat right through; it was his way of showing the Steels his appreciation of all the extra hours she worked without complaint.

The warmer weather came and the practice went quiet; so Richard went to Lindley with various instruments he wanted repairing or sharpening and brought back a supply of teat bougies which David's staff made, a lamb size Holborn bloodless castrator and more clinical thermometers. While he was there, David suggested that he should have his holiday soon—one year had gone and Mr White would run the Holme practice while he was away. So he went home for three days. On the Saturday he telephoned Joan and he was lucky she was also home. He invited her out to dinner, but she refused and said she would like to go to the pictures to see Greta Garbo in *The Painted Veil*, and they arranged a time. His father told him to take the car, and when he called for Joan at 6 o'clock, he was very happy and gave her a box of chocolates. They enjoyed the film, ate the chocolates, and smoked, occasionally holding hands. Joan invited him in when they arrived back in Weston; the maid brought the coffee, after which they chatted, and they kissed when he left at 11.30 p.m. He lay awake in bed at home thinking how much he loved her and wanted her; he knew that whatever happened she would reign in his heart for always. He took stock: he had no house, no car, really no secure job and £570 in the bank. How could he ask her to marry him? They were a wealthy family owning an estate, businesses, and shops with a magnificent house which had a ballroom and tennis courts, so he decided it would have to wait no matter how amorous he felt.

After talking to his Uncle Dick on the telephone he accepted his invitation to go and spend a few days with them, and at the last moment put his old clothes and rubber boots in his suitcase. Alice and Dick were pleased to see him; Tom the shepherd was still there, but Walter had left and been replaced by a nineteen-year-old Scot called George Greaves. The next day Dick said they were going to gather the flock and separate out the ram lambs for cutting and docking; he hoped they wouldn't lose as many from fly strike as they had last year. Richard at once said there was no need to lose any and explained about the bloodless castrator, but regretted that he hadn't one with him.

"Where do you get them?" asked Dick and when Richard replied "London", he told him to get one ordered at once for urgent delivery. He soon convinced the girl on the end of the telephone in London that he wanted the castrator sent to Holden, Higher Hindshead Farm, and not Lewis Duncan and Holden in Lindley. It was sent express on the first available train and they received it next morning from the stationmaster in Ashton. They soon brought in the ram lambs they had separated on the Monday and Richard showed Dick and Tom how to pull the jaws of the instrument away from the lamb and then to feel that the cords were broken properly; then the instrument was closed on the tail which was twisted off and dipped in anti-fly oil. It was the middle of the afternoon before they were finished, and Tom made them all laugh when he said, "We won't be eating shepherd's pie for the next fortnight this year," but the lamb losses were in fact very few that year. Then they started to clip, and Dick said he was trying to get other farmers in the area to have electricity laid on to their premises; that way he could afford it, if eight of them shared the installation costs. As it was it was hand clipping and Richard too wished they had electricity and that he had Cooper Stewart clippers in his hand. Soon it was Wednesday and he had to leave but not before he had promised to send his uncle some anti-fly oil and some soap for obstetrical work.

When he arrived back at his digs, Mrs Sykes the landlady said she was pleased to see him, because Mrs Steel had rung up twice to see if he were back and she told him that she had had difficulty in getting Mr White to attend to cases. This annoyed him, so next morning he rang David and let him know that he would be taking morning surgery, so there was no need for Mr White to come over.

"But he will come over to bring your car back; we had to borrow it, he will tell you why."

The entries in the day book for the previous week were only half of what he had expected, and Mrs Steel said that Mr White had only come to the surgery when she telephoned him so people had to wait a long time. By now Richard was really annoyed, and when Jimmy White finally arrived Richard started to tell him off in no uncertain manner but Jimmy stopped him and said:

"Cool down a bit, you don't know half of it. You see, Mrs Lewis fell down the stairs and broke her leg last Friday morning so David has done hardly any work for a week. I spent all last Sunday doing non-urgent jobs and then on Monday morning I parked my car outside the cattle market and when I came out a cattle wagon had backed into it and smashed the front in and the engine. I've never had a bloody minute. I'm fed up with my uncle and his practice."

Richard got Mrs Steel to make some tea and toast and apologised for being angry, but Jimmy laughed it off, saying he had a right to be annoyed and then explained that Mrs Lewis was his aunt.

"So that's it, and both of you come from Scotland."

"Oh yes, Uncle David met Jenny when he was an assistant in Scotland years ago. I like them both, but he treats me like a servant and pays me very little. We had a row last night and I told him that I was not his skivvy."

Richard quickly drove him back to Lindley, and then got on with his day's work, but Jimmy's remark that his uncle paid him very little worried him. He had noticed that David and Alastair watched every penny and that their only expense at Holme had been the first Austin car and the conversion of the stable. Everything else had been paid for out of the Holme earnings and there was nearly £800 in the bank account.

That evening he bought some flowers and went to Lindley to see Jenny who was very cheerful and thanked him for the flowers. She had broken her ankle and was sitting up on a day bed with the plastered leg stretched out in front of her. David fussed round her like a worried hen, and Richard realised that this couple were still very much in love, and what an attractive pair they still were, Jenny with her pale skin and deep gold coloured hair and David with his black mane of hair, really like a younger Lloyd George.

With the approach of autumn the practice became busier; the Steels had a week's holiday during which Mrs Steel's sister stayed in the flat and acted as surgery assistant and was very helpful, but she irritated Richard by fussing over him, making tea and trying to anticipate his every need. At odd times he caught her eyeing him, when she would smile and turn away and he thought, what's wrong with the woman?—I wish Mrs Steel were back. When they returned, Will Steel asked Richard if they could have a dog because Will's firm were starting a night shift. Will would have to work at nights one in three, and he didn't want his wife to be alone in the building. She was nervous when late at night people tried to open the front, or more often the cellar, door. Richard found them one for nothing, a six-month-old wire-haired fox terrier called Roy which immediately became Mrs Steel's guard dog, and could quickly show it by growling and threatening to bite. Soon at night he had the run of the whole building, but in the daytime was upstairs in the flat. While he was there he always barked if the telephone or door bell rang, and he hated cats. Richard gave him the virus serum treatment for distemper and did not charge Will Steel. He was glad he had done so when distemper appeared that autumn and rapidly spread, so surgeries were busier than normal with dogs in all stages of the disease.

He received a telephone call from the accountant one morning, informing him that they would collect the books and ledgers one day soon as it was the financial year end for the practice. Some weeks later the three partners met in the offices of the accountants, and the profit and loss account and the balance sheet were explained and considered. Richard was congratulated because the turnover in the last twelve months had been £1,278; after all expenses had been paid the profit for distribution among the partners was £428.

When they started to discuss the balance sheet Richard suggested that new practice premises be found, because the present ones were very inconvenient, being on three floors, and in spite of the stable conversion, working conditions were cramped. David said it was a good idea and would be examined, but reminded Richard that his own premises were also on three floors, to which Richard replied that David's rooms were twice the size. Car repairs also came in for consideration, and Richard explained that the very rough roads up to some of the hill farms caused many broken springs and punctured tyres. It was a friendly meeting and Richard was pleased to know he would have £107 profits to come. He never examined the figures closely, or he would have discovered that he had received no payment for all the work he had done for Alastair and David or that among miscellaneous expenses, like repairs, decorations and so on, the partners had got the accountant to include £50. They had got back half the expense of buying the new car.

The weather turned wet and cold; and husk, foul in the foot, ringworm, lice, sore teats, and all the troubles associated with calving increased in number. At the railway stables, and all the commercial stables there was much to do, with an outbreak of strangles and rarer cases, one of azoturia and another of purpura haemorrhagica. Richard found husk in sheep; a bad outbreak of foot-rot; then fluke and gid; he began to see so many conditions he bought a Black's Veterinary Dictionary as a quick reference book. He was so busy that he forgot his mother's birthday on November 20th and Joan's on the 22nd; but telephoned his mother and wished her all happiness. He was glad to get home on Christmas Eve with presents for his parents and Mary, but Mary was staying in London with her fiancé's parents, having recently got engaged. Jim White covered for him on Christmas Day and Boxing Day and Richard reciprocated when being a true Scot he went "hame for Hogmanay", but Jim's uncle was very annoyed when he did not return until the 3rd January, looking worse for wear.

Tom Dickenson was a dentist with a large practice in the town who lived at Hill Cottage, an enormous house in Valley View. It had been built by a wealthy industrialist, Ebenezer Hall, at the turn of the century and was two houses behind one façade with communication between the two. Originally Mr Hall's staff of butler, maids and cooks lived in one half ruled over by the housekeeper, and the Halls lived in style in the other half. Now, Tom Dickenson lived in one half with his wife Jean and his three children, Flora, Mary and William; while his sister, Mrs Lawson, her husband and a large brood of children lived in the other half. Richard was a client of Tom's but even so was surprised to receive an invitation to a New Years Eve party printed on a white card with gold edging. It was a great party, with a lovely buffet supper and plenty of drinks both soft and alcoholic. A large room with a parquet floor had been cleared of furniture and carpets and they danced to music played on a radiogram. Richard was introduced to Flora and was at once attracted to her, with her blonde hair and ready smile; her figure was shown off to advantage by a tight fitting red jumper and royal blue skirt, but he excused himself later and circulated among all the other men and women, talking, getting them drinks and having the odd dance.

Nevertheless at supper time he found himself again with Flora as, balancing plates on their knees, they ate, talked and joked together. Then the games began: the animal game; treasure hunt; singing for your supper; and spot prizes given during the dancing. Tom and Jean Dickenson and the Lawsons came and joined them at five minutes to twelve, and to the chimes of Big Ben Auld Lang Syne was sung. Flora gave Richard a firm, hot kiss full on the lips with her arms clasped tightly round his neck, and Jean Dickenson noticed this happen. Robin, the teacher, and Richard walked home, saying what a good party it had been. When Robin told Richard that he had made quite a hit with Flora he was a little embarrassed, but secretly had really enjoyed the last few minutes when he had a vibrant young woman's body pressed so close to him that passion stirred.

After a typical February day of driving sleet and a bitter south-east wind Richard felt he was developing a sore throat, but in spite of using an antiseptic gargle, it was worse next day and his chest felt sore as a cough developed. Mrs Sykes made him a hot toddy at bedtime and after taking a dose of cough medicine he went to sleep, but he awoke at six with difficult breathing. He felt really ill, so when Mrs Sykes gave him a call later, he asked her to get a doctor and to ring David Lewis and tell him that he was ill. It was an attack of bronchitis which took three days to abate under a treatment of a febrifuge and an expectorant medicine, and he did not smoke cigarettes for some time because they made him cough.

At Fisher's the tailors he bought a cashmere scarf and some warm leather gloves, but in spite of keeping warm did not feel well for a fortnight. Flora was waiting at the bus stop one Saturday morning, so he gave her a lift into town and arranged to take her to the second house of the pictures that evening. Sitting in the semi-darkness at the back of the stalls, they held hands and ate chocolates all through the main film which did not finish until 11 o'clock. When they drove up to Hill Cottage Flora invited him in for cocoa. He refused, saying that he must go back to digs because Mrs Sykes had not a telephone number to ring, in case any messages came in, but she told him to ring from her house. Tom and Jean Dickenson welcomed him again but after they had finished their drink they went out. He put his arms round Flora and kissed her, and quickly she flung her arms round his neck and they kissed repeatedly as she pressed closer to him. When she fell back dragging him on top of her, he became embarrassed and extricating himself said that he must go because he was on duty in the morning. Really, he did not know what to do, because he had little experience of women, and vaguely wondered what would happen if when he got very randy things got out of hand. On the other hand she did not object when he was on top of her, and so this courting went on every Saturday when he was off duty, and he became more and more enamoured of her.

It was a misty night when Tom Dickenson caught the night sleeper train to London so that he could attend a meeting next morning. The mist became fog in the Midlands, but the train was travelling fast when it crashed into some derailed wagons. Tom was one of nine persons killed. This caused a harrowing time for the family, and distressed Richard, who accompanied Flora to the funeral, and so it was some weeks before the Saturday routine was re-established. He took her for dinner to the Sitting Goose, where they were welcomed by Miss Ruth Haworth, and after a lovely meal drank two whiskies each in the bar. Flora decided not to go to the pictures but to go home instead, and as they were leaving they met Mary and Bill, her sister and brother, with their respective escorts just coming in, who being hungry just waved to them and went on into the dining room.

In the lounge at the cottage a standard lamp cast a soft light across the beautifully warm room, which was heated by the bright coal fire. They soon were on the couch kissing and cuddling, their hands exploring more and more as they became bolder with each other. Richard became more excited when his hand touched the silk of her stocking. Flora sighed and pressed harder against him, but suddenly sat up and said, "I must go for a minute," and, getting up, left the room. She returned wearing a silk dressing gown, and said, "I'll switch off this light; it is nicer in the firelight," and at once sat down beside him. As they kissed their hands explored each other gently and she undid his braces and then his trouser buttons, and then pushed her hands round behind his back and stroked it up and down. As his hand stroked her thigh and slowly moved higher he realised he was sexually very excited but didn't care if she felt it against her. Slowly she withdrew her hands and opened her dressing gown revealing to Richard's adoring gaze that she was naked. When she held out her arms to him, he pushed down his trousers, and lowered himself onto her saying, "Oh darling, this is heaven." Flora repeatedly kissed him; wrapped her arms round his neck and her legs round his body. Gently he sank down and his hard hot, erect penis slid into her warmth and wetness. She sighed and tightened her grip, and then began to move vigorously, and Richard responding drove harder and harder into her until the wave of burning throbbing overwhelmed them; they stopped and he gently collapsed on to her, murmuring, "Darling that was wonderful. I love you so."

Flora replied, "I love you too, but did you use a safe?"

"A what?" asked Richard.

"A safe, silly; you know, a French letter, so I won't have a baby."

Jerked back to reality, he said, "No, I didn't."

"Really, Richard, what am I going to do?"

He thought furiously for a moment and, quickly dressing, said, "I know," and ran out to the car. He scrabbled round in the dark until he found a box and rushed back into the house.

"Look, Flora, this is a new Higginson syringe, you put this rubber extension piece on the nozzle, put the end into salt solution and syringe it out; put two teaspoonfuls of salt in a pint of warm water."

Flora ran from the room and he sat on the couch and wiped the perspiration from his forehead, still dazed by a glowing happiness but feeling sleepy. Flora was fully dressed when she returned and gave him the box, and then sat down beside him and kissed his neck. He put his arm round her and held her tightly to him for a long time until she finally said she was sleepy and after a long lingering kiss they said "Goodnight". Lying in bed later Richard at last understood what his father had been trying to tell him after he failed his examination, and idly wondered how Flora knew about contraceptives but he never reached a conclusion because he sank into a deep sleep. They met regularly but only kissed and held hands, and were both very relieved when Flora's period came. When next he wanted his hair cut he went to a barber's on the other side of the town and on overhearing a man ask for a packet of three, when he had his trim he asked for packet also, and secretly felt a real devil; and thought, now we can enjoy ourselves.

But they didn't because Flora had a recurrence of tonsillitis and the doctor advised the removal of her tonsils. On the day of the operation Richard sent flowers to the hospital. The next day he visited her, taking a bunch of red roses and a box of sugar sweets, and when the nurse left the room for a moment he kissed her, feeling very protective towards her. Mrs Dickenson arrived and Richard greeted her, but when Bill and Mary also came, he said goodbye and left. Flora was home in two days and he telephoned her daily until she felt well enough to go out. He bought her lunch and a drink and soon she was back to her happy smiling self, and Richard found that he was jealous when he saw other men looking at her. Happily in love he went into a jeweller's having decided to buy an engagement ring. Though he had plenty of money he was a bit taken aback by the price of lovely diamond rings, and the jeweller sensed this, and said:

"I realise they are expensive, would you consider a ring which has been returned?"

Not thinking of it being second hand, Richard bought the ring, a lovely emerald between two diamonds, with a promise that it would be made to fit free of charge if necessary, and it looked lovely against the white velvet lining of the little blue box.

He arrived back in the surgery in the middle of the afternoon and telephoned Flora at the dental surgery where she still worked and asked if he could see her.

"Yes, come round here. What's wrong? You sound upset?"

"Oh nothing's wrong. I'll be there in five minutes," he replied.

He had the ring box open when he went into the reception room and Flora stood up behind the desk.

"What is it, Richard?" she asked.

"It is this, darling, will you marry me?" and he showed her the ring.

"Oh, it's beautiful," she said and coming round the desk flung her arms round his neck and kissed him and said, "Yes, of course I will, we won't tell anyone now, but come for dinner at 7.30 tonight."

Bill was talking to Richard, and Mrs Dickenson and Mary were pouring out the pre-dinner drinks when Flora came into the room. Richard went across and stood besides her and she said, "Listen everybody, I'm engaged," and flung her arms round Richard and kissed him and then stretched out her left hand with the ring sparkling on her third finger.

"Congratulations!" They all crowded round, and many kisses were exchanged and toasts drunk before they went in for dinner. Richard telephoned his father and mother and broke the news and was told to come for lunch on Sunday. Late that night, with a slight feeling of guilt, he wondered what to say to Joan. The finished letter's message was direct and a little abrupt but said that as he had become engaged he did not think it correct to continue to see Joan and so he must say goodbye. After sealing and addressing it, he sat very still, ignoring the voice which told him he was wrong, but it was very late that evening before he posted it. Later he tore up every letter she had ever written to him together with her photograph, and went to sleep to dream not of Flora but of Joan.

It was a glorious April day when Flora and Richard arrived at Bowland, and were met by Ted who escorted Flora into the house where Richard also introduced her to his mother and Mary, and they all went into the lounge to have coffee. Flora looked radiant, she was wearing a striking yellow and blue dress and Mary looked dowdy besides her. Mary was a little quiet during the traditional Sunday lunch, but he was not prepared for her attack when he went into his study to find a book; he turned round to find she had followed him into the room and closed the door.

"What do you want, Mary?" he asked.

In a threatening tone she said, "What do you think we want? I'll tell you, an explanation of your conduct, getting engaged and never bringing the girl over so we could see her, you have no thought for your family." By now her voice was loud and shrill as she continued, "And anyway who is she? We know nothing about her or her family, and coming dressed like that in that revealing dress."

Richard's anger was rising but still under control, "Please shut up, Mary, what the devil's got into you? I'm almost twenty-six; do you expect me to come running to you like a little boy to ask your permission? I've never even seen your fiancé, some long-haired fiddler with a slate off, I suppose."

"You leave him out of it, your mother's in tears in the kitchen, you casual devil."

Richard in a rage shouted, "Shut up and get out, Mary, or I'll throw you out," and flung open the door to find his mother there looking very anxious and saying, "What on earth is going on? We can hear you two all over the house!" but Mary continued to shout, "She can get out of here!" and began to run down the stairs. Flora, who was standing with Ted in the hall, opened the front door and ran outside. Victoria shouted, "Stop him, Ted!" as Richard in a blind rage rushed up to his sister who raised her hand to strike him. Ted stepped in between and hurled Richard aside, and in his best barrack square voice bellowed, "Stop this, you two, at once!" Mary turned away and Richard ran out of the house to find Flora.

When he caught up with her, tears were streaming down her white face and she looked very young and vulnerable. He put his arm round her to comfort her, but she still sobbed, "Please, please, Richard, take me home, I can't stand it, I never thought this would happen, you'd better have your ring back."

They stood still looking at each other and Richard said, "Flora, I love you and that ring stays on your finger whatever happens–to hell with our Mary," and he slowly pushed the ring back into place on her finger. Linking arms they walked slowly back to the house and Flora got into the car. He went into the house to get their coats and Flora's bag. Ted and Victoria apologised and his mother kissed him, then they came out to the car and said goodbye to Flora, and Richard realised that he was close to tears. He had tea with Flora and her mother and then went to his digs, where he sat in his room reliving the events of the day. He was overwhelmed by the realization that in his blind rage as he rushed down the stairs he wanted to murder Mary. Thank God his father had been there. He then telephoned home, and thanked his father for his intervention and then his mother for lunch and she replied:

"Richard, I think she is a lovely warm-hearted girl. Don't worry about us, you go on and get married and my blessing will be with you when that day comes. God bless you my boy. Good night."

Richard stood stock still as the icy shiver of premonition ran through him, and then he replaced the receiver on the hook.

He spent most evenings that week with Flora, either going for walks or sitting in the lounge in the cottage. He comforted Flora, who had been dreadfully upset by the events of Sunday, never having experienced anything like it before. She had been brought up in a very happy family, had been to a children's private school, and then to the Girls Grammar School. By the end of the week though her depression was gone, she assured him that did not want to break off the engagement and they became a loving couple again. The emotional wound his sister had inflicted on Richard was very severe and never healed throughout his life.

Alastair now arranged more work and more horse work for Richard to do. As well as the usual castrations and dockings, he did two difficult hernia operations which were successful, and foaled a mare after embryotomy on the foal. It was a lovely morning after a very stormy night when Bob Mattinson rang to say that he had found some sheep dead. Bob met him in the yard and he said he was certain that it was lightning but the Insurance Company wanted a vet's certificate. He got his crook off a nail on the shed wall and then opened the door. Out came three collies, and Richard noticed the one with only three legs.

"So he gets around well, Bob?"

"Oh yes, he keeps up with the others, even over walls."

"Never," said Richard.

"Oh yes, you'll soon see." He said "stay" to the dogs and then opened the field gate. The two men walked through and closed it behind them and then walked on a short way. Bob put his fingers in his mouth and whistled and the three dogs came over the wall and raced towards them, and three-legs was second.

"What did I tell you, Richard—he's a great dog."

They walked on for a mile and finally reached a walled field in which many ewes and lambs were grazing. Inside the walls a single strand of barbed wire was nailed on posts level with the top of the wall to stop sheep getting over.

One wall ran from the gate straight up to the top of the fell, and beside it lay the carcases of many sheep. The wool had burn marks on it, and the distinctive smell of burnt wool was present around the carcases. The position of the posts was marked by heaps of matchstick-sized splinters of wood at intervals along the wall, and here and there were shiny blobs of metal. Richard, in spite of this evidence, decided to skin one ewe, and was doing so when the agent for the insurance company arrived, so that he was able to show him the lightning marks on the flesh and in the joints of the carcase. Richard wrote out the certificate certifying the death of 23 ewes and lambs from lightning when they were back in the farm house. Bob's father remarked, "I don't mind any calamity so long as it's outside; you can stand that, but not when it comes inside the house."

Years later Richard remembered the saying of the old man. On the smaller farms and smallholdings, there was little assistance, so Richard used to take Willie with him. They arrived at the small farm in the early afternoon on a very hot day to remove angleberries and extra setts from the young cattle. The yearlings had been brought in and tied up, so Richard soon nipped the extra setts with the little castrator then cut the rudimentary teat off with scissors. There were four twenty-month-old heifers tied up, so one at a time they were led out on a halter, roped and cast. The searing irons were put in the brazier, and while Willie sat on the heifer's head the farmer held the rope tight. When the local anaesthetic had taken effect Richard cut off the angleberries, lightly seared the bleeding points and then spread anti-fly oil over the area. The extra setts were removed and the heifer allowed to rise and wander off. Willie and Richard were so hot and sweating, that they took off their shirts and laid them on the hedge. They were dealing with the fourth heifer, when the farmer suddenly shouted, "Quick, get your shirts," but by the time Richard reached the hedge one had disappeared and when he tugged the other free from the mouth of the cow on the other side of the fence there was less than half a shirt. After they had finished with the heifer they went into the next field, but a neckband and a cuff of some torn material was all that was left. Mrs Steel laughed until she cried at the sight of Willie and Richard driving into the yard naked to the waist with half a shirt between them.

Later another spell of very hot weather developed, and it was during this time that Richard arrived at a farm to investigate the cause of death of a heifer. The farmer, his man and Richard found the heifers in an overgrazed field; it was getting brown from the sun's heat.

"Were they well yesterday?" he asked the farmer.

"Oh yes. I counted that fourteen were all here and seemed all right."

"But did you go up to them?"

"No, just looked from the gate." The dead heifer was lying not far from the gate, one or two were grazing, but others were standing or lying and paying little attention to anything.

"They are far too quiet," said Richard, "Are you giving them any cake?"

"No," was the reply, "I think they are fit enough."

"Where's the trough?"

It was up at the top end, and they walked up to it, to find that it was empty.

"No wonder they look hollow and quiet with no water in this heat. When was water brought to the trough last?"

"Four days ago," was the labourer's reply. "I don't see how they can have drunk all that so soon."

"Well, fourteen need a lot of water, it would soon go."

The farmer leant over the trough and when he touched the metal plug it was obvious that it was not properly seated in the outlet and so the water had dribbled away. They made the cattle rise. Many of them had a watery diarrhoea and two would not rise but grunted with pain and the diarrhoea was running from them.

"It looks as though they have been poisoned with something, but what can it be?" said Richard.

"There's no poison in here," said the farmer.

"Right then, it must be a plant poison in the hedges. Come on, we must walk right round and look out for deadly nightshade, foxglove or yew."

This they did and reached the far corner where the hedge was overgrown. Some of it had been trampled down, revealing a sheep-dipping tank with a lid half off on the other side of the four strands of barbed wire.

"What's in that tank?" asked Richard.

"Why, sheep dip," was the reply.

"I know," said Richard, "It's sheep dip; but what sort?"

"Arsenic," said the farmer.

"Of course it is!" said Richard, "Acute death pain and watery diarrhoea with jelly in it."

"Ay, I can see they've reached through and knocked the lid back."

There were two down, one dead, six ill and five apparently all right.

"Get them out of this field, I'll take a smear from the dead one, though I'm certain there's no anthrax; and get those ill ones tied up. I'll go back to the surgery for an antidote, but in the meantime have you got any slaked lime?"

"Yes,"

"Then put a big tablespoonful into a gallon of water, stir it up well and drench each one with a whisky bottle full. I'll be back within an hour."

Back in the surgery the smear was negative; he consulted his book on poisons and then got Jim Lord to make up packets of an iron compound which was an antidote. Back at the farm another had died and another would soon.

"Have they drunk any water?"

"Yes, five of them have, but the end one hasn't yet."

Richard gave him the powder and told him to dose them according to the instructions. In the end ten survived the poisoning and slowly put on flesh again, grazing aftermath and being given cake.

At Berry's yard he watched two dead heifers dragged out of the truck and waited until they were cut open and the stomachs and intestines pulled out. When these were opened up they were blood-raw inside; the tissue looked like a red velvet in some places. As Mr Berry said, these poor devils must have suffered terribly.

While he was there Richard noticed the number of carcases which were affected with bovine tuberculosis, and which Berry said the vet never saw. The farmers just milked them as long as they gave any milk and then asked him to collect them. He expected more if the new schemes which were being talked about came into effect, but Captain Munn, the Veterinary Officer for Holme Corporation had an uphill battle against TB.

Jean Dickenson, Flora's mother, had a brother, Jerry Lawson, who lived in Llandudno in North Wales and was a solicitor by profession. He with his wife and four children did not fill the large house which was at the west end of the Promenade. It was here that Richard and Flora stayed for five days after they had made a quick visit to Droughton where the atmosphere was almost pleasant. During the day they went swimming or walking, but the best day was when the six young ones had a picnic on the Great Orme, taking Pip, the Lawson's dog, with them. He once got into the hamper but was driven off before he ate any of the tongue and ham sandwiches and couldn't touch the lettuce, radishes and hard-boiled eggs which were in a bag. With lemonade and bottled beer they made shandy and all had a happy old time. It was during the holiday that the lovers decided to get married in a year's time, "because by then I'll be an old man of twenty-seven," but Flora said that he didn't show any signs of that yet.

Back in Holme Jim White had managed very well, Richard thanked him, and to show his appreciation took him with Flora to dinner at the Sitting Goose. During the meal Jim revealed that he was going to leave the Lindley practice the next year and hoped to join the Ministry of Agriculture and Fisheries, but made them swear to keep this a secret because he had not told his uncle. The autumn came and with it the seasonal diseases, the calving cases, mastitis and husk. Some of the horses in the LMS stables had been replaced after the strangles outbreak had ended and the horses were in better condition following the appointment of a new horse foreman. One animal soon became well known in the area.

A horse and lorry were outside the station when Richard bought his evening paper in the shop opposite. As he left the shop the Town Hall clock struck the first note of 5 o'clock. The horse raised his head, pricked his ears, and moved off; though the brake was on, it was not tight enough and the back wheels turned. Going down the slope towards the town centre the horse began to trot. Richard jumped into his car and followed, trying to get nearer to the runaway in the evening traffic, expecting there would be an accident. By now the horse was cantering along, straw blowing off the lorry, coming up to the policeman on point duty at the bottom of Leeds Road. He was quick-witted and stopped the traffic and the runaway thundered past down High Street. The policeman joined two more men who ran after the horse in a vain attempt to catch it. Richard expected a crash at the end of the street, where the horse would have to turn right into Stanley Road which led up to the stables and the goods yard, but the horse slowed down and round he went just missing a parked car. His pursuers had almost reached him, but he accelerated and did not stop until he reached the trough in the stable yard. Richard had picked up the out-of-breath policeman and they were both relieved to see the horse safe and sound; but the foreman swore to sack the driver who had been told to brake and scotch the wheels if he had to leave the horse, which had done this twice before. Richard examined the horse and found no injuries, but the policeman and the foreman soon found that the connecting rod to the brake shoes had snapped and they all wondered who had done it, the horse or the driver.

The year seemed to have passed very quickly to Richard, when the accountant arrived one morning and collected all the books and the ledger. During the year Richard had kept a diary of all the work he had done for David and especially for Alastair, with all the mileage. This he now priced and added to the daily totals he had kept from the day book, which he had priced also and added up every night, because somehow he was suspicious that he was not being treated fairly, that £300 profits was too much money to be taken out of a one man practice which he was working so hard to increase in size. He felt that David's financial control was too tight and too self-centred. As all the purchases for drugs, equipment, stationery and dressings were made from Lindley, that practice had the benefit of all the discounts.

It was in this doubting frame of mind that Richard went to the finance meeting which was held this year in the afternoon in the Lindley house.

The accountant produced the profit and loss account which showed that the turnover had increased to £1,490, but with a rise in expenses to £879. The profit was therefore £611 which meant Richard would receive £175.95 as his share and they all agreed that it had been a satisfactory year. Here Richard commented that he knew it had been a good year, but thought he had done better than the figures showed, because by his reckoning the gross figure should be £1,660. David asked him how he knew that, so Richard showed him his financial summary of every week's receipts and expenses and remarked that when £879 was deducted the profit was £781, of which 2/7 was £222, and how did they explain the difference? The accountant, David and Alastair looked at each other, and then the accountant asked if Richard was disputing his figures. He replied that he was not, but wanted to know where the £170 was. David asked where he got the figure of £170 from, to which he replied, for the work that he had done both for him and for Alastair. David said that was not included, to which Richard asked why not? David explained that he had been ordered to do the work and that he had to obey orders was written in the agreement and he would go and get it; and left the room. It was obvious that he told Jenny to take in the afternoon tea; be a good hostess and keep the conversation going for as long as necessary.

On his return he opened the document and said, "Here it is; '...and the said Richard Baden Holden will be obedient to the senior partner's orders, and instructions.'" Richard replied that Alastair was not the senior partner, but ran his practice in the same way as Richard ran his, and so he did not see why he should work for Alastair for nothing, and that the £170 should be added to make his share £222. He also asked why he should have 2/7 of the Holme practice profits, when he did not supply any capital. David was getting rather flustered and said that what Alastair did or did not do was immaterial, that they had made an agreement, Richard had read his copy and signed it and that was the basis they were working on and so the £170 stayed out.

"Well, in that case I will not do any more work for Alastair, but will concentrate on my own end of the practice."

David reminded him that under the agreement he had to obey his orders, and Richard said he always had done so but would not take orders from Alastair in future because he had been putting on him for two years and so he wanted that £170 included. David said that Jenny had taken messages for visits to be made by all of them and that they would have to stop now and have a further meeting, and with that they all left.

When November came and nothing had happened, Richard rang David and asked what he was going to do, but David said that Alastair would not agree to the £170 being added to the Holme account; but when Richard rang Alastair, he said it was David who would not agree. Richard again rang David and when he refused to add on the £170, Richard replied that as they were sticking rigidly to the agreement he would do the same and give one month's notice of his intention to leave David's employment on Friday 8 December. David protested that he had been in practice for 41 years and was wanting to retire and hoped Richard and Alastair would buy the practice, but Richard said that he would leave on that day if he had not received a cheque for the full amount of the profit, and hung up the receiver.

A fortnight later he and Jim White met on a country road. They both stopped their cars, and began to chat, Jim wanting to know if it were true that Richard was leaving. When Richard said that he was, Jim said that he was leaving also, having got a position with the Ministry of Agriculture and Fisheries, and that he would start work in the laboratory, at New Haw, Weybridge, near London in the New Year. Richard asked Jim if he knew what the partners were going to do, and Jim said that they were advertising for an assistant under a box number in the *Veterinary Record*. They both wondered why only one assistant was required.

Flora on the Saturday night asked Richard what was wrong and so, sitting in the firelight on the couch in the lounge at the cottage, he told her the whole story. She asked if he had received the cheque and when he said no, she was anxious to know what he was going to do, to which he replied that he would have to get another post. When she realised that he could be leaving in two weeks to work anywhere in the country Flora was upset, and asked him not to leave her, but he said he could not stay and work with people who exploited him and whom he did not trust. Fed up with the subject he steered the conversation round to their wedding and they finally decided it would be in July next year. After supper and many kisses he finally went back to his digs and found that week's issue of the *Veterinary Record* in which there were only two "Appointments Vacant" advertised. He wrote a letter to the one which said "Experienced assistant required in mainly cattle and horse practice, Welsh Border, immediately, live out, Box No. 109." and enclosed the references from Major Gilmour and Walter Buxton. The Town Hall clock struck eleven as he posted the letter, and felt depressed and a little lonely when later he drifted off to sleep.

On the Sunday morning he told Will and Mrs Steel that in twelve days time, he would be leaving. Will said that he thought he was a fool, after more than two years' hard work building up the practice to leave it all for somebody else to reap the benefit. He told Richard to go and offer to stay if they would add half of the £170 to the accounts, but Richard refused to go. On the Tuesday he went to Jim Benson's to a cow down with the milk fever and he injected her and soon she got up. When they were having mugs of tea in the farm kitchen he told Jim that he was leaving, but gave as the reason that there had been a disagreement over the running of the practice. Jim was annoyed.

"I don't know what's wrong, but surely there's no need to leave; it's the first time for years we've had a good vet here in Holme and everybody likes you. You stay and brazen it out. Whatever it is, you've nothing to lose, Mr Holden."

Richard said he would consider it, thanked him for the tea and went off on his morning's work.

He had just finished the evening surgery on Thursday when George Smith from Intack Farm rang up and asked if he could call in to see Richard in about ten minutes. This was agreed, and when George Smith walked into the waiting room he was followed by Jim Benson, Bob Mattinson, Charlie Dean, Bill Bond and John Gardner.

"Good evening, gentlemen, this is a nice surprise. What can I do for you?"

"Nay," said George Smith, "It's what we want to do for you. We're committee members of our local branch of the NFU and I'm chairman this year. We've decided to come and ask you to put your plate up here and we will back you—I'll go further than that and say I'm certain nearly all the farmers round here will come to you, and you have all the stables as it is, now what do you say?"

Richard looked at their cheerful expectant faces, the faces of men he considered almost his friends now, and was deeply sorry when he refused their offer, but explained that he was bound out from practising within an area over a radius of 10 miles from Holme Town Hall, by the partnership agreement.

"Look, Mr Holden," said Charlie Dean, "You can put your plate up in Whitley; that's near enough ten miles away and though it's only half the size of Holme, it's growing and our Lawrence has got a useful house empty at the moment, you could go there for a start."

The discussion went on for some time until Richard said he would consider their proposition and let George Smith know fairly soon. But the letter he received on Saturday morning made him give up the idea of staying in the Holme district, because it was from Captain George Black Gillmour, the Major's brother, offering him the post of assistant in Melbury in Herefordshire. He offered £400 a year live out, and said though he trusted his elder brother's judgement he would like to see him and would pay all the expenses this might incur. Richard took Flora to the Sitting Goose for dinner and later when they were having coffee, gave her the letter, which she read and then said that it appeared very good and that if he went she would not be marrying a vet on the dole. They laughed at this, and drank a toast in brandy to a happy new post and then went to the cottage to tell Mrs Dickenson.

On Thursday the 8th he rang David and said that as he had not received his cheque for the share of the profits the accountant had calculated, he having worked his notice would be leaving at 4.30 p.m. the next day. David said that he didn't want him to leave; it was all Alastair's fault, and that he would come to see him on Sunday. Richard just said, "Well, that's it; my best wishes to you and Jenny. Goodbye." The taxi took him to Flora's at half past four. Over tea they had a long talk, and tried to plan for the future, and he decided to keep his digs at Mrs Sykes for the time being; visit his parents for a few days; go to Melbury; and come back and spend Christmas with her at the cottage.

Melbury was a delightful town of black and white houses and inns, bordering each side of the very long High Street in which there was an old timbered Market Hall, and a large Norman church. Leaving the station, he walked along this street, and by the time he had arrived at The Corrie, Captain Gillmour's house, he had fallen in love with the town, so attractive in the pale light of a December afternoon. While they were having afternoon tea, George explained that his assistant had married the daughter of a veterinary surgeon in Somerset, and had gone there to work with him. The

Captain was physically very like John his elder brother, with red hair and blue eyes, but there the resemblance ended. He was easy-going, always pleasant, and quick to laughter. His wife Mary reminded Richard of a younger Jenny Lewis. She had gold-coloured hair and a pale skin, and both she and her husband spoke quietly with a slight Scottish accent. Richard took to them both immediately. Behind the house the practice buildings comprised one block with waiting room, consulting room, dispensary, small operating room, and the usual store rooms, in one of which Richard met Pat Magaritty, a small, thin Irishman with a mop of black, curly hair who volubly welcomed him like a long lost brother. The Captain finally stopped him and explained that he was always like this, a very good worker but a terrible man for the drink. Pat replied that that made two of them and went on cleaning saddlery. The other was a stable block, and from the boxes two horses watched them. The Captain explained that one was Blackthorn, a lovely horse, and the other Boxer, which had a fiery temperament; he asked Richard if he rode and when he replied that he did, George said he would like him to go with him some mornings to give the horses a little exercise and that at this time of the year, he went with the local hunt regularly. Richard was very impressed by the place; everything was of the very best, immaculate and well painted.

The next morning Richard accompanied the Captain who was driving a big Armstrong Siddeley car, on his morning visits, going through a gentle countryside, with red cattle with white faces in the fields and the red earth of the ploughed fields throwing the green pastures into bright relief. The farms were large and well kept, some had hop yards and all had cattle and sheep, the latter a small breed which Richard did not know and which the Captain said were Clun sheep. Before lunch George asked Richard if he would start work on 3 January. They shook hands and drank each other's health in a lovely sherry; and Richard thanked him for giving him the job.

After lunch there was just time to inspect the digs which the Captain had found for Richard before he caught his train home, breaking his journey in Droughton to see his family, and to tell them his news. Flora was very curious to learn all about the new post, and about Melbury and said that from all he had told her, it would be a lovely place in which to settle down. He had a very happy Christmas with the Dickenson family and the Lawsons, but Flora was in tears when he left on the 8.10 a.m. train on 2nd January. He made her promise, however, to come to Melbury at Easter.

V

Melbury proved to be just as attractive when he arrived for the second time. The Captain met him at the station and on the way to The Corrie said he had forgotten to mention a car at the interview. Though the practice had an old Austin, this was kept mainly as a relief car in case of breakdowns. The previous assistant had his own car and the practice paid all its expenses, and would Richard like to do the same? Richard said he would, but until he had bought a car he would drive the Austin. He would like a Ford Popular which had proved reliable in the Lindley practice.

He and Pat loaded up the old Austin and next morning he was away working by nine o'clock, very happy to be again among horses and cattle; and though it took him some time to find the farms he did seven visits during the day. After all the industry and traffic in Droughton and Holme, Richard found it a pleasure to drive on roads with little traffic in this pleasant countryside. The first week ended with a surprise when he received a letter from David Lewis which had been forwarded by his father, and in it was a cheque for £175 9s. George took him to Hereford, and he bought a two door Ford Popular with sunshine roof and leather upholstery for £110. This was his first car and he was very proud and delighted with it. He carefully ran it in for the first 500 miles even though he was very busy all the next week because George went hunting with the Melbury and Pat went with him to stay with the spare horse.

He went early one morning to calve a cow in a village five miles away. It was a large, well-kept farm with a pedigree Hereford herd, and a breed new to Richard: Friesians, a black and white breed known for their good milking qualities. He had just delivered a live calf when the owner walked into the box and Richard was surprised to see that he was wearing a scarlet jacket, leather breeches, and boots and wore a clerical collar—he was a farming vicar who rode to hounds. He introduced himself and thanked Richard for being so prompt and getting the calf alive because he was building up a pedigree herd. But though George went hunting he still worked hard, for on that day he arrived back at The Corrie wet to the skin, but had a bath and changed into dry clothes, after which he drove away to do three farm visits.

Richard was the only paying guest in the digs, and was really waited on hand and foot. His meals were served in a small morning room, his bath run in a morning, and a stone hot water bottle placed in his bed at night. At least twice a week he wrote a love letter to Flora before he went to bed, and unlike

Holme there was little night work to be done which was surprising in view of the large amount of livestock in the area.

Sometimes at 7 a.m. he rode Blackthorn, and George rode Boxer and they trotted them on the grass verge of a country lane until they reached a field which belonged to George. Here Richard experienced the thrill of galloping Blackthorn, and beating Boxer back to the field gate. On most mornings however it was Pat who rode out with the Captain, who was always very well dressed, while Pat wore an old cap back to front, a thick-knit jersey, and blue serge trousers. As he was an ex-jockey he could control Boxer better than the Captain, and he was always sober, in spite of his reputation for the drink.

He remained sober until one morning when the Captain asked Richard to be back in the surgery before 11.30 because that was the time when the drugs hampers would be delivered, and to take out the methylated spirits and lock it up in the dangerous drugs cupboard. Richard was delayed at the last farm and in spite of driving fast did not reach the farm until a quarter to twelve. He walked into the store room, and found the two wicker hampers had been opened and partially unpacked, and straw was scattered everywhere and there was no methylated spirits to be found, though 1 gallon was on the delivery note. He walked round the stables, calling for Pat but he had disappeared. The Captain arrived and Richard told him what had happened.

"Oh, it's not your fault," said George. "It's that devil of an Irishman; now he's got the spirits we won't see him for weeks."

"You don't mean to tell me he drinks it!" exclaimed Richard.

"Yes I do, and he causes nothing but trouble when he does this. Now I've no groom, yardman or driver for the horse trailer, but we will manage somehow." They did, and it was days before Pat returned, the white muffler he had tied round his neck accentuating the pallor of his face. When Richard asked him why he had been absent for a fortnight, he never forgot the reply: "Ah, sure and begorra, but I've had a bit of indigestion!"

And so Easter came and on a cold snowy morning Richard met Flora at the station and was delighted to see her, giving her a good kiss before taking her in his car to the Crown Hotel in the High Street, where later he joined her for lunch in the dining room, with its beamed ceiling, oak panelled walls, and huge fireplace where a big fire burned brightly. After lunch he took her to The Corrie and introduced her to Mary and George, who immediately invited her to dinner that evening. The light from the candles in the Georgian candelabra shone and sparkled on the glass and silver of the place settings on the highly polished mahogany dining table, and illuminated the lovely faces of the two ladies and the handsome men. The maid filled the glasses and they drank a toast to Flora after which they enjoyed a very good dinner. In the lounge they drank their coffee and listened to the wireless and the worrying

news of Chancellor Hitler's threat to take back German lands by force.
George rose and turned off the set, remarking that he thought the man spelt
out trouble for all Europe, and they chatted until it was time for Richard to
take Flora back to the hotel.

On Good Friday afternoon Richard took Flora to his digs for lunch and
then out by car to show her some of the lovely countryside. It was near
Marcle that they stopped, got out of the car, and looked over the hedge
surrounding an orchard which was carpeted with daffodils, thousands of
them in the pale spring sunshine. Then they went on to Ross on Wye, hand
in hand, exploring the town. After going to church on Sunday morning, they
drove over British camp to Great Malvern and had lunch, and walked along
the hillside arm in arm talking about future plans. For Richard the highlight
of the weekend was reached after dinner on Monday when they spent an
hour happily making love in the big bed in Flora's hotel room. He never
forgot the joy and exquisite pleasure of their loving, and life was drab and he
felt a little sad after she left on the Tuesday.

As George had let Richard have Easter Sunday and Monday off work, he
decided early in April to go from Friday night to Monday morning with a
friend fishing in Wales because the practice had gone quiet. On Saturday
there was little work until early evening when, assisted by Pat, he set a dog's
broken foreleg, and then had to go to a colic case in a hunter, to which he
had to return at 10 p.m.

Arriving at the digs at midnight he found a message on the pad by the
telephone, and went a long way south-east to a cow unable to calve. It took
him some time to realise that he was not dealing with a case of twins but with
a condition called schistosomus reflexus which he had never met before,
though he had read about it in a book on veterinary obstetrics. Fortunately
he could reach parts of the calf, and perform an embryotomy, but it was
some hours later before he delivered the malformed remnant. At 6 a.m. he
was awakened by Mary telephoning him a milk fever case, and that began a
busy Sunday. At night he went to an acute mastitis case in a cow, followed by
a case of milk fever and then at 1 a.m. a case of a cow straining to calve at the
vicar's farm. When he arrived there was plenty of assistance, which was just
as well because on examination the cow had a twisted vagina and so could
not calve. She was a very big, full pedigree Hereford with massive horns and
resented being handled, but finally was roped and cast and rolled. The first
roll was in the wrong direction but Richard quickly realised his mistake and
the cow was rolled twice in the opposite direction. With a flood of fluid the
water bag burst and then a live mahogany-coloured bull calf was delivered.
The vicar was delighted and when he had washed and dressed took Richard
to the house and gave him a hot toddy. Slightly tipsy and dreadfully tired he
just flopped into bed at daybreak. He had written "don't disturb" on the

telephone pad so his landlady let him sleep on. The phone rang at 9 a.m. and when he answered it George's cheery voice said, "Hello, that you, Richard, have you gone on strike?"

"No, I'm trying to catch up on my sleep–I'll tell you all about it in an hour." he replied. Richard sat in the office and wrote up the day book for Saturday and the night's work and then Sunday and that night's work. George looked at the entries later and said, "I am really sorry I wakened you. In all the years I have been here I have never known 48 hours as busy as that."

Though Mary had two maids, only one lived in and on her night off Mary answered the door and the telephone, and even helped Richard when required. After dark the two big gates which opened into the yard were closed and all callers rang the house bell. After his dinner Richard had returned to the surgery to write up the day book, and do some dispensing. George was out at a case, and Mary was repairing an electric table-lamp. Mary came into the surgery, collected some medicine for which a farmer had called, entered it in the day book and went out. A few minutes later all the lights went out. Richard made his way to the car, found his torch and shining it before him went into the house shouting, "Mrs Gillmour, what's wrong with the lights?" He heard a moan and ran into the lounge and found Mrs. Gillmour on the floor barely conscious. He at once rang the local doctor and was kneeling beside Mrs Gillmour when George arrived wanting to know why the lights were out. Richard called him and while he stayed with Mary, Richard found the fuse box, put a new wire in the pot fuse holder and switched on the lights. At this moment the doctor arrived and after examining Mary and bandaging her right hand helped George and Richard lift her onto the settee. What had happened was now revealed. Mary had been ready to shorten the flex which led to the lamp when the farmer called. After she had attended to him, she came back to the lamp, picked up her dressmaking scissors and cut through the cable, having forgotten to pull out the mains plug. There was a flash of light and Mary remembered a dreadful pain in her hand before she blacked out. She was confined to bed for two days and said she realised how lucky she was to be alive after receiving such a shock: it took weeks for the burnt flesh on her hand to heal. George never left her for some days, so Richard had to shoulder all the work.

At Easter he and Flora had decided to get married in the summer, but had not fixed a date. A letter arrived from her one morning asking him to go and see her at Whitsuntide, because she had chosen Friday 29th July for the wedding day, and they had a lot to discuss and decide. George gave Richard the time of the Whitsun holiday off duty. In pencil he ringed 29th July on the calendar, crossed out the week following, and asked him where he was going

to live after the wedding. Richard said that he had had a look at a
semi-detached house in Abbey Lane, which would be coming up for auction
in June, and had also got the addresses of two flats. When the holiday
weekend arrived he went straight to Holme to the Dickensons, and was very
happy to be with Flora, but unprepared for a hectic time. They had an
appointment with the Suffragan Bishop and booked the day, the church, the
choir and the organist. Flora was very efficient, and with Jean her mother
had all arrangements well in hand; the guest lists prepared; the lunch
provisionally arranged at the Sitting Goose in the banqueting room; and the
wedding dress ordered. The morning room was really an office manned by
the Dickensons and the Lawsons, so Richard had little to do except ask Bill
to be his best man. Bill was so pleased with the invitation that he took them
out to dinner and Joan his girl friend made up the four. On the Sunday Flora
asked Richard if he would ask his sister to be a bridesmaid and thus repair
the broken bridges. The other bridesmaids would be Mary Dickenson and
Brenda Lawson, and the three Lawson boys would be ushers. By afternoon
they had chosen the hymns for the service and the invitation cards and then
Jean and the Lawsons joined them and they all went to Evensong.

On the Monday they began trying to decide what sort of house they would
like, but also considered alternatives because not many houses came up for
sale in a town as small as Melbury. He broke his return journey at Bowland
and told them all the news and the date of the wedding, but was disappointed
when Mary refused to be a bridesmaid. He had a talk with his mother who
told him not to be upset over Mary's refusal and to go on with the
arrangements for what she was sure would be a very happy day. She kissed
him goodbye and his father drove him to the station and in fun told Richard
to get a ring of the right size and not to drop it on the 29th and wished him all
the best, and on this pleasant note they parted.

It was a month later when his father spoke to him again on the telephone
to say that Victoria had had a slight stroke, and would have to take things
easily for a bit, so Connie Heald had come to stay and help because Mary
was in France playing at four concerts. Richard telephoned three nights running and learnt that his mother was rapidly improving, but early on Tuesday morning Connie Heald rang to say that Victoria had had another stroke
and would he go home at once. He caught the first available train and arrived home at four o'clock to find his mother propped up by pillows in bed
having suffered a severe stroke of the right side of her body, but mentally she
was alert though speech was difficult. Mary had also just arrived and, after
talking to their mother, had a meal with Richard, but somehow he did not
feel at ease with her. Later the three sat talking with Victoria who, when the
grandfather clock chimed a quarter past six, asked them all to kiss her, because she said, "This is goodbye. I will go when the clock strikes half past."
They all kissed her, Mary began to cry, and they watched as slowly Victoria

closed her eyes. As her head fell to one side and she died the clock struck the half hour. Mary sobbed; the two men began to cry and supported her until Connie and the doctor came into the room. After assuring himself that Victoria had died, the doctor very gently led them from the room.

There were many people at the funeral, the Bradshaws walking behind Ted and Mary, Richard was with Flora and Auntie Nellie, then Tom and Frank and all the Holdens, as they gathered at the graveside, shielded from the heat of the summer sun by a magnificent beech tree, and watched Victoria laid to rest.

To Richard the 3rd July was of no special importance until in the evening. George came into the surgery, gave him a large envelope, and asked him to read the contents, and let him have his comments the next day. As soon as he had had dinner, he opened the envelope, and found the draft agreement for a half share in a partnership to commence on January 1st next—he was thrilled because he liked the Gillmours, the practice and the town where by then he would have Flora with him. It was a very different agreement from the one of Lewis and Duncan, and as Richard read it through for the second time he noticed how fair all the proposals were; that an independent accountant would value the partnership and a surveyor the practice buildings. He was impressed by the fact that all the books of the practice and a copy of the agreement would be provided for Richard's solicitor and accountant. He sat at the dinner table and considered that as he was to be married in a month he had better get a solicitor and an accountant, and take out a life insurance policy as well, even though the agreement said that each partner would insure the other against death and dissolution of the partnership. Next morning he thanked George, saying it had been a thrilling surprise, and that he would be very willing to become a partner in the New Year. George replied that he was glad that Richard had agreed because they got on so well together. He and Mary could not get to the wedding and would be really sorry to miss it, but would celebrate later.

Wearing morning dress and sporting red carnation buttonholes, Bill and Richard walked up the aisle of St. John's Church. Richard noticed that the nave was full, that all the family were present, and that many of his farmer friends in Holme winked or waved as he walked past. Richard spoke to his father who looked very distinguished and immaculate, but Mary, who was wearing a black toque and black coat, looked away. As the music rang through the church, Bill said, "Now's your last chance, Richard, out quick through the vestry." Richard looked round to see Flora wearing a lovely white wedding dress, her face covered by the veil used by her mother at her wedding, walking up the aisle holding Jack Lawson's arm, accompanied by her three bridesmaids, who were wearing powder blue lace dresses. They were Mary Dickenson, Brenda Lawson and Annie Holden, his Uncle

Harry's daughter.

As Flora took her place besides him she smiled and said that she could not stop her knees shaking, but her hand was very steady when he pushed the platinum ring onto the third finger of her left hand. When the Bishop gave the Blessing, Richard for a second recalled his mother's words, and he realised that she had known that she would not be at his wedding. Any momentary sadness he felt was buried under the tide of good wishes which swept over the newly married pair. During the reception Miss Ruth Howarth informed Richard that Mr Kerr, a cousin of Alastair's, was running the Holme practice and that he had arrived on the Monday as Richard had left on the Friday. Richard wondered if it had all been done to make him leave. The platform at the station was full of well-wishers so they left for London smothered in confetti. They were glad to relax in the first class compartment, and pick up all the confetti, and throw it through the open window. They were idyllically happy as the sunny summer days allowed them to explore London, and each evening they went to a different show. Richard telephoned his landlady to tell her of their plans, and to say that they would arrive on Saturday afternoon. This they did, having collected in Holme the Ford 8, which was packed with all the presents they could possibly get into it, although they had to leave some behind.

Richard collected the keys to the flat and on Sunday they went to see it. Flora liked it at once. From the lounge window she could see some of the High Street, and the kitchen window looked onto a garden, part of which was a lawn. Together they made up the bed, and then enjoyed themselves looking at all the presents again and identifying the senders. Jean had made a list of them all, so they decided that soon they would send thank-you letters. They formally occupied the flat on the Monday, and soon began to make contacts both in the house and in the town because Flora was very gregarious and easily made friends, so much so, that it was not long before Jean Gillmour invited her to make up a four for bridge once a week. During his time off-duty Richard took Flora shopping for articles they required for the flat, because it was only part furnished. In this way they discovered that they both had expensive tastes and loved old things such as silver, pictures and furniture. They nearly lost all their treasured possessions, however, early one evening, when Richard arrived at the flat, the day's work done and began to help Flora by putting the tablecloth and the cutlery on the table. When she came in carrying the glasses, he put his arms round her and they kissed and held each other close until she suddenly said, "Let me go! the dinner!" and she rushed into the kitchen with Richard close behind her. The chip pan was blazing and black smoke spreading across the room, though the door into the garden was open. Richard grabbed a teatowel and hurled the blazing pan outside, the flames singeing his eyebrows and hair. Flora was very upset, so they went to the Crown for a meal, and then spent the rest of the evening washing the greasy black film off the walls and ceiling of the kitchen, while thanking their lucky stars it had not been worse, for them and all the other people in the house.

The occupants of the other ground floor flat were an elderly business man called Watson and his wife. She suffered from a heart condition and was regularly visited by her doctor, but in spite of her illness she was a pleasant, cheerful woman. She and Flora soon became friends and unknown to their respective husbands helped each other in many ways. Again it was early evening and Flora and Richard were relaxing in their lounge having eaten dinner and washed the pots. Suddenly there was a furious knocking on their front door. They both rushed and opened it to find Mr Watson standing there shouting, "Do come quick, my wife's dying!"

They both ran behind him into the flat to find Mrs Watson sitting in a chair, her face blue, her breathing stertorous, and she was reaching into her mouth with her fingers.

"Please do something, she's swallowed a piece of chop bone," .

Richard, without stopping to think, pulled her hand away and pushed his finger into her mouth at the back of which he could feel a curved piece of bone. He pushed his finger under it at one end and pulled and the bone slid past his finger, to come into his hand as Mrs Watson vomited and coughed blood-stained saliva and food, all over his sleeve.

"It's here, I've got it; hold her up so she can breathe."

At this moment the doctor arrived and took charge, and Flora and Richard went back to their flat. Some time later, Mr Watson and the doctor came in. The latter thanked Richard for his timely intervention, but said it would have been different if Mrs Watson had died while he was removing the bone. Mr Watson scoffed at the idea, and said that Richard had done a wonderful act of kindness, and he would always be in his debt. A week later Mr and Mrs Watson gave them what Mr Watson called a late wedding present—a pair of Georgian silver serving spoons. They were saying that they were lovely and how much they appreciated their gift, when the telephone rang and Richard had to leave and go to the Hunt kennels.

These were a few miles from Melbury, pleasantly situated, surrounded by two fields and an orchard. Two cows were kept, looked after by the feeder and one was having difficulty calving on this hot humid autumn night. The kennel huntsman met Richard in the yard; Richard's examination revealed a calf in the breech position. The big Hereford cow strained with all her power and even with John pinching her back to prevent her, Richard had to use all his strength to repel the calf and reach the legs. Soon he was sweating and perspiration running into his eyes. In time he brought one leg back, having got a calving rope on to it, and then the other. John and he now pulled with all their power to move the bull calf, which finally came with a rush so that all three fell in a heap onto the straw. The men got to their feet.

"By jove, that took some getting." said John. "Lucky it's alive. I'm absolutely boiling. I'll go and get us both a drink."

Richard enjoyed the pint of thirst-quenching, cold, red cider and asked John if he had made it and how it got its colour. John showed Richard the stone cider-making mill and told him that he added beetroot to give it more "kick". Richard downed his second pint, thanked John and set off home. On the way he passed a very fat boy on a bicycle riding quickly towards Melbury. By the time he reached the surgery he was half drunk. George asked him where he had been and when Richard replied that he had been to the kennels, George immediately said that he knew that he had been drinking John's red cider and Richard wasn't used to it. He brought Richard some black coffee and when he arrived back at the flat an hour later, he had sobered up, but vowed never to drink red cider again!

Next morning George asked Richard if he saw the fire at Well Farm as he was coming home, to which he replied that he hadn't seen it, only one or two cars and a fat boy on a bicycle. A week later another farm fire occurred, which destroyed two stacks, and it was obvious that they had been deliberately set on fire. A few days after, the sergeant of police called to see George and Richard and asked them to report anything suspicious they might see while driving round the countryside in the early evening. George said that he hadn't seen anything he could remember, but Richard had seen a fat boy on a bicycle late in the evening not far from Well Farm on the night that they had a barn burnt down. The sergeant said that they were thinking of the culprit as being some adult with a grudge, rather than children, but would tell the firemen to look out for the fat boy because he could not think of one in Melbury, and he thanked them for the information.

He must have been annoyed and felt very frustrated when another fire broke out that night. That year George had taken a hay crop off the field which he used for exercising his horses and it was stored in a Dutch barn at Oakfield Farm nearby. Driving home one evening he saw thick smoke in the direction of the farm and, suspicious that it was coming from another stack fire, at once drove at top speed the three miles or so until he reached the road up to the farm. He swung in without slowing down very much and within a short distance met head on the fat boy on his bicycle, who swerved and crashed into the ditch. In a moment George, swearing at the lad, had skidded to a stop, and was out of the car running to try and catch him as he struggled out of the ditch and remounted his bike. The fire tender turned into the drive and jerked to a stop, blocking the youth's escape route and the firemen dismounted as George ran towards them shouting, "Stop him, stop him!"

One of them brought the boy down with a rugby style tackle and then sat on him. George immediately drove into the yard, followed by the fire tender and they were confronted with three bays of the barn blazing. Mr Twine and his men were valiantly trying to stop the fire spreading along under the roof using hosepipes and with the assistance of the water from the five hoses soon had the third bay fire out and began to throw down the steaming hay and corn sheaves to make a fire break, but in spite of all their efforts, the first two bays were so badly burnt as to be useless, and all George's hay was in the first bay. The police took the fat boy into custody, but it was soon discovered that he was mentally defective, having the mental age of a five-year-old child. He had come to stay with relatives near Melbury but he was sent back to an asylum in the Midlands. Flora said that her ideas of living quietly in the country were changing rapidly because there was never a dull moment; it was more exciting than living in Holme.

Richard, returning from an early morning call on a very wet cold November morning, saw George on Boxer ride away to the second meeting of the Hunt.

He had ridden Blackthorn at the first meeting, and was giving the older horse a rest. Most of the visits that morning were in the northern area. By lunch time he had done them, and called at the post office in a village to collect any messages. The post mistress said that there was only one, saying that he had to go back to Melbury at once as it was urgent. He set off at once, but was delayed because he had a puncture, and had to change the wheel in the pouring rain. This annoyed him because he had to stop again at the station garage to leave the wheel to have the puncture repaired.

As he drove up he saw a lot of cars outside The Corrie, and was dismayed to see the doctor's, the Vicar's, and a police Wolseley among them. It was with a feeling bordering on panic that he hurried into the surgery, and on into the house where in the kitchen Edith the maid and Pat were sitting at the table and she was softly sobbing.

"Whatever's happened, Pat?" said Richard.

Pat, who had obviously had a drink or two, replied that he didn't really know because he had been waiting with the horse box at the pub when the police car and the doctor's roared past up the Worcester Road, to come back a bit later with the doctor sitting in a Morris Isis attending to somebody. Then some of the hunt had arrived and told him that the Captain had been badly hurt in a fall and Boxer had broken a leg and been shot. He had immediately come back to the surgery and Betty Rose, Mary Gillmour's sister, had just told them that the Captain had died in the Cottage Hospital. Stunned by the news, Richard just said, "Poor Mary," and sat down, feeling again that awful sense of isolation and finality, such as he had felt before in other jobs when he had been given his notice—he saw his future here disappearing before his eyes.

Dr Wells came into the room and said to Edith that they would want tea for at least ten people and would she brew some at once and, turning to Richard, said:

"Well, Mr Holden, we meet again. I am sorry that George has died but he had sustained a large depressed fracture of the skull and stopped breathing just as we arrived at the hospital. I have given Mrs Gillmour a sedative and Mrs Rose is taking charge."

Richard, recovering from the shock, thanked the doctor and then asked Pat if there were any messages. When he said there were none he got to his feet and walked through to the lounge which was full of people. When Mrs Rose saw him, she asked him to go and have his lunch and come back as soon as possible.

He walked into the flat, poured brandy into one glass and whisky into another, added the mixer, picked them up and turned round to face Flora who was coming into the lounge saying, "Why didn't you call 'it's me' when you came in?" Then seeing the look on Richard's face she ran to him and asked, "Oh love, what's the matter?" He handed the whisky to her and said, "Drink this," and took a big drink of his brandy. They both sat down and he told her the tragic story, and when he had finished neither had much appetite for lunch.

By the time Richard and Flora arrived back at the surgery most of the people and cars had departed, so they went into the house to see Mary and to try and comfort her. In spite of the sedative she was distraught. Flora sat down beside her and put her arms round her. When Betty Rose, who had been talking to a reporter, came in, she said to Richard that he was in charge of the practice and she hoped it wouldn't be too busy until Elizabeth and the Major arrived to help. She asked Flora to stay and help with all the details which would have to be arranged.

Richard was busy, and very relieved the next day when Elizabeth and the Major arrived in their new Chrysler Ascot 23 horsepower motor car. By early afternoon John was with Richard in the surgery. They divided the work between them and soon John had taken over the responsibility for the running of the practice. That evening they worked together removing a tumour from a dog. John said that he was going to stay for some days, until he could find out what Mary wanted to do, but as the practice would have to go on he would send Terry Allen, the junior assistant in Corchester, to come and assist Richard. Trying to plan their future, he and Flora talked until it was quite late, and finally decided that there was no way by which they could buy the Melbury practice even if it were offered to them, and so they would have to leave. At the thought of turning their backs on this town and county which they both loved, Flora began to cry, upset by the thought that she would have to leave the first home they had shared together in their married life, and they were both depressed when they went to bed.

Two days after the funeral, a meeting was held at The Corrie. Mary was there with Betty Rose, Elizabeth, Flora, John and Richard. John took charge and in a business-like manner said that Mary wanted to leave the house and go and live with her sister. This meant that the practice, house, buildings and fields were to be sold, and he gave the provisional figure the surveyor and solicitor had arrived at as to their value. He asked Richard if he wanted to buy it lock, stock and barrel, but Richard replied that though he and Flora would love to buy it they had not got that amount of money, and would have to refuse, but were grateful for their consideration in offering it to them. John said, that being the case, they would have to consider offering it to Harry Walker, who wanted to buy a practice in the area, and whose mother had approached Betty. Mrs Walker was the Chairman of T.H. Walker Ltd., the cider makers, and he was certain that a sale could be made quite quickly. In the meantime would Richard, with a salary increase, continue to run the practice until the end of the year, with Terry Allen to assist him. All were agreed and it was also decided that the practice would buy a Ford 8 for Terry to use, he living in Richard's old digs.

Back at the flat, knowing now that he had to get another job, Richard found the last few issues of the *Veterinary Record* which he had not had time to read. He replied to two box numbers enclosing copies of his references. In one issue he read under Deaths "Evan David Jones on Oct 23rd at Llanon, North Wales" and details of his career. He said to Flora that he would be glad when the New Year came, because this had been a miserable one with three deaths in the last five months. A reply to one of his applications came from Yorkshire and returned his references. He was asked to telephone Kirkireton 308 to arrange an expenses-paid interview, which he did and took Flora with him travelling by train. It proved to be a pleasant stone-built market town and they quickly found the big gloomy Victorian practice house. The interview with John Good was a waste of time from their point of view; Richard would receive a lower salary, less mileage allowance, fewer holidays and the promise of a partnership agreement was very vague; they would also live in a flat over the stable block and Flora would be expected to be available to answer the telephone and help with the cleaning, but would not be paid for doing so. Richard had agreed with everything which had been said, but the idea of his wife cleaning the front steps and the floor made his blood boil. While Mr Good was still talking, Richard rose to his feet and, interrupting, said that he had listened in silence to all the vague proposals, but found them completely unacceptable, being a veterinary surgeon not a slave, and that his wife was a dentist's surgery assistant and not a damned housemaid, so he would not waste any more of Mr Good's time and his expenses were £5. Mr Good replied that if that was Richard's attitude he would not employ him, quickly gave him the money and they left. Walking down the street, Flora began to laugh and said:

"Richard. I am proud of you. the way you told off the bombastic skinflint. I should not have let you take that job. if it were the very last you could find." In a good humour and in spite of having no job. they had a meal and caught the train back to Melbury.

There things were now moving quite quickly and Mary asked if Richard could leave on the Friday before Christmas. because she would be leaving and Harry Walker arriving. So the next weekend they packed up all the small objects and the silver they had acquired. filled the back of the car and took them to Hill Cottage in Holme. telling Jean that they would be there for Christmas. The parting was sad but very friendly. and to show her gratitude for all they had done Mary Gillmour gave Flora a beautiful pure silk scarf, and Richard six antique silver teaspoons. Feeling a little sad they drove out of Melbury in their overloaded car on that Friday morning. in a rainstorm. After twenty miles. they were on the outskirts of a small town when there was a grating noise from the back of the car. then a loud bang and it stopped. Richard tried everything he knew. but could not get the car to go; then Flora burst into tears so he put his arms round her and tried to console her. though he was feeling very miserable himself. When she stopped crying. he put on his cap. then his oilskin coat and rubber boots. and hurried off through the driving rain to find a garage. He was very wet when he found one. but luckily the owner was helpful. listened to Richard's tale of woe. and said he would tow the car in. but advised him first to throw away his green cap. because green was an unlucky colour.

He took it off and dropped it into the cokestove. By evening a new half shaft had been fitted and Richard joined Flora in the hotel. She telephoned her mother and explained the reason for their non-arrival and promised to be home the next day. In after years Richard considered that morning to be one of the blackest moments of his life when. utterly depressed. with his wife sitting in a broken down car half a mile away and no job. he had walked into Thornton's garage almost soaked to the skin.

Jean was glad to see them and made them very welcome. helping them to unload the car and storing their belongings in an empty room. There were only two "Situations Vacant" in the *Veterinary Record* which had been sent on from Melbury. and he replied to them. He and Flora had a long discussion on what he should do. She said that they had got to try and decide a strategy for the future.

"Richard. what do you really want to do?" asked Flora. "Stay in private practice. work for the Local Authority. or join the Ministry of Agriculture and Fisheries?"

"Really. I want to stay in practice; I know that you have more security working for the last two; but I want to be my own boss and I enjoy working among animals in the countryside." Richard replied.

"Well then. you had better begin writing after a job. because it will be weeks before you draw a wage again, and we can't live here with Mum for ever."

Such was Flora's advice and Richard took it. He wrote letters applying for both situations, one in north-west England and another in the south.

Two days before Christmas they went to Droughton taking presents for Ted and Mary, and were surprised to find that very few preparations had been made at Bowland to celebrate the festival; there was no holly, and dust showed on the furniture; the house both inside and out was dingy. Ted explained that he had suffered an attack of angina pectoris, for which the doctor had prescribed tablets to be taken daily, and capsules to be used when an attack commenced, and said that he was going to have a good rest over the holiday period. When Richard asked Mary if she enjoyed being home from London for Christmas, she replied that she was now at home permanently, but gave no explanation as to why she had suddenly changed her plans. They noticed that she began every sentence with the words "I have" and it was obvious that she was now the dominant person at Bowland and was making all the decisions. She replied to every question which Richard addressed to his father, and later, barely hiding her animosity, she made them a cup of weak tea. So they left their presents, and after exchanging seasonal greetings, Flora and Richard drove away, the latter thinking that after six months, he knew nothing about the life of his father and sister, that they ignored Flora, and treated him as though he were a distant relative making a courtesy call. Basically, though he was hurt by this treatment he was not surprised, because Mary and Ted had always gone to the Methodist Church together, while both he and Victoria had gone to the Church of England, because Victoria loved the singing and the Order of Service. They were more liberal, more worldly, and enjoyed the luxuries of life. His mother had always been ready to help anyone, and throughout her life was the unofficial midwife in the area, though she had no formal training. She was also much in demand to "lay out" a person who had died. For a few moments a huge wave of sadness swept over him and he was conscious of how much he missed his mother, especially her cheerfulness and love. He glanced sideways at Flora, appreciating that she had taken his mother's place in his life, and that he loved her more deeply than he could ever tell.

On Christmas Eve it was open house at Hill Cottage, which was crowded with the Dickensons, the Lawsons, and all their relatives, as well as neighbours, including Mrs Sykes and Robin Bull from the digs. They had decorated the house; Bill had three crates of beer stacked in the kitchen, and in the dining room a large buffet supper had been prepared. It was a happy get-together, which ended at 10.30, the female members of the household washing up, while the males put away chairs and tables, and took out all the empties. Then in five cars they went to St. John's Church to take their first Communion of Christmas. The candle-lit ancient church was crowded, and the spirited singing of the Christmas hymns by the choir and congregation, accompanied by the Holme Brass Band, was most inspiring. After the service ended they spent a short time talking to friends and to farmers who were former clients, but this was stopped by a renewed snowfall.

After Christmas Day lunch at the Dawsons the presents were distributed and Richard received as many as the others. He was very happy because he had Flora beside him; the Dickensons and the Dawsons had taken him to their hearts, and he was treated as one of the family.

The first reply to his letters came from Bridgwater, and he was asked to attend an expenses-paid interview, but given little information as to the actual work of the practice. It was a long train journey, but they both agreed it was well worth it, because they immediately liked the small town with its Georgian houses in the High Street, and the water meadows near the river. Major Godfrey, a pleasant man in his forties, explained that he wanted an experienced salaried partner until his two sons had grown up and qualified, which would be ten to twelve years in the future. Then he wanted to take a back seat and leave the partner and his two sons to run the practice. He offered an excellent salary, good holidays and provided a car, but there was no accommodation. It was obvious that this was a thriving practice offering a permanent position, and with the salary they could enjoy a nice life here. Major Godfrey thanked them for coming, and explained that there were three more applicants to be interviewed, so it would be a week or two before a decision could be made. Going home on the train they agreed it was a good position; the only drawback they could see was that it was so far away from their families.

In the middle of January he got the second reply, including his references, requesting him to ring Sandhaven 264, to arrange an expenses-paid interview. They were both excited by the thought of living in Sandhaven so he telephoned the number at once. When they went there they found Charles Parsons MRCVS, a white-faced old man, who obviously had been ill, and was not yet fully recovered. Speaking slowly he asked Richard about his practical experience and his reasons for moving from one place to another. He said that he could not afford to pay a big salary. He explained that his previous assistant had "put his plate up" four miles away contrary to his binding out agreement and the rules of the Royal College, but he was certain that it would come to nothing. The successful applicant would also be offered an agreement with an option to buy within two years time. He said he would write soon to let Richard know the outcome and paid him his expenses. They set off in the car to explore the town, and going south soon arrived at the fish dock and boat yards and then returned along the promenade for some miles and reached the park at the north end. They stopped here and watched the trawlers going up the channel to the dock, and they talked about the job.

They both thought that Mr Parsons looked so ill, that he could die soon, or else it could mean the assistant would be overworked. This fact did not daunt Richard, and as they both liked the town they drove back until they reached the main street, and found an estate agent's office. They soon found out the price of flats and houses for sale, and also the rents charged for flats.

Passing through Droughton on their way to Holme they called at the Healds who made them afternoon tea. They gave them all news, because Ted had not been to see them since Ezra died, and they had only seen him briefly at Victoria's funeral. Then they went to see Uncle Tom, who was in good form and said business was brisk, but he thought Ted was going peculiar, because he had not been asked in for a cup of tea and a chat, last time he delivered a ton of coal. When Nellie and Frank arrived Richard had to bring them up to date with all the family news, and a history of his movements. At six o'clock Nellie made them stay for the evening meal, and Tom wanted to know why they were in Holme. Richard told them the Melbury story, and then said that they had been to Sandhaven for an interview for an assistantship that day. Tom was very interested, because he knew a lot of farmers around Sandhaven, having bought hay and straw for the horses from them for years.

"I hope you get the job, Richard, because it is a good farming district, and you would be near enough to see to my horses." said Tom.

"Thank you, Uncle Tom; let's not count our chickens before they are hatched though."

Tom laughed and said, "I've heard you are a good horse vet and that's what we want in Droughton; the fellow we have here now doesn't seem to know much about them; so if you get the job let me know."

Richard promised to do so and he did get the job, Mr Parsons asking him to start work on 1st February, which was only a fortnight away. The very next morning he was offered the post in Bridgwater, and for twenty-four hours he and Flora talked over which they should accept. It was an agonising choice and instead of considering their own future, they were influenced by consideration for their respective families and so chose Sandhaven. Soon Richard began to think that he had made the wrong choice, but kept these thoughts to himself, and with the greatest determination worked to make Sandhaven a thriving practice, against Mr Parsons' lack of enthusiasm.

VI

Mr Bolton the Estate Agent soon found them a first floor flat to rent, which was over a high class ladies dress shop in High Street and they had use of a wooden garage near by. Richard wanted to buy a house, but Flora resisted the idea vigorously, saying that if Mr Parsons died suddenly before they had any agreement signed, they would be in the same position as they had been in Melbury, only this time they might be forced to sell the house at a loss. They were happy together, and worked hard distempering the lounge and the bedroom in the flat. Jean gave Flora a Singer hand sewing machine; on it she made all the curtains though often Richard had to turn the handle, while Flora fed the material under the needle. From Maurice Reed in Holme they bought some furniture, which included a new bed, a Georgian chest and a bureau, two lovely small tables, a grandfather clock, and a brass warming pan with a mahogany handle. Flora had good taste, and was very definite in what she wanted to complete the furnishing of the flat. She bought good pieces at the local auction room of Joe Bolton for weeks after they had moved in and so made a pleasant comfortable home they both liked. Her best buy was four H. Alken prints which she got very cheaply; and later a Cecil Aldin. Richard was very pleasantly surprised when his father gave him the dining table and four chairs from Bowland, and with this gesture he hoped the past was forgotten, but time soon proved him wrong.

On the first of February, everything was white with frost, and shrouded in freezing fog, which froze onto the windscreen of Richard's car when he drove to The Elms–the practice house. The sign "surgery" pointed to the rear of the building, so he walked past the garage, and finding a glazed door pressed the bell push. When Mr Parsons opened the door, he was wiping his mouth with a table napkin; he apologised for not having finished his breakfast and asked Richard to come in and wait. He sat down on a bench in this gas-lit narrow room which had a quarry tiled floor, and was very cold. A door led into the house, another was at the top of a flight of steps at one end of the room, in the centre of which was a strongly made kitchen table, while under the window was a sink with a draining board. Richard, looking round, experienced a feeling of mild panic, and asked himself what was he doing here? Had he chosen the right situation? and why was everything so cold, scruffy, and old fashioned? He now remembered that he had never been shown the surgery and other rooms when he came for the interview, and considered this place a hovel when compared with Melbury or Corchester. Then as the feeling of disappointment diminished, he became more rational and realised that he had accepted this situation because it gave him the opportunity to have his own practice in two years; that both Flora and he liked Sandhaven, and that it was a good agricultural area with horses, cattle, sheep and pigs.

This train of thought was interrupted by Mr Parsons coming down the steps carrying a leather bag. He asked Richard to drive the Vauxhall Six saloon, which he did very slowly, because though the fog had cleared the roads were very slippery. As they drove along Mr Parsons explained that taking Sandhaven as the centre of half a circle whose diameter was the river, the radius of the practice extended into the country for approximately twelve miles, though there were a few farms further away than this. At each farm Richard was introduced as the new assistant and examined and treated the animals; and by lunch time they had done five visits. In the afternoon they went to a pig farm where Richard farrowed a sow, the first in his veterinary career, and he was very pleased to have delivered nine live piglets, pedigree Large Whites. Back at the Elms, they went up the stairs into a very large room which had been made by converting two bedrooms into one. The two pendant gas lights illuminated a veritable Aladdin's cave of veterinary instruments and drugs, which were ranged on shelves all round the walls, with some standing on the floor. In the centre of the room was a large table on which stood a pair of highly polished brass scales, and an apothecary's balance. A microscope was on a small table near the window beneath which was a square yellow sink. Many of the two, four, and eight ounce bottles of medicines and lotions were already dispensed and wrapped in shiny white paper, the ends being closed with sealing wax; each was labelled according to the contents—the Mixture; the Medicine; the Lotion etc., and directions were given as to their use—Richard at once thought of the meticulous dispensing of Willie Wilcock in Holme.

After three days Mr Parsons began giving Richard a list of visits a good distance from Sandhaven while he did the ones near to the Elms. Mr Parsons ran his practice in a leisurely manner, and there was not enough work for two men, so often Richard had little to do in an afternoon. He was off duty on alternate weekends, and sometimes took Flora to Holme to see her mother. For use in the practice Mr Parsons bought all the powders ready made up in bulk, so the correct amount was measured into an envelope and sealed; six powders being wrapped in white paper and labelled. All medicines were bought in one gallon glass Winchester bottles, and dispensed in two, four, eight, or sixteen ounce bottles. Richard could do in one hour the dispensing which would have taken all morning at Corchester, and soon realised that Mr Parsons did not need a dispenser. His wife and daughter answered the telephone and the door, and Marjorie the daughter was the book-keeper. From them he learnt that Charles had been ill most of the previous year with stones in the kidney, and had only recently recovered. During his illness the assistant had run the practice, had become weary of having to do all the work, and finally had become so exasperated that he walked out after giving a week's notice, and "put up his plate" in a village four miles away.

In spite of what Charles had said about the previous assistant, this worried Richard because there was so little work to do for two men, and though Charles attended to any small animals brought to the surgery he never had any operations to do. When Richard asked him why this was so, Charles replied that he did not like small animal work, and any cases requiring surgery he sent to a colleague eight miles away; serious cases he destroyed. Richard told Charles that he had done a lot of small animal surgery at Holme, and had bought a case of veterinary instruments three years ago, and since then bought the instruments necessary for more difficult operations. He asked to be allowed to operate on any surgical cases which were brought in. Charles agreed to this, and for the consulting room to be used for surgery. So Richard brought all his instruments from the flat and they were put in a cupboard. His fish kettle which he used as a sterilizer was put on a gas ring on the long draining board along with his anaesthetic box with its graduated chloroform container and air pump. In the upstairs room he found braided silk suture and tubes of surgeons' catgut, which he put in the instrument cupboard. Charles brought a large Valor paraffin room heater from the house, and also bought a gallon tin of the new Dettol antiseptic, and Richard was very pleased with the progress he had made. Charles was completely up to date with all the advances being made in veterinary medicine and surgery, being an avid reader of all the professional publications, especially the *Veterinary Journal*, the American magazine *Veterinary Medicine*, and papers presented to Congress. Again after reading all the relevant literature he was keen to use any new drug which was produced.

With the advent of spring, there was more work to do with cattle and sheep—calving and lambing cases with all their attendant troubles. The milk fever cases were treated with the safer calcium-borogluconate which Richard injected intravenously using a neo-injector, but Charles gave it subcutaneously saying that given intravenously it might cause the heart to fail. Richard replied that his cases got up a lot sooner which pleased the farmers. Though more motor lorries were being used, there were plenty of heavy horses in the Railway stables, and in the stables on the docks. When they had colic Richard administered his medicines by stomach tube and was nicknamed the "Hosepipe Vet" by the stable men but he also used acetyle-choline, a new drug which worked well on cases of impaction of the large bowel, and he much preferred it to physostigmine and pilocarpine which he had used previously. As this was an area where the Shire horse was bred, there were plenty on the farms, as many as sixteen horses on the larger ones.

After Easter the representative of the German drug firm Bayer–a Mr Dalrymple–arrived one day and soon had Charles and Richard so very interested in a new drug called "Prontosil", which in trials had proved a successful treatment for streptococcal infections in animals, that a dozen bottles were ordered there and then. It was first used on a big pedigree red Shorthorn cow which had an acute mastitis, but though the cow recovered, she gave very little milk afterwards from the quarter which had been affected. The farmer was pleased that the cow lived, but Charles was disappointed that the drug had not saved the quarter.

Joe Fowler owned the Abbey Stud of pedigree Shires which was three miles from Sandhaven. He was a big man in every way, with a reputation for working hard, plain speaking and he had a quick temper. It was 7.00 a.m. when Richard took a telephone call from him, which was abrupt and to the point.

"Is that the vet? Joe Fowler here; the Abbey Stud. I've a newly foaled mare in a bad way. I want Mr Parsons here immediately," and he rang off.

When Richard arrived at the surgery to get some sterile cheese cloths and pessaries, Charles said they would go together, as Fowler could be an awkward customer, and Richard had never met him. He put the steriliser and some bottles of Prontosil into the car, and Richard drove him quickly to the farm. The mare was a 17 hands dapple grey with a foal at foot; she looked dejected, was sweating slightly and did not move. Charles looked at her and then asked Joe when she had foaled.

"Yesterday morning, Mr Parsons."

"Did she cleanse properly?" asked Charles.

"Yes, I think so," said Joe.

"Then I want to see it, so go and get it, and bring back a bucket of hot water, soap, and a towel," said Charles.

Joe went out of the loose box shouting orders to his men, while Charles examined the mare, and found her temperature 105.2°F and her heart rate 100 a minute. With difficulty they made her walk on a few steps, and after Charles had felt the pulse above the fetlock and the warmth of her feet, he said to Richard that she had laminitis developing. Carrying the towel and the bucket Joe came back with one of his men, who was pushing a barrow in which was the placenta. Charles laid this out on the floor, and the small blind end was missing.

"Joe," he said "she's got a piece of afterbirth inside her and she's going septic with founder starting in all her feet."

Joe swung round to face Charles and shouted at him. "Oh blast it, I don't want to lose this mare like I did "Fell Foot" two years ago."

Charles quickly said, "I don't want to lose her, either, Joe, so Mr Holden is going to get that piece of afterbirth out of her, and then we are going to give her a new treatment. It's expensive, but it works."

"I don't care what it costs, but get that mare better, Mr Parsons. I want to show her at Derby this year."

After soaking his arm in Dettol solution, Richard examined the mare *per vaginum*, and found the piece of placenta. He withdrew it and when this was added to that on the floor it made up the complete placenta. He then mopped out the uterus with the sterile cloths, and put in four Acriflavine pessaries. Charles had filled a 50 c.c. glass syringe with Prontosil and injected this subcutaneously at the base of the neck, and repeated it on the other side.

"That's it, Joe," said Charles. "Offer her a bucket of water and get that foal fed."

"Oh, he's not taking any harm," said Joe. "He's had a belly full off another mare that was running her milk."

"Then we'll be off and be back this afternoon."

Richard had just finished his lunch when Charles arrived and said:

"Come on, drive me quickly to Joe Fowler's. He says that mare is passing blood, and dying."

Richard got into the Vauxhall and drove very fast to the farm, into the yard and up to the door of the box. Joe came running from the house and roared:

"Hell, you've been quick, Mr Parsons."

"Don't blame me," said Charles, "Blame Campbell here, he was trying to break the land speed record coming here. Anyway, where's the blood, Joe?"

"There, that puddle on the floor, her water is pure blood."

Mr Parsons dipped a piece of white bandage into the puddle, and when he withdrew it, it was stained a brilliant red. Looking at Joe he said, "This is not blood, it's the drug I've injected into her which is coming out in her water."

"Are you sure, Mr Parsons?" said Joe.

"Yes, I am," said Charles, "and while Mr Holden examines her I will get some more from the car."

Now her temperature was 104.4°F and her pulse 96.

"She has slightly improved since this morning Joe, so I am going to repeat the treatment," and he injected another syringeful into the mare. Driving down the road from the farm Richard asked:

"Don't you think you've given her too big a dose of the drug?"

"Yes," said Charles, "because I think it didn't work too well in that mastitis case, because I gave too small doses too far apart. You know the speeds with which bacteria multiply, it's astronomical; so I've formed the idea of drowning them before they get too many to handle."

"Yes, I know that," replied Richard, "but aren't you worried about the effect it may have on the heart or kidneys?"

"No, I'm not worried at the moment because the drug appears to be very rapidly excreted, and there have been no after effects in Billy Hancock's cow. Also I want that mare to get better because Joe Fowler is a terrible talker, and whether she lives or dies he'll praise or blame me to everybody at the next horse sale."

When they revisited the mare at 6 o'clock they were both astonished to see the grey mare had turned faintly pink, and her eyes were bright-red. Fortunately Joe thought a pink mare funny. "Aye, when I came in an hour ago and looked at her I thought I'd better go and sign the pledge never to touch whisky again. It's queer stuff you are giving her," said Joe.

"Yes, it's new; you could say we are experimenting on her," said Charles, "but it is working, her temperature and pulse rate are still falling, and I see she's drunk some water."

"Oh yes, that's her second bucket."

Richard injected another 50 c.c. into the mare, and during the next day she received another 150 c.c. and was even pinker in colour. On the fourth morning, a beautiful spring day, wearing a rug she was turned out with her foal which she was soon feeding, while she nibbled at the first patches of new grass. The three men stood watching her, and Joe was in a good humour saying:

"You know, Mr Parsons, I still think I'll write to the Society and tell them to alter the colour of that mare to dapple pink."

"Yes, I'd do that because her description is not right at the moment," said Charles, "I'll bet they would be tickled pink."

Joe roared with laughter, while Charles continued. "But seriously, without that Prontosil I am certain that mare would be dead in Bob Whiteside's yard!"

It was a bad season for foalings, because the stallion had left deformed foals behind him and Charles had to shoot eleven mares because it was impossible for the foal to be delivered, or it had done irrepairable damage to the dam as she tried to expel it. Yet each mare they treated for metritis recovered; foals with joint ills were in some cases cured, though others failed to respond, and it had good results in cases of strangles and pneumonia.

Charles was still white faced and thin, but getting stronger and more active with every week which passed and was beginning to encourage Richard's small animals work, now that he had spayed two kittens and castrated a few cats, one for Miss Bishop who owned the Market Café and was extremely fond of her cats. The café was the information centre of Sandhaven and the three sisters had a great reputation as bakers, confectioners and chocolate makers. So for bread, cakes, chocolates and coffee it was the place to patronise, the shop being next door to the café, which was on the corner of

King Street and High Street. It was here that in the mid-morning the clerks
and housewives called to drink the lovely coffee Miss Bishop made and to
gossip – which was the *raison d'être* of her existence.

Duke, Son and King were an old established firm of solicitors in Victoria
Street and Mr Duke Senior took his dog for a walk along the Promenade on
most mornings during the week. It was he who, after ringing the bell, walked
into the surgery in the middle of the afternoon. Richard came down the
stairs and Mr Duke introduced himself and said that his red setter had
vomited a few times during the day, the last time in the car as he was coming
to the surgery and it smelt foul. Richard found that the dog had a slightly
raised temperature and a rapid pulse, but while he was making an examination of the dog's abdomen, he felt a hard lump and the dog growled and tried
to jump off the table. He put a muzzle on the dog and carefully palpated its
abdomen again and found that the hard lump was movable.
    "Mr Duke, I have found a foreign body in your dog's bowel, which is
obviously causing all the trouble and the only answer is an immediate
operation."
    "What are the chances, Mr Holden?" asked Mr Duke.
    "I would say better than evens," said Richard.
    "Then in that case you have my permission to operate on Rusty," said Mr
Duke.
    "Yes, I'll do that as soon as possible, Mr Duke."
    "What time shall I ring up to see how Rusty has gone on?"
    "Say eight o'clock tonight." said Richard.
    Mr Duke stroked Rusty's head, turned quickly and went out.
    Richard tied the dog to the table leg and then knocked on the door and
went into the kitchen. He awakened Charles who was asleep in a chair by the
fire, told him the position and asked him if he would give the anaesthetic. To
Richard's surprise he was enthusiastic and they soon had the dog on its back,
tied to the table. Its abdomen was shaved and washed with diluted Dettol.
The sterilizer which had been bubbling away was now opened, the tray lifted
out and everything made ready. Charles slowly anaesthetised the dog with
chloroform. Richard put on brown rubber surgeon's gloves and with the
Bard Parker scalpel made a mid-line incision through the hole in the drape.
He quickly found the area of bowel containing the lump and drew it carefully
through the wound and packed boiled cotton wool all round it. He pushed
the lump along the bowel for a couple of inches and then cut down onto it
and took out a stone. Richard carefully sutured the bowel using gut, and then
the peritoneum. The administration of chloroform was stopped and the
muscle layer and then the skin were closed using interrupted silk sutures.
Between them, they bandaged the dog's abdomen with open wove white
bandage and then with Elastoplast. Tom Wilson at Corchester had advised

injecting isotonic sterile saline solution into the radial vein where a lot of fluid had been lost by vomiting. Richard did this, and also injected Prontosil into the dog to try to prevent peritonitis.

They carried the unconscious dog over to the stove, laid it on a sack and covered it with a piece of an old rug. Charles congratulated Richard on doing the operation so quickly and so well, while he in turn thanked Charles for being the anaesthetist. Charles asked Richard if he had heard of the new drug "Nembutal", which was being used in America and if he had seen the report on its use intraveneously in the dog, by the surgeons at the Royal Veterinary College. Richard said he had but not having any of the drug had not been able to use it. Charles then said that he did not like chloroform for dogs or cats and so would order this new drug from Abbott Laboratories at once.

By evening the dog had recovered consciousness and drunk two tablespoonsful of glucose water, so when Mr Duke telephoned to ask how the operation had gone, he was very pleased to be told that he could come and take Rusty home. It made a good recovery, the wound healed by First Intention and Miss Bishop and Mr Duke had a lot to talk about and to tell their respective animal-loving clients.

Later that year they were introduced to another new drug, "Phenothiazine", which was very effective against worms in the bowels of horses, gastro-enteritis in cattle and goats, and black rush in sheep–called winter scour. Charles was very enthusiastic to use it and dispensed dozens of powders of the drug for use on mares and foals, because so many paddocks on the stud farms were heavily infected, the horses were always exposed to infestation and foals sometimes died.

When the cows were turned out, work became less and so Richard and Flora often had breakfast together. She enjoyed this because she so often ate her meal alone when he was out on an early morning call. They were doing the washing up in the kitchen, when she suddenly said:

"Oh, Richard, I do feel queer," and as he turned towards her she fainted and he had to fling his arms round her to stop her crashing to the floor. He carried her and sat her on a kitchen chair. She quickly came round as he waved the smelling salts under her nose, then he made her go and lie on the couch in the lounge. She was almost her normal self when he went to the surgery and at lunch time told him that it must have been something she had eaten which had upset her, because she had vomited. But when this had occurred three mornings running, it dawned upon her that she was pregnant and a few days later this was confirmed by their doctor, "Bill" McConnell, a charming softly-spoken Derry man. They were both very happy that this had happened. On the telephone Jean Dickenson said she was thrilled and would let the Lawsons know.

Richard wondered what had happened at Bowland because there was no reply each time he telephoned them and he and Flora were very disappointed when they drove there on the next Sunday and found the house empty and a "For Sale" notice in one of the windows. The mystery was solved when he received a letter from Mary informing him that she had obtained the post of music mistress in a girls' grammar school in Stroud in Gloucestershire and had commenced her duties on the first day of the summer term. Richard and Flora both wondered what had happened to the fiancé in London and if a breaking off of the engagement had been the reason for this sudden move. They realised now that Ted and Mary were not being altruistic when they had given them the mahogany table; obviously it would have been much too big to go into the bungalow which they had rented and which she described in her letter. Almost as an afterthought she added that her father was well and was happy with the move south, but she did not give their new telephone number.

In his reply he gave an outline of what had happened since Christmas but did not mention Flora's pregnancy. Her state of health was beginning to worry Richard, because the flat was very inconvenient in many ways, all the shopping and the coal having to be carried up two flights of wooden stairs. The day she slipped and fell on the wet wood of the stairs he went to see Joe Bolton in spite of her objections. He was pleased to see Richard again and all attention when he announced that he wanted to buy a house. He was a bit dismayed when Joe asked him what size of house he wanted, and whereabouts in the town. Did he want a terraced house or detached, with a garage and with land? Richard said he would go and make a list of what he wanted, but obtained the prices of various types of house. That evening he and Flora discussed the question at length and they decided that a house like the one in Melbury would be a very conveniently planned one from which to run a practice. This had six rooms on the ground floor, two each side of a central passage which extended from the front door to the end of the second room back, where the stairs went up to the first floor. Doors on each side of the passage at the foot of the stairs led into rooms five and six. The house would stand detached on a small amount of land which could be used for expansion in the future and would have a garage. When he went to see Joe again, Richard explained why he wanted a big house with room for expansion.

"So you are the vet who operated on Tommy Duke's red setter?"

"Yes," said Richard, "I am Mr Parsons' assistant and he wants to retire in about eighteen months because he has been ill on and off for a long time."

"I know that," replied Joe, "he wouldn't come to see my dogs–you see I breed black Labrador retrievers and I'm a member of the Club. I'm glad you're going to stay, we need a good vet here now."

"Yes. I want to stay but what about a house?"

"I've nothing suitable at the moment, but I'll let you know if any suitable house comes up for sale," said Joe.

"Really, I would like to be at the top end of Hall Road, or on Nelson Crescent if possible."

"Maybe, but don't forget, Mr Holden, those houses cost from one to two thousand pounds or more."

"Very well, Joe, I'll just have to wait for a bit and see what turns up," and with that Richard went off to the surgery, where he found Bill Meadows from Whingate Farm waiting.

"Hello, Bill, how are you?" asked Richard.

"I'm all right, thanks," said Bill, "but I'm very worried about two heifers I've bought. One of them "picked" last night and the other is showing a bit of a bag."

"When were they due to calve?"

"September was the date given at the sale and the auctioneer said they had been vaccinated against abortion but I don't like it. What can you do?"

"First of all, Bill, where are they?"

"Oh they're both in boxes. I've kept them away from the herd, as soon as I saw the first one bagging up a bit."

"So they've not been out in the fields?"

"No, they've only been in the paddock with our Mary's pony."

"Then first of all put sacks soaked in strong disinfectant outside the doors of the boxes. See that only one man has to deal with these two heifers. What did you do with the calf?"

"It's still in the box and I'm the only one whose been looking after these two. I did wash with disinfectant after I'd been into them both last night and this morning."

"Where did they come from, Bill?"

Bill gave the name of a well known Jersey herd in the south of England, and said that he had bought from them before and not had any trouble.

"Well, in that case, let them know what has happened right away, and I'll come and take blood samples and swabs and send them off to the Pathology Lab. in Liverpool."

Richard later in the day went to Whingate Farm, and was glad to see the boxes were on the other side of the house from the shippons. Nevertheless, he gave instructions for Bill to keep one lot of buckets and shovels for the two animals, and for the straw dung and the calf to be burnt. He soaked his arm in Dettol and then put two pessaries into the heifer, also he gave her an injection to make her cleanse.

"Bill, I don't like the look of the discharge from this heifer. It does look like contagious abortion to me. Have you anywhere further away you could put them?" asked Richard.

"Not here, Mr Holden, but our George could take them; he's only got store cattle on his place at the moment and of course his horses."

"Bill, I'd like you to get them over there in his horse box; and then completely clean and soak in disinfectant these boxes and everything you've used including your rubber boots and even your jacket, because the last thing we want is an abortion storm."

Bill was most careful to carry out all Richard's instructions, and then all they could do was hope for the best. The results from the Laboratory were positive for infection with brucella abortus, which were sent to the seller at once; he ordered both heifers to be slaughtered, and said he would stand any loss and expense which Bill had suffered. Bill was lucky because as the weeks turned into months, no sign of infection occurred and the Brownlow herd of Jerseys steadily grew in size, but it had been a near miss, because Jerseys are very susceptible to the disease. Bill had started the herd the year before, buying only cattle which had passed the Tuberculin test, and from breeders who had a good reputation for their pedigree stock. Richard had treated three cases of milk fever for Bill in the spring, and they were fast becoming friends.

That spring and summer Charles and Richard decided to try and reduce the amount of navel ill and joint ill in foals, by the preventative innoculation of the pregnant mare and the foal. Breeders were advised to let the mare foal in a field, not in a box, and to dress the foal's navel with a dressing which they dispensed. This was made up of equal parts of tannic acid, aluminium sulphate and zinc oxide. Charles kept a record of all joint ill and navel ill cases seen from 1st April and compared it month by month with the cases recorded the previous year and they were pleased to see that the number of cases had declined. Richard began to advise all horse owners to have their animals vaccinated against tetanus, navel ill and joint ill, but it was hard work to persuade them to have this done.

For a few days Flora had said she did not feel too well, but refused to go to the doctor, telling Richard to stop fussing over her. But early one morning he awoke to find Flora walking around the bedroom, and he was immediately anxious.

"Flora, what's the matter?" he asked.

"I don't know really, Richard, I've got stomach ache and can't sleep," she replied.

"Look, you get back into bed or you'll catch a cold, and I'll go and make you a cup of tea, and bring you a hot water bottle."

When he came back, she sat up in bed and slowly drank the tea, and put the hot water bottle across her abdomen. Richard went and had a shave, and heard Flora go into the lavatory; then heard her come out and she opened the bathroom door, and said:

"Richard, will you ring the doctor, quick, I'm bleeding."

He went down the stairs three at a time, and was relieved when Dr McConnell answered the phone, and said he would be there in five minutes. He was as good as his word. He quickly examined Flora and said:

"Mr Holden, I am sorry to say that your wife is aborting and she must go to hospital at once."

"Right," said Richard, "Flora, can you walk down to the car?"

"I don't think so, Richard."

"Well then, put my thick dressing gown on over yours and I'll carry you down."

He picked her up in his arms, and carried her down to the car and drove her to the Memorial Hospital. He saw her taken into the labour ward and told Dr McConnell to get the best gynaecologist as soon as possible, and it didn't matter what it cost. He said he would go and do this at once and then told Richard to go home as he could not do anything by waiting. As he drove back to the flat he suddenly realised how much he longed for them to have a family of two or three children. Arriving home, he made more tea and drank it, and wandered up and down feeling very restless and miserable, recalling Bob Matinson's words those years ago: "I can stand any trouble as long as it stays outside the back door." Richard dreaded to think how bad the trouble would be which had come into the house and struck his wife. He rang Charles and told him what had happened, at which Charles said that as there was little work in that day, to stay at home so that he could receive any telephone calls from the hospital. The call came after lunch from the Memorial Hospital asking Richard to go there at once. At reception he was directed to a waiting room, and it was here that Mr Graham the gynaecologist told Richard that Flora had lost the baby; she had also lost a lot of blood, and would have to stay in hospital for four days. The nurse led Richard into the ward, and held aside a screen to let him reach the bedside, and he was almost in tears as he looked at Flora's white face. He leaned over and kissed her, and with tears running down her face she quietly said, "Oh Richard, I've lost our baby, I'm so sorry, so sorry."

He found and held her hand, and replied:

"Flora, I'm sorry too, but don't blame yourself, it was not your fault. I think it was your falling on the stairs, you mustn't blame yourself."

"I'll try not to, Richard."

He spent some time comforting her until he had to leave when a young doctor and a nurse came to give her a check-up. On reaching the flat, Richard telephoned Jean, who said she would come at once though he told her that Flora was all right, but she was adamant and said she would ring back when she knew what time the train would arrive at Sandhaven. This proved to be at a quarter to five, so he met her then at the station. She was carrying a bunch of flowers, and anxiously asked many questions as he drove her to the hospital on Rydal Road. Because it was not visiting hours there was a conversation between the nurse at reception and the Matron before permission was given for them to see Flora. She told them that she was feeling better and had drunk some tea, but would like an orange because she was so thirsty. Richard asked the nurse to bring one and when it arrived he was pleased to see her eat it. Mother and daughter talked a little longer until the nurse asked them to leave. On the way back to the flat Richard stopped at Harold Marsden's the florist and bought a dozen red roses, then again asked Jean to wait when he pulled up outside Joe Bolton's. From his desk, Joe looked up and said:

"Hello, Mr Holden, nothing yet suitable for you, but I might have something soon."

"Oh, I'm not bothered about the house at the moment, but I want a ground floor flat now—as soon as possible," said Richard.

"Well, why didn't you let me know?" said Joe. "I've a good one on the Promenade. It was Mrs Dryden's, but now she is eighty she has left it, and gone to live with her daughter."

"Right, I'll have it now, but I'll still want a house. Can you arrange it for this week?"

"That's a bit short notice, Mr Holden, but I'll do my best."

"I know it is," said Richard, "but I'm not having my wife falling on those damned stairs again, so be as quick as you can. I'll be in tomorrow and tell you why. Cheerio."

At the flat Jean quickly took over and began to issue orders.

"Richard, get a suitcase and put in it two nightdresses for Flora, and a bed jacket, and soap and a face flannel and a towel, and find her hairbrush and comb. She'll want some handkerchiefs too and something to eat."

When Richard had done this, Jean had tea ready—cold mutton and chutney; bread and butter; cake and tea; which they rapidly ate. After washing up they went back to the hospital because visiting hours began at 6.30 p.m. and they spent the hour with Flora who was pleased with the roses, and liked the idea of the new flat. Sister escorted Mr Graham to Flora's bedside, and Richard introduced him to Jean. When Sister asked them to leave, he said it was not necessary; he took Flora's pulse, and asked her if she was comfortable. When she said that she was, he told them that she was now out of danger from further haemorrhage, and tomorrow could go into one of the side rooms, which were more private. After Richard had thanked him for his attention he left, and the three of them talked together until it was time for Jean to leave to catch the 8.40 train.

Back at the flat, Richard poured himself a brandy, and sat down reflecting on the events of the day. He was very sad when he thought that there would be no baby next Christmas, but he was grateful to Mr Graham that Flora was now out of danger, and would be home in a few days time. He wondered how he could have managed if he had been running his own practice, because without Flora, who would have answered the door and the telephone? So it would be impossible for just the two of them to run the practice. He would have to employ someone–but who could it be? Mr Parson's daughter Marjorie would be the obvious choice, but her mother had poor health so she might not be available. He ruled out his father, and then thought that out of the two Lawson families' nine children there should be someone suitable. But how would they get a holiday? He had heard that *locum tenens* were not very reliable, yet if he became ill he realised he would have to employ one; but as the practice did not appear to be getting any bigger, probably he would be able to get by.

Feeling hungry, he went into the kitchen to make his supper. He found there was no milk, so he was feeling really annoyed with himself because he had not thought to do any shopping that morning. Supper was Crawford's cream crackers and cheese washed down with milkless tea.

Next morning he rang Dr McConnell and thanked him and then telephoned the hospital and was cheered to be told Flora was doing fine and had had breakfast. He told the Parsons the story, and they were very sympathetic, but they did not send any flowers to Flora or visit her; they gave him the odd cup of tea, but he was not invited to a meal. For the next three days he had his meals at the Market Café, and told Miss Bishop why he had to do this. She listened attentively to all he had to say, and fed him well. She also wanted to know what she could do for her cats now that an epidemic of cat flu had broken out. He advised her to have her three cats injected with Wellcome feline distemper prophylactic vaccine at once, and did this the next week. When he had finished his work that afternoon he went to see Joe Bolton who had arranged for Richard to take possession of the flat on the Promenade on 1st August. They went together to see it. It was modern and had electricity for lighting and heating; it was light and spacious; the views from the lounge were lovely, because they looked out to sea, and one could watch the shipping and the trawlers coming and going. That evening he found Flora sitting up in bed in a private room, which was nice and warm and had a good fire burning in the grate. She was almost back to normal, and listened to all Richard had to say with growing amusement.

"Well, I hope you have done the shopping today; get two bottles of milk tomorrow morning and then go to the butcher's for some eggs and order a small loin of pork for the weekend," said Flora. "I want something to eat on Friday.'

"Yes, I'll do that," replied Richard, "but I must tell you that I have got a ground floor flat; it's on the Promenade, and provisionally we move in on August 1st. It's a nice flat, and has electric light which will be a blessing after the gas we have had to put up with for the last six months."

He described it to her, and so they spent the rest of the visiting hour planning how to arrange the furniture, and how to lengthen the curtains to fill the tall windows.

The Memorial Hospital was so named because of all the money subscribed for a War Memorial in 1919. Only a small amount was used for a stone Cenotaph which was erected in the Town Hall gardens which were on the corner of High Street and King Street. The remainder of the money was used to double the size of the old Cottage Hospital, and re-equip it. In the entrance hall were two large white marble squares which were fixed on the left and right walls respectively, and carved on them were the names of all the local men who died in the Great War of 1914-1918. There were many names recorded there, because the local battalion was almost wiped out in the fighting on the Somme on 1st July 1916; while many others perished serving in the minesweepers of the Royal Navy which were based in Sandhaven. As he was leaving he stopped and read some of the names: Pte. Collinson, Pte. Griffin, Lieut. Laycarte-Porter, Corpl. Meadows, Sgt. Roberts, 2nd Lieut. Vickers and Pte. Young, and recognised the names of the farmers, and even that of the son of the owner of the Hall.

On Friday Richard brought Flora home. She walked round the flat and commented that she would be glad to get to the new one, and that tomorrow she would start packing. But by Saturday afternoon Richard noticed that she had not packed anything, and had not paid any attention to the *Daily Telegraph* of which she was usually an avid reader. On Sunday Richard was on duty, and had to go out early to a cow having difficulty calving. When he arrived back at the flat he found Flora still in bed, so he made breakfast for the two of them and then put it on a tray and carried it into the bedroom.

"Come on, Flora, and have some breakfast. It's half past nine," said Richard.

"Yes I'll have a cup of tea," she replied and sat up in bed and watched Richard eating rapidly.

"You're not eating anything, Flora, is anything wrong?"

"Oh I don't know," she replied, "I'm so depressed; I don't seem to have any interest in anything."

"Flora darling, don't be depressed, it was not your fault. I am certain that awkward fall on the stairs was the cause of all the trouble."

"But Richard, you don't understand, I've lost my baby, I've lost part of us, and I wanted it so much" and she suddenly burst into tears.

He hurriedly moved the tray, and sitting down beside her on the bed, put his arms round her, and hugged her, and kissed her gently.

"Don't cry, love, I'm dreadfully sorry too, but it's happened, and we must just hope things will be better. Now go and have your bath and I'll light the lounge fire, and make some more tea." When he left to do his morning visits Flora had cheered up, but occasionally during the week she would suddenly have a bout of crying. He did everything he could to stop her being depressed. One night he took her to the Theatre Royal in Droughton to see the film of Ginger Rogers and Fred Astaire; on others he played her favourite records on the gramophone, and he even remembered to buy flowers. Flora now began to take an interest in things, and to help Richard with the packing, but it was the letter she received on the Thursday morning which cured her depression. It was from Annie Holden, Uncle Harry's daughter, inviting them to her wedding in September. Jean had been invited along with all the family, and so Flora, Jean and Mary were soon telephoning each other to talk of dresses and costumes, hats and gloves.

The Promenade, Sandhaven, was two miles long, and divided into the West and East Promenade at Queen Street. Going west most of the houses were detached, standing in their own grounds, and many wealthy people lived here. To the east of Queen Street there were long terraces of three-storey brick-built Victorian houses, which were raised above the level of the road, and had a pavement edged by a low wall in front of them. This prevented them being flooded when a high spring tide driven by a south-westerly gale forced the waves over the sea wall. Each of the three terraces had a name: Waterloo, Balaklava, Ladysmith, and it was in the latter at number four that the ground floor flat was situated. They moved in on 1st August and Flora was occupied with arranging the furniture and altering the curtains; but whatever she did could not disguise the fact that the big rooms were sparsely furnished. They had a battery wireless set, which was relegated to the rear of the house when Richard bought a six valve Marconi wireless set which had a brown Bakelite case and two illuminated panels showing the names of English and Continental stations. It was second hand and using it Flora loved to listen to the dance bands of Henry Hall, Jack Hylton, Ambrose or Joe Loss at 10.30 at night. Richard was more interested in the news which was becoming more ominous as Hitler threatened war if his territorial ambitions in Europe were not satisfied.

The message was: "A horse with colic at Boundary Farm", and Richard was soon there to be met by George Meadows.

"Good morning, George," said Richard, "Where's the horse?"

"In that big end box. It's a big gelding and it's got worse rapidly this last hour."

"When did it start?"

"I don't know really, Mr Holden. It was our Tom who found it when he went to bring two of them in about 8 o'clock."

The horse was sweating profusely and kicking at its belly with its hind legs. Richard immediately said to himself that it looked a bad case; they often were when they occurred in a horse at grass. Its temperature was raised, its pulse fast and hard, and it was breathing heavily. When Richard noticed the trickle of green fluid from the horse's nostrils, he began to consider a twist of the small bowel, or a distended stomach, so he immediately tried to pass the stomach tube but it proved difficult, the horse making expulsive movements and resenting the attempts to pass the tube. Richard finally accomplished this but it did not help the diagnosis, because only a little gas came through the tube. He administered chloral hydrate in a saline solution, telling George that it would ease the symptoms because he now thought the diagnosis was an intussusception. He withdrew the tube and watched the horse for some minutes. It did appear easier, so he told George he would be back about lunch time. As he drove away from the farm he worried about the diagnosis, and decided to go and find Charles because Meadows was a good client. He rang the surgery and Mrs Parsons told him that Charles had gone to two farms over Southall way, and that he should be back by eleven o'clock. Richard told Mrs Parsons about the case, and asked her to tell Charles to meet him at 11.30 at Boundary Farm. He was delayed at the last farm he visited that morning, so Charles arrived first and was examining the horse when Richard walked into the box. The horse was plainly worse; it was sweating hard and had more green discharge about its nostrils.

"Richard, I was just telling Mr Meadows that this horse is dying of an obscure colic, what did you diagnose?"

"An intussusception, but it was not as bad as this two hours ago, and it has had chloral and saline."

"Good. It was a rational treatment, but I have been reading Professor Gaiger's article about Grass disease and this case fits the very acute form he describes. George I am sorry, but very little is known about the disease, and I think the horse will be dead in an hour."

"Mr Parsons, I would rather you shot it than let it go on like this, the poor devil is black with sweat and it's been up and down non stop."

"Right, I'll do that now, but tell Bob Whiteside, I want to see it opened at his place and to let me know when it is ready."

The horse had gone down again when Charles returned carrying the loaded Greener's and while Richard steadied its head Charles put the muzzle just below the forelock and fired. The horse fell over dead and the three men, all rather dejected, left the box. The post mortem gave the negative evidence associated with Grass disease, which was unusual as the disease appeared more in the south of England. Richard later learned from George that it had been brought there six weeks before. That evening he went to The Elms and read the article by Professor Gaiger and another by Dr Gordon on various aspects of Grass disease, so that he could recognise the disease and its various forms next time he met it among the large horse population in and around Sandhaven; but it was the usual cases of lameness and injuries which occupied his time on the farms and in the commercial area around and in the docks. Beyond the station in the east end of Sandhaven the Borough council had built an extensive council estate to house the growing population, and

Richard wondered why with so many cats and dogs in the area so few came to the surgery.

The reason for this was the behaviour of Charles who only saw animals by appointment at The Elms at 2.00 p.m. or 5.00 p.m. and, unknown to Richard, did his best to discourage them from coming again. He advised destruction of any animal needing an operation for a pathological condition, or wanting a long course of treatment. This deprived Richard of many surgical opportunities, and accounted for the fact that many an afternoon he had no work to do. He felt frustrated because the practice was not getting busier, because he was trying to use the most up-to-date methods. Recently he had pursuaded Charles to buy Solila stainless steel needles and 2, 5 and 10 cc. Record hypodermic syringes. Charles refused to buy the new drug Sulphanilamide, saying that the farmers would not pay for such expensive drugs, though Richard argued to the contrary. It was true that many farmers still ploughed using horses, and hand-milked their cows, and only two miles from Sandhaven farms were lit with oil lamps, because there was no gas or electricity available. There was no street lighting in the villages and they were very isolated in a bad winter.

Some of the farmers were great characters, none more so than Jack Clough who farmed Leach House at Marthorpe. He was probably in his late sixties, but was a powerfully built man with bright blue eyes, a huge moustache, and a voice to match. A flat cap covered his thick white hair and he always wore a heavy, big, black overcoat which was going green with age; big clogs completed his outfit when he went off to plough with his team of two black Shire horses.

Richard never forgot the afternoon he went to Leach House to treat a cow down with milk fever. It was about half past four and as the semi-conscious cow had been in danger of hanging herself the tie had been cut. She had slid backwards and was now on her side in the dung channel. Richard told Jack to bring a bale of straw, and then when Jack pulled the cow partly upright Richard jammed the bale behind her shoulder. As he was putting the rope round the cow's neck with which to raise the vein, Jack went out of the shippon but was back in a minute saying in broad dialect:

"I wonder where she is? She isn't back yet."

"Who isn't back?" asked Richard.

"My little lass," said Jack.

Richard thought he was making a big fuss about the little girl and said, "Don't bother about her, Jack, but hold this rope tight while I get the needle in the vein."

When the blood flowed freely from the needle he attached the milk fever apparatus and began the injection and Jack went out again quickly to return in a minute.

"She's still not here. Is cow all right, Mr Holden?"

"Yes. I've nearly finished injecting her, now, just stay here and hold her head still." Richard disconnected the apparatus and withdrew the needle.

"Right, Jack, you can let go." This he did and almost ran out of the ship-pon, to return, saying:

"I'm fair worried, my little lass should be here by now."

Richard, getting a bit exasperated, said, "Jack, will you get some ashes and straw and scatter it round her and in the channel, and we will see if she can get up."

After this had been done, Richard gave her a hard smack on her back and she rose to her feet, with Jack holding her tail to steady her. He then fitted a new tie, secured the cow, and went out again. Richard washed and dried his hands, put away his equipment and Jack returned and said, "She's still not here, my little lass, but cow looks right."

"Yes, she is, but don't milk her tonight and go easy on the milking for two days."

"Aye, I'll do that, Mr Holden."

By now they had reached the car and Jack, looking up the drive, said, "I wonder where my little lass is."

At that very moment a very fat, middle-aged woman riding a "sit up and beg" bicycle turned into the drive. She was wearing a big hat which was held in place by two tapes tied under her chin and the voluminous coat accen-tuated her size. Jack walked towards her. "It's my little lass, my Ruby, she's all right." Richard, flabbergasted at the size of the "little girl", quickly got into his car and drove down the drive, so that Jack would not see him laughing heartily.

"Ye Gods! What a little girl!" he shouted.

Marthorpe was surrounded by marsh land, which had been reclaimed in the early eighteenth century, by digging straight channels called "drains" which finally emptied the water into the sea near the docks. It was peaty soil, and grew good potato crops, but in very wet weather soon became unwork-able. For stock, liver fluke was an ever present danger in damp autumn weather. This year proved no exception and cattle and sheep were affected, so Richard spent some afternoons dispensing *Ext. Filicis Maris*, the requisite dose to be given to the animal after twelve hours starvation. In the late summer husk appeared again among stock, and so Richard spent some hours injecting heifers and sometimes adult animals intratracheally, a slow job as each animal had to be caught and injected individually. One lowland flock of sheep became affected and the owner collected two gallons of husk medicine and spent two days dosing all the animals.

Charles gave Richard four days holiday in September so that he could attend Annie's wedding. Flora and he met Jean, Mary and Bill at the railway station in Droughton and they had a good journey to Winchester, changing trains at Oxford. They spent the night in a hotel in Winchester and next morning went to Alresford. Here they met Dick and Alice, and Richard met his cousins Annie, Harry and Ezra for the first time, and Auntie Jane again having last seen her at his mother Victoria's funeral. Uncle Harry and Auntie Joan made them all very welcome until it was time to go to the service which was held in St. Mary's Church where Annie Holden married Thomas Ryde Facer. It was a very fashionable wedding held on a glorious sunny day, followed by an excellent lunch in a nearby hotel. After the meal ended Richard and Flora had a very pleasant time talking to their relations and meeting Joan's family, Madge and Bert Gould and their two children Madge and Harry. Uncle Bert was a wholesale butcher and soon he and Richard were talking about cattle and the meat industry. Uncle Harry joined them for a short time, and they both asked Richard why he was staying in Lancashire, waiting as Bert said "almost for dead men's shoes". They pointed out the better climate in Hampshire, and the flourishing agriculture, and advised Richard to think about it. After spending the next day in Winchester Richard and Flora left Jean, Mary and Bill to continue their holiday, while they returned home. Richard had been disturbed by his uncle's advice and he and Flora began to wonder if they were doing the right thing staying in Sandhaven on a small salary waiting for another year and a half to take over the practice. In the end they decided to stay in Sandhaven because Flora's family was not too far away and Richard felt that his roots were in Droughton.

They broke their journey at Morton to go and visit Flora's Aunt Winnie, her late father's sister. Her husband had died three years earlier, having been the Chief Inspector of Taxes for the area. He had left Winnie a fortune in houses, Government securities, equities and a sizeable income from money left in trust. She had become eccentric, rarely leaving the big house where she lived with a cook and housemaid to see to her wants. When Flora told the maid that she had come to see her aunt, the maid told her to wait and after a moment invited them into the house and they were shown into the morning room. It was beautifully furnished with walnut antique furniture; there were several lovely old paintings and Richard guessed that Flora got her love of antiques from her father's family, the Dickensons. Winnie was delighted to see Flora and meet Richard and they told her all their news, but she still wanted to know more and chattered on until Flora and Richard said it was time for them to leave. She hugged and kissed Flora and then the maid showed them out. As they made their way back to the station Richard grumbled that Winnie should have offered them afternoon tea, but Flora laughed and told him he did not know Winnie's funny ways, they were lucky to have been invited in and she never sent letters or Christmas cards. Richard remarked that there was one in every family; his father and sister were like

Winnie and he was very disappointed that they had not gone to the wedding as they had not heard from them for five months. Flora did not reply.

They arrived back just in time for Richard to take over the running of the practice single-handed because Charles had become ill again and the doctor had ordered him to bed that day. Richard spent that evening making two visits to a horse with colic down on the docks; it was one of thirty that Harrisons, the haulage contractors, kept for work in the docks, though for deliveries elsewhere they used motor lorries. The motors were getting bigger in size and numbers as more Foden and Leyland lorries were purchased, but for the short journeys in the docks, the horse transport was ideal. Nevertheless, they were in constant danger of being involved in accidents with shunting engines and lorries, they had shoes torn off when caught in the points on the railway lines and they were worked hard. When they were taken out to drink at the horse troughs by their drivers at 7 a.m. the horse which was a shy drinker might drink very little and then eat a big meal of dry food. This was the type of horse, which began to show signs of colic in the early evening as it developed an impaction of the large bowel. At each visit that evening Richard administered medicine in three gallons of water via the stomach tube. After he had done this at the second visit he waited until he could hear intestinal movements taking place before he went home at 11 p.m; it had been a long day.

The next morning he took his two rolls of film to the chemists to be developed, and his Kodak Box Brownie camera to have a new film put in it. Situated just past the Town Hall on the High Street, the chemist's shop was large and had a central door with large windows for displaying goods on either side. As Richard pushed the door open, the bell rang. When he entered, the chemist walked towards him behind the counter and the instant recognition was mutual.

"Well, Jim Lord, fancy seeing you here. This is a nice surprise." said Richard.

"I can reciprocate those sentiments gladly." Jim replied.

"And what are you doing here, Jim? Are you helping out?"

"No, Richard, I have bought the business and moved in last weekend."

"I've been to a wedding in Hampshire, so that's why I didn't see you before, but what's brought you here?"

"It's a long story. I got married two years ago, just about when you left Holme and then my father died suddenly leaving me the business. At the beginning of this year my wife started to have asthma attacks. We have tried everything, but they have become more frequent and our doctor advised moving to the seaside, because my wife came from Whitby and he is certain the smoky air in Holme is the main cause. My cousin Dick Harrison is the manager of the District Bank here, so he arranged the purchase of this business, while I sold the one in Holme, and here I am."

"So that's it. Well, we live on the Promenade at No 4, Ladysmith Walk; you must come and see us as soon as you get settled."

"Thank you, Richard, I would like that."

At that another customer entered the shop and so Richard left his camera and films very cheered up by finding that he had a friend who was almost a confidant in the town, and knowing his connection with his bank manager could be very useful in the future when he wanted to buy a house.

When Charles recovered he looked very frail, but at once began his work as a Veterinary Inspector for the County Council, a position he had filled for many years. Owing to the Acts passed by Parliament, there was more work to do. Charles went to farms at 8.00 a.m. or 6.00 p.m., when the milking was usually finished and examined the animals for certain pathological conditions such as tuberculosis in any form, anthrax, foot and mouth disease, mastitis, and other conditions which were likely to convey disease in the milk as detailed in the Milk Order of 1936. As all the milch cows had to be examined and their udders palpated, this duty was soon called "bag punching"; in carrying out his inspection the Inspector got splattered with dung especially in summer, and had to avoid being kicked, or hiked by the cows horns. If there was any abnormality in the udder, a milk sample was collected in a screw-capped bottle, and if the cow had a cough a search was made for any sputum on the wall in front of the animal. The inspection completed, the owner was given the relevant form, usually a blue one if the herd was producing accredited milk, or a white one if it were a non-designated herd. Back in the surgery the milk samples were centrifuged and the sediment was smeared onto a glass slide to which it was fixed by heat and then stained using the Ziehl-Neelsen method. The slide was examined using a microscope with a one twelfth objective. Samples of discharges from the uterus or of sputum were smeared directly on to the slide, stained and then examined. This work kept Charles busy in the morning or evening on many days and often Richard had to examine slides when Charles said his eyes had got too tired. It did cause eyestrain, examining slides for long periods by gas-light using a monocular microscope. If an animal was found with suspicious or definite clinical symptoms of tuberculosis, or if a sample proved positive, a form A was served. Later many other forms had to be completed and copies had to be given to the owner; the other copies along with the account form had to be sent to the County Public Health Dept., the County Offices, Droughton. Many tubercular cows were found during these inspections and so Charles devoted most of his time to dealing with them, while Richard did all the other work and Richard sometimes found one, when asked to examine an animal which was "not doing", or had a bad cough.

Some of the more progressive farmers, disturbed by these losses, disposed of their herds and restocked with cattle which had passed the Tuberculin

Test; more were asking what it entailed and how much it cost. Jack Booth at Intack Farm, on taking over from his father, lost many cows with TB and came to see Charles one day for advice. As a result he sold his herd and decided to alter his buildings, which included installing a milking machine and also building a ramp to make it easier to load the milk lorry, because ten gallons of milk in a steel can is very heavy to move about or lift. All the buildings were cleaned and disinfected, and two weeks later he began to restock with pedigree Friesian cows which had passed the test, some of which came from a famous herd in Cheshire which Richard knew. In the way of business, Uncle Harry telephoned Richard one evening, wanting information about Jack Booth and if his credit was good. Richard was able to reassure him and then Harry invited him and Flora to join them and Uncle Dick and Alice in Alresford at Christmas. Richard was sorry to have to refuse the invitation, but explained that he only had Christmas Day and Boxing Day off for the holiday.

The photographs of the wedding were very good, so Richard asked Jim Lord to make two more sets of prints, one set for Jean and the other for Uncle Harry. When she received them Flora took one set to her mother, leaving Richard to have his lunch at Miss Bishop's café that day. It had been a cold, stormy morning and the wind was still getting stronger by the hour when Richard walked into the café. He expected it to be cheerful and warm, which it was, but he did not expect the nice surprise of finding Tom Seed sitting at one of the tables. Richard immediately joined him and as they ate, they brought each other up to date as to what had happened to them during the last few years. Tom had sold his hay and straw business in Droughton and was now the chief representative of the Droughton Farmers Ltd. About every three months he toured the area to visit the farmers who were bad payers and to sort out any problems. His daughter Doris had married Bill Bainbridge of Duckworth Hall, which was between Wyreham and Droughton and their vet was Mr Townsend from Wilton.

It was blowing a gale when Richard arrived at The Elms. Charles sent him to the docks immediately because a horse had been injured, giving him the humane killer as he left. The dock policeman at the gate told him that the horse was on the South Quay, where Richard found a group of men and Syd, the foreman of Harrison's waiting. The latter told Richard that the accident had happened about twenty minutes before and that their insurance agent would arrive soon. A lorry had been driven alongside the horse, which was being held upright by leaning on a wheel. One leg was protruding from under its body at a peculiar angle while the other was stretched straight out behind it. The shafts of the lorry were smashed, and Richard stepped over them to examine the off hind leg which he found was broken above the stifle, where the bone was protruding through the skin on the inner side of the thigh. The horse did not feel his examination, which told Richard that its back must be injured or broken. To confirm his suspicions, he got a needle out of his instrument case and began to prick the horse's skin going forwards from the tail. When he reached the loin the skin twitched and the horse tried to drag itself along.

"Syd, I am going to shoot it at once on humane grounds, it's got a broken back and a compound fracture of the leg," said Richard.

"Aye, I thought it was hopeless," Syd replied.

The agent from the insurance company arrived and immediately agreed to the destruction of the horse. After the dock police had moved the men back to a safe position Richard shot the horse. As he was walking with Syd back to Harrison's office, he noticed the driver of the dead horse and another man pull a tarpaulin over it. On the telephone he told Bob Whiteside to come and remove the carcase, but not to dress it until he had made a post mortem so that he could complete the Veterinary Certificate of the insurance company.

"Now Syd, how did it happen?" asked Richard.

"It was like this, Mr Holden," said Syd. "The lorry was ready for that container to be lowered on to it. It had a chain hooked onto each corner and was swinging in the wind, but the gang were trying to hold it steady with the ropes. Suddenly a chain broke, the container keeled over sideways and then fell like a stone. The driver and the gang were lucky it missed them as it landed half on the cart and half on the horse which went down with a squeal as a wood flew everywhere. There was nothing anybody could do about it, I suppose it was an act of God as they say."

Richard thought, surely God would never inflict such suffering as that on a dumb animal; it was more likely some fool had not made the chain properly and he was surprised by the intensity of his anger against that unknown individual. Following the accident, he advised that all the horses be injected with tetanus antitoxin, and this he did during the next week. He still tried to extend the amount of preventative medicine undertaken in the practice, in spite of the reluctance of Charles. He did manage to persuade him to stock packets of powder for the treatment of warble fly, though getting the farmers to buy it was hard work. So many grumbled that it was no use dressing their stock between March and June when their neighbours did not; the newly hatched out fly would fly into their fields and lay eggs on their cattle. But that year he had convinced some of the sheep farmers of the value of using lamb dysentery serum. In the district some farmers bought ewes at the autumn sheep sales in Scotland and let them graze the stubble, catch crops, and clover leys. Then the tups were put in, so that the lambs would be born in March of the following year. John Huddlestone at Red Barn had done this, but was certain that the ewes had brought infection with them, because lambs began to die. Richard diagnosed lamb dysentery and obtained serum at once, so that every lamb could be injected as soon as possible after it was born, and this stopped the outbreak.

On a slight hill at the corner of West Promenade and Church Road stood St. Lukes, the Parish Church of Sandhaven. An ancient foundation, which was mentioned in the Domesday Book, it had been rebuilt in the thirteenth century, but retained a lovely Norman door with carved tympanum. Flora went fairly regularly to the 8.30 a.m. service of Holy Communion but Richard did not go with her because he had not been confirmed. The reason for this was that Ted and Mary were Methodists while Victoria and Richard went to the Church of England. Neither parent would allow Richard to be confirmed in the other's faith and so it was never done. But he wanted to go with Flora and so asked the Vicar if a confirmation class would beheld. No class was being held because he was retiring at the end of the year, but his replacement would begin a class as soon as he arrived.

At church meetings Flora had met Betty Heyes and they had become friends. Dick was Betty's husband and was the greengrocer in Sandhaven, having been brought up in the business, and inherited it when his father had died in his early fifties the year before. He sold only the best fruit and vegetables and supplied the Porter Arms Hotel, the Memorial Hospital, the Grammar School and much of the town. The opposition from the two stalls in the Market Hall in Victoria Street was negligible. His Morris van, made into a travelling shop, toured the suburbs and the surrounding villages twice a week selling produce. He was going to buy a second van, because of increasing demand caused by the growth in the population. Houses were being built along Woodfield Lane, which was an extension of Church Road, The Borough Council had begun to build another estate on the land between Station Road and London Road in the east end of the town and beyond the gas works a big factory was being built for the Government.

At Christmas Flora and Richard decided to ask their friends and acquaintances to the flat for drinks. Flora rang Jean and asked if she and Mary would come and bring some cutlery and glasses. Jean said that Mary had bought an Austin Seven saloon car and so they would come in it. Flora soon drew up a list of names: Jim and Isabel Lord; Dick and Betty Heyes; Tommy and Edna Duke, Joe Bolton and Mary; Bill Meadows and Elizabeth; and Dr McConnell the handsome batchelor. Richard and Flora decorated the flat with holly, ivy, and paper decorations coloured green and yellow. The Christmas cards on the mantlepiece, the window seats and the lounge coffee table added to the festive appearance. Big fires were made in the lounge and diningroom and with all the lights and lamps switched on the flat was warm and bright. Mary made ham sandwiches, while Jean cut up the Christmas cake which Flora had made, while her mince pies were put into the gas oven to warm. Richard carried all the plates, serviettes, and cutlery into the dining room, and arranged them on the mahogany table, and then polished the glasses and checked his bottles of sherry, gin and whisky; tonics and ginger ale, and the lemon slices.

Their guests were reasonably punctual except Bill McConnell who telephoned to say he was detained at the hospital, but would be along in half an
hour. Flora introduced her friends to each other and to Jean and Mary,
and quickly two groups were found, each holding animated conversations.
Richard was working on the principle that to get a party going, give one or
two strong big drinks at the beginning. It was certainly effective today, and
he was most efficient at filling up half-empty glasses. When Bill McConnell
arrived, he entered into the party spirit immediately, kissed Flora under the
mistletoe and then circulated with her and Jean, finally joining the group of
the Boltons and the Dukes who were discussing whether or not Mr Chamberlain was right with his policy of appeasement. Richard had listened to this
with interest, but was amused to find the Heyes, Lords and Meadows
discussing the local woman who had had a win on the football pools. The
party went very well, the mince pies and the cake were praised and Flora,
who had been very nervous before the guests arrived at midday, was very
happy and pleased when they left from about three until almost four o'clock.
Jean asked Richard and Flora to spend Christmas Day and if possible Boxing
Day with her, and they accepted at once; so again they spent the holiday at
Holme, and on Christmas Day after lunch listened to the new King's speech
on the wireless.

For the milk their cows produced, the farmers received a cheque each
month from the Milk Marketing Board and this regular income was directly
proportional to the amount of milk produced; the bigger the milking herd the
bigger the income. The animal which gave the greatest amount of milk was
the black and white Friesian, which was rapidly replacing the Ayrshire, Dairy
Shorthorn and other breeds. When a herd composed of one of the latter
breeds failed the Tuberculin Test, a few farmers, after cleansing and disin-
fecting their premises, restocked with attested Friesian cattle. Both Richard
and the farmers soon realised that there were going to be difficulties with the
breed, because their large udders were prone to injury and mastitis, and the
number of cases of milk fever began to increase, but in addition to these
troubles was the difficulty encountered in trying to deliver a very large calf
when the cow was calving.

The worst cases were often the result of any Ayrshire-Friesian mating.
Calving ropes were attached to the two legs of the calf which were presented
and two men pulled on each rope. They often broke under the strain, so
stronger ropes were attached and tied to pulley blocks and finally the calf was
delivered. As a result of the excessive force used, the cow often was unable to
rise for a day or two and sometimes never did and had to be destroyed.
Charles bought steel obstetric chains, but Richard argued that they were not
the answer to the problem, because when they were used instead of ropes the
cow appeared to suffer greater damage. With more valuable calves being

born, Richard used more white scour vaccine and serum, to try and prevent
the disease, and advised that calves should have separate buckets and pens
but even so some cases occurred, often where the calves had been purchased.
Some farmers were buying packets of warble fly dressing to treat their cattle;
others said it was a waste of time and money and would not do it, until their
neighbours dressed their cattle. Wanting to discuss many problems, Richard
went to a meeting of the Veterinary Society, which involved a round trip of
eighty miles, but was stimulated by the informed opinions expressed and by
listening to the experience of other veterinary surgeons. On the outward
journey the car did not go very well, but coming home it lost so much power,
that it only just reached Dock Garage. Gordon Hindle the owner was still
working and so the Ford 8 got immediate attention. Gordon put the starting
handle in position and turned it.

"Mr Holden, the car has no compression on one cylinder and very little on
the other three."

"Is it as bad as that, Gordon?" asked Richard.

"Yes, have you had it from new?" asked Gordon.

"Yes, I bought it when I was in Herefordshire last year, Gordon, and it's
gone very well except for a half shaft breaking and the odd rear spring."

"But you haven't had it decarbonised?"

"No, I haven't," said Richard.

"In that case you will have to leave it. I'll decarbonise it and grind in the
valves and it will need a new gasket and fan belt," was Gordon's reply.

"Right, make a good job of it," said Richard, "and let me know as soon as
it's ready; have you a car I could borrow?"

"Not tonight, but come in the morning and we'll arrange the insurance and
you can take the old Minx."

"Thank you and good night," said Richard and walked home, now tired
and depressed. This was aggravated by the scolding he got from an anxious
Flora, who had become worried when he was so late arriving home. To be
at The Elms next morning driving the Minx was the response he got from
Charles.

Charles had plenty of work to do for the County Council so, though the
practice was quiet, Richard found himself doing more laboratory work,
which he enjoyed, especially when a slide proved positive for the causal
organisms of TB, anthrax or the streptococci and staphylococci from cases of
mastitis. Charles would not buy a better centrifuge than the two-tube model
they had, but gave way over the drug Sulphanilanide, when he found out that
some farmers had obtained it. Very quickly they were selling packets which
contained six one-ounce powders, for use in horses and cattle. When Charles
was carrying out the Tuberculin Test in a herd, Richard went with him and
wrote down the animal's particulars and the skin measurements. As the
animal had a number tattooed in the ear it had to be caught and held, and

after the grease was wiped away, the number was read. Animals which had been born since the last test had to be marked, so the marking ink was rubbed on the inside of the ear, then the tattooing forceps put in position and as they were closed the number was punched into the skin, indelibly marking the animals. So the test took a long time and, starting at 8.00 a.m., they were often still testing as lunch-time approached.

Though the Tuberculin Test benefited the farmer, some of them wanted it done as quickly as possible so that their men could get on with routine work. So after three or four hours testing some men became impatient and short-tempered and told their men to get a move on. Of this ilk was Tom Priestly of Beech Tree Farm, a handsome black-haired man aged forty-five, of good physique, who worked hard himself and expected his sons Smith and John and his men to do likewise, and he brooked no delay. The cows and heifers had been tested and as they walked across the yard to the calf house, Tom told his two men to take an early meal break and to be back within the hour.

Following Richard's advice, each calf was in a separate pen with a door, and most of these were held shut by loops of baling wire. Smith went into the first pen and caught the calf, while John went into pen number two. Tom had tattooed all his stock, so he read out the number. They had worked in this way until they were about halfway along the row of pens and Smith was trying to untwist the wire which was holding the door shut.

"Come on, Smith, get that door open," said Tom brusquely.

"I'm trying to, but the wire's got twisted up," replied Smith.

"Here, take my knife and cut it; hurry up!"

Instead of taking the knife, Smith seized the door and tried to wrench it open but it refused to budge. On the second attempt the wire broke as the door flew open; one piece hit him in the face and he yelled.

"Hell, it's my eye! Oh, my eye!"

"What have you done, you clumsy devil; come on, let's have a look," and Tom pulled his son's hands away. A little blood-stained watery fluid was running down his face and Richard could see that the cornea was torn and that there was a lot of blood behind it. From the wound in the centre a piece of black tissue was protruding from which a little blood was dripping.

"Don't touch your eye, Smith," shouted Richard. "I'll get a dressing from the car."

He knew the sterilizer was on the back seat and from it he took a large piece of boiled cottonwool and picked up a white bandage. He ran back to Smith, covered the damaged eye with the dressing and bandaged it in place.

"Tom," said Charles, "Take Smith at once to the hospital to have that eye seen to; we three can manage here and get finished."

"Right, Mr Parsons," said Tom, "Come on, Smith," and he took him by the arm and they left the shippon.

John was still standing in the next pen holding a calf, aghast at what had happened.

"By jove, that's a bad do for your brother," said Charles, "being hit in the eye like that."

"Really, Mr Parsons, I hope they can save it for him; he's getting engaged in a few weeks time to Betty Whitehead from Far Parkside."

"I don't know what they will be able to do," said Charles, "but let's get on and finish these calves," and they were all very quiet and disheartened until the job was done.

Richard telephoned Tom Priestley towards the end of the week and was dismayed to learn that the surgeon had excised the eye because it was hopelessly infected and he feared that meningitis might develop. Later, Smith had a glass eye fitted and duly became engaged to Betty; while Tom became less domineering and it was more pleasant to work for or with him.

At the month end Richard paid his account at the garage and later found that his bank balance was down to £320. He became depressed, because though the car was going well, it was one and a half years old, and showing signs of wear and tear. His salary of £5 a week was barely adequate to cover all the calls made on it. Richard had to buy new rubber boots, a rubber apron to wear when carrying out obstetrical work in large animals, and a warehouse coat which he wore over his jacket to try and keep it and his trousers clean. Charles never helped financially. So Flora and Richard had a heart to heart talk one evening, because they were uncertain that they were doing the right thing staying in Sandhaven. In the end they decided to stay, because they would be taking over the practice in twelve months time and they were certain they could do well. They did not want to go to the south of England, because the papers said that war could break out, with Hitler threatening Austria, and if war did come Sandhaven would be as safe as anywhere. Above all, they liked the area very much. On these bright spring days Richard loved the countryside awakening from winter, and was thoroughly happy driving through it doing a job which gave him great satisfaction. Flora liked the town and after shopping used to walk along the Promenade, invigorated by the keen wind off the sea; or sometimes go into Miss Bishop's café and drink coffee and gossip with her circle of friends.

It was while walking along the Promenade one morning, carrying a heavy shopping bag, that Flora began to have pains in her abdomen. Arriving at the flat she made a cup of tea and drank it, all the time considering the likelihood that she was pregnant again. As the pain became worse she decided she was not, and went and lay on the bed. It was there that Richard found her when he arrived at lunch time. He was worried immediately and wanted to telephone the doctor, but Flora insisted that there was no need to do so, as the pain was passing. She drank a cup of coffee to which he had added a little brandy and when he left her at two o'clock the pain had stopped. The second attack began on a Saturday evening while they were in the cinema watching the Pathé News showing the German Army marching into Austria, and accompanying Hitler who, having displaced Schuschnig by force, proclaimed the *Anschluss* the next day, 13th March.

"Richard, I want to go outside, that pain has started again," said Flora, and he held her arm, as they descended the three flights of stairs to reach the street.

"That's a bit easier," she said. "I think sitting in a cramped position in that circle seat must have set it off."

Back home he made her drink coffee laced with brandy, to wash down two aspirin tablets, but the pain persisted for some hours. The attacks became more frequent and in the end Richard said that she had to see the doctor in spite of her objections. Dr McConnell in a few minutes arrived at the provisional diagnosis of a grumbling appendix. Quietly speaking, he deprecated his own diagnosis and proposed they had a second opinion from the surgeon, Mr Tennant. When that consultation took place Dr McConnell's diagnosis was confirmed and to Richard's surprise the attacks almost ceased in the time that elapsed from then until the date arrived for her admission to the hospital. Flora was admitted at lunchtime on Monday. Richard saw her for a short time that evening, and at seven o'clock it was a very emotional parting for them both.

The flat was cold because the fire had died out; his doubts and depression returned, but he remade the fire, lit it and put the blower to it. In the kitchen he brewed a pot of tea, made cold beef sandwiches and returned to the lounge, to find a roaring fire when he removed the blower. As he ate his meal he wondered what he would do if the operation was not a success because a malignant growth was found; what if Flora died? He remained sitting in front of the fire for a long time pondering the questions and then went into the bedroom and knelt down and prayed to God for help. So, lonely, cold and depressed he undressed, got into bed and a long time later slept.

The next day at lunch time he went to the chip shop, bought a pie and chips and was eating them in the flat when the telephone rang. He was trembling slightly as he put the receiver to his ear.

"Is that Mr Holden?" was the enquiry.

"Yes, speaking," he replied.

"This is the secretary of the Memorial Hospital. I have to inform you that Mrs Holden has had her operation and her condition is very satisfactory."

"Oh, thank you so much for ringing; when can I see her?"

"Between five and six o'clock this afternoon. Goodbye now."

His eyes filled with tears of relief as he put the receiver down and he said, "Oh God, Thank you for your help and mercy", and then he remembered that he had not let Jean know.

She was annoyed because he had not telephoned her earlier, and said she was coming at once. This she did and for a week made Richard's meals and cleaned the flat. Each evening they spent with Flora in the daffodil-decorated room until they brought her home. They all laughed heartily when, on pushing back the settee, they found half a pie and some chips, now slightly mouldy, the remains of the unfinished lunch.

One Thursday evening the parishioners filled St. Lukes Church for the institution of the Reverend Thomas Griffith Evans, MA as the Vicar of Sandhaven. Among the congregation were the mayor and mayoress, some members of the Town Council and the governors and masters from the Grammar School, and all was most efficiently organised by Alan Laycarte-Porter and Tom Collinson, the two churchwardens. Flora was quite excited and keen to meet the Vicar, because Jean had told her that he was the brother of Gladys, Jerry Lawson's wife who lived in Llandudno. After the service, tea was served in the Parish Hall and the Vicar and his wife met and mixed with the parishioners. Flora introduced herself to this tall, black-haired priest with the deep-toned clear voice and then Richard, who liked him at once, though they only chatted for a few minutes. He was obviously pleased to meet members of his own family, before he moved away among the people. Richard hàd learnt from him that the confirmation classes would begin in about three months time, so he dismissed them from his mind and concentrated on his professional work.

It had been a good lambing season, with mild weather and few difficult lambing cases. The use of lamb dysentry antiserum ensured that more lambs had survived and fewer ewes had udder disease. Charles had bought an emasculator to use when castrating horses, because the operation was completed in one visit. The horses had to be operated on before the flies arrived and so Richard was busy on many days, castrating, and also docking foals. Some farmers still preferred clamps to be used, but George Meadows asked for the emasculator to be used on his colts, both of which were well grown. After injecting the local anaesthetic Richard waited a few minutes and then operated on the nearest testicle, squeezing the instrument shut for a minute and then releasing it. He repeated the procedure on the other testicle and there was little bleeding. Nevertheless he got a bucket full of clean cold water, poured into it some Dettol and then splashed the operation site. When the second colt was brought out Richard noticed that it had a swollen knee and George said that it had had a clout off the other one. Richard operated exactly as before, but there was more bleeding, even after it had been splashed with cold water. He waited some time and again used the cold water. He talked to George until the bleeding was reduced to the odd drop falling and then left the farm, telling George to put the colt in a box on its own and to have a look at it in an hour. When Richard arrived at the surgery at midday, Charles was putting the sterilizer and the chloroform mask into his car and told Richard to get in quickly.

"What's the matter, Charles?" he asked.

"One of the colts you cut at George Meadows' is bleeding," replied Charles.

"That's strange, I waited until they had stopped bleeding, though the second was dripping a little, but had almost dried up."

"Well, it isn't now. Did you use the emasculator?"

"Yes, it's the fourteenth time I've used it with no trouble," said Richard and wondered what had gone wrong.

Arriving at the farm they found the second colt in a box and from the operation wounds blood was dripping quickly. Charles looked at the pale mucous membranes of the mouth and at the blood on the floor and said:

"George, the only way to stop this haemorrhage will be to cast and chloroform this colt and ligature the cords, so I want two side lines and some men."

The colt was speedily cast, Richard administered the chloroform, and when it was unconscious it was rolled onto its back.

After swabbing the site with Dettol, Charles got a pair of long rat-toothed forceps and tried to find the ends of the cords, but it proved impossible so the scrotum was tightly packed with boiled cotton wool and then the wounds stitched. They waited for half an hour and finally the colt got to its feet, so they told George that they would be back later in the afternoon and left.

Richard drove the car and Charles said:

"I don't like the look of that colt, it will be lucky to pull through. You know how quickly horse blood coagulates, well, its blood didn't stick to my fingers and that on the floor was not properly coagulated, it was like thin porridge."

"What do you think is wrong?"

"Either some failure of the lining of the artery to retract and close the hole, or it's got some blood disease," Charles replied.

When Richard got back to the farm about five o'clock, George Meadows was standing by the door of the box. He came over to the car and said,

"There's no need to get out, Richard, it's just died."

"That is a pity. I am sorry it's died, George, but neither Mr Parsons nor I can understand why it has kept on bleeding, so I will go to Southall to see if we can find out the reason. Have you rung Bob Whiteside?"

"Not yet," said Charles.

"Right, then tell him I want to see it opened and to let me know when he's got it there," was Richard's reply.

The next day they went together to the horse slaughterer's yard and on examining the carcase found the scrotum distended with watery blood. In the abdomen there was more than half a gallon of blood, and more ran out as the butcher eviscerated it. Charles found signs of strongyle damage to the aorta and took scrapings from the lining of the intestines. At the surgery he made preparations from the samples, examined them under the microscope and found strongyle worms and eggs. He decided that the failure of the blood to clot properly was caused by a reaction to the worm infestation. Richard said he thought the worm infestation was secondary to a primary haemophilia. Charles replied that you only got that condition in racehorses. Nevertheless, Richard found Charles one day preparing clamps, because he was going to Joe Fowler's to castrate a big colt, and so the emasculator was put in the instrument cupboard and only used for castrating bull calves, when the owner wanted them clean cut.

Tom Bishop's bread was sold all over Sandhaven, being delivered in a horse-drawn van, but in the countryside a Morris motor car was now used. The bakery was behind the Market Café and shop, but even so was not big enough to cope with the increasing demand for its products. In 1937 Tom and his three sisters formed a private company whose object was to expand the business. The confectionary and chocolate making was continued in the old bakery in King Street, but a new bakery for bread and related products was built, using part of the old Rope Mill in Wharf Street. He had chosen a good site close to the docks and the railway station, which gave easy access to Droughton Road. As far as was possible it was a self-contained unit, with offices, staff canteen, stores, garage and stables. The production line was mechanised and though originally only two shifts were worked, later a night shift from 10 p.m. until 6 a.m. was introduced. The company prospered and soon vans were delivering bread daily to Droughton and Southall and local pig farmers collected stale bread to supplement the rations fed to their stock.

Though there was not a big dog population in Sandhaven, cases of hysteria did occur and if they did not respond to the treatment of morphia and valerian root which Charles prescribed, he destroyed them. George Hindle had an Alsatian dog called Blackie, which was his mother's companion and guard dog for his baby son and the garage.

If the dog was loose, no stranger dared to approach the pram or enter the garage. One day it had an attack of hysteria and, barking frantically, ran off into the council estate on Broad Lane, where it was found by Gordon and brought back to the garage. It was excited and trembling slightly when Richard examined it and he gave it four sedative tablets as one dose.

"Well, Gordon, what set this off?" said Richard.

"I don't know, Mr Holden. I had just let it loose and was going to walk it down to the beach when it began to bark and howl and then ran off."

"It's typical of hysteria; what do you feed him?"

"Since the bakery started across the road, I get a two pound loaf for him every day and he gets this with half a pound of scrap meat from Wood's the butcher's. I pour the gravy over it and chop it all up with any household scraps. He soon gobbles that lot down," said Gordon.

"I think he is getting too much bread. You know they are really only meat eaters, Gordon, so cut out the bread and give him only meat and give him these sedative tablets, one three times a day."

Blackie continued to have the odd attack, but they were less severe and suddenly ceased. Richard was getting petrol one day and he asked Gordon how the dog was now.

"Oh, he's back to normal; by the way, is baker's yeast bad for dogs?"

Richard considered the question for a moment and then replied,

"In small amounts I would say No, but I am certain a piece the size of your thumb would swell up in a dog's stomach and cause him distress, and finally vomiting would begin. Why do you want to know?"

"It's like this, though the bakery is across the road, I only got stale bread for Blackie there, because my mother still makes bread twice a week. Some time ago she dropped some yeast and the dog ate it before she could stop him. Now she gives him little bits when she is baking and you know, he hasn't had a do for some time."

"You still feed him only meat, don't you?"

"Oh yes, and if he gets a bit worked up, I give him a couple of tablets."

"Well, there's no reason not to give him a little as a tit-bit, because it's not done him any harm."

Charles believed the condition was caused by a mutant of the distemper virus and he and Richard often argued as to its cause, because the condition was on the increase. The meat diet with a yeast additive was prescribed for any affected dog; some recovered, but many were destroyed.

Though Richard and Mr Parsons got on very well professionally Flora and he were never treated as friends. Flora was disappointed that after a year she had never met Mrs Parsons or been invited to tea, and Richard replied that he could count on one hand the number of cups of tea he had had from Mrs Parsons.

The message asked Mr Holden to visit a sick horse for Tom Bradshaw, Coal Merchant, Droughton. Charles was curious to know why Richard had been asked for, until he explained that Tom was his uncle, Victoria's brother. Then he made him telephone Tom to make certain that the animal had not been seen by another veterinary surgeon. Tom told Richard that he had sacked Mr Kennedy, who had been treating his horse. Charles advised Richard to telephone Mr Kennedy and explain that he had been asked to visit the animal. Mr Kennedy gave an outline of the history of the case, told Richard that he was glad to be rid of Mr Bradshaw as a client and rang off.

Richard took with him the tooth rasps and a gag and all the powders and medicines he thought he might need, because it was a thirty mile return trip to Droughton. He was pleased to see Uncle Tom, who went into the stable and led out a Shire gelding which was in poor condition. He told Richard that for three months it had slowly lost flesh, and he had not worked it for a fortnight. Now it ate half a feed and played about with its hay, wasting more than it ate. Richard carried out a careful clinical examination, finding the animal's heart rate, pulse, temperature and mucous membranes were all normal. With Tom's help he put a gag in the horse's mouth, examined its palate and teeth and found some of its molars were sharp, so he rasped them. Tom told him that he had given it alterative powders and condition balls and then worm powders, but they had had no effect. He asked for a bucket of warm water, soap and a towel and soaped his arm and while Tom held up a fore leg examined the horse *per rectum*. He found nothing abnormal, except that the sloppy dung contained a lot of undigested oats, so he put a little dung into a tin.

"Well, Richard, what's wrong with it?" asked Tom.

"Uncle, I've ruled out the obvious things like tooth trouble, jaundice and chronic grass disease, and I can't feel anything wrong with its guts. Does it ever get a bit blown up after eating?"

"No, Richard, it doesn't eat enough."

"Then I am certain it is some form of stomach trouble, so I am going to wash it out and then give a worm dose."

"How are you going to do that?"

"I'll soon show you."

He passed the stomach tube, which amazed Tom, and then administered half a gallon of sodium bicarbonate solution. He disconnected the pump but no fluid came out.

"You can see its stomach must be emptying properly, so I'm going to give it this oily worm dose."

He pushed the funnel into the end of the tube, climbed onto the wall of the coal store and slowly poured the pint of medicine into the funnel.

He withdrew the tube and Tom put the horse back in its stall.

"See how it goes on for a few days, Uncle, and then let me know, will you?"

"Yes I will, Richard; now come on into the house and have a proper wash and Nellie will make you a drink of tea."

This he did and enjoyed talking to them both and telling them how things were going for Flora and himself. He missed seeing his cousin Frank, who was on a long distance trip driving one of the steam wagons.

In the dung sample an insignificant number of worm eggs were found. He decided that if the treatment did not improve the horse's appetite, he would ask Charles to visit it. This proved unnecessary because Tom reported in a week that the horse was improving but not right. Richard visited it again and repeated the treatment, after which it made a complete recovery, and he decided that it had been a case of gastric catarrh, probably caused by an infestation of bots.

In May the funeral of Mrs Laycarte-Porter, the mother of the Colonel, took place at St. Lukes Church. During her eighty-five years of life, she had seen Sandhaven grow from a fishing village which had a harbour, to a seaside resort with docks, from which trawlers and pleasure steamers sailed. In the twentieth century the east end of the town was becoming increasingly industrialised. For many years she had been one of the leading personalities in the town and had lived in a mansion called The Rookery in the countryside behind the town. When Richard heard it was for sale he went to see Joe Bolton who told him the price and it was out of his reach. However, Joe suggested that he considered a house in the town which would be for sale soon. It was a detached house: Number 2 Cross Street which, though it faced into Cross Street, was the first in Victoria Road. Between numbers 2 and 4 Cross Street was a large yard in which was a disused stable block of two storeys. It had obviously been the first house built there in the 1840s and now was not far from the bus station, the market and the Market Hotel, and it was easy to get from Victoria Road to the west and north, and to Droughton in the east.

Accompanied by Flora, Richard drove to Cross Street and sat in the car looking at the house. It was soundly built of brick, with a stone doorway, stone quoins and large Georgian style windows. It was very neglected, wanted painting and the garden in front of the house was overgrown. Even so they both liked it and after assessing its possibilities drove back to Joe's office. He told them that it was owned by the very old former manager of the gas works who, having had a severe stroke, was a patient in the Memorial Hospital. His wife wanted the house sold quickly without too many prospective purchasers coming to view it. Joe arranged for them to go through it one evening and they soon realised it was very suitable. The vestibule led into a long hall which had two rooms on the left and three on the right and at the end the stairs led to the first floor. Beneath the stairs was a toilet. Upstairs were four large rooms, bathroom and toilet. The building in the yard was made up of a two-stall stable and a coach house, over which were a loft and a tack room in which was a fireplace. Inside, the house was well decorated and painted and by the time they left it Flora was suggesting how they could furnish it and Richard was planning where he would have his consulting room and operating theatre. But money was the big headache; how much Mrs Walker would want for the property was the crucial question.

The next time Richard went to see one of Uncle Tom's horses he visited an estate agent's in Droughton. There he soon discovered that a house similar to

Mrs Walker's would cost about £1,000. and more if situated in a superior area on the outskirts of the town. On the return journey, he went to see Bob Townsend who lived at Ashfield in Wilton Village. "Bob" was the abbreviation used by all the vets in the area for Robert Naylor Richard Townsend, a bachelor and a good veterinary surgeon who ran his practice singlehanded. Sarah, an elderly lady and a distant relative, kept house for him. Just after Christmas, at the Veterinary Meeting Richard had met Bob, who invited him to call if ever he were near Wilton. Richard parked his car behind three others and noticed that they were all dirty, then he rang the door bell, but did not enter though the door was open. "Come on in," someone shouted, so Richard walked into the hall and turned right into a large room, along one wall of which were stacked wooden crates containing beer bottles. In the middle of the wall above the crates a dart board was fixed.

Glass in hand, Bob Townsend rose to his feet and, shaking hands, said: "Hello, Holden, nice to see you again, now what was your Christian name?"

"Richard."

"Yes, of course it was," said Bob. "Let me introduce you to these three ne'er-do-wells; they are Tony Smith from Ridgeton, Bert Woods from Southall and Peter Baird from Corchester."

With shouts of "You are a lazy beggar yourself," and "Shut up Bob," followed by a lot of laughter, Bob blithely continued,

"They are all taking a few moments off from the rigours of our busy life and relaxing. Have a beer, Richard."

"Thank you," said Richard and while having his drink asked Peter Baird how Major John and Bill MacDonald were getting on.

"Oh they are just the same. Edwards and Allen have both left, so now I'm senior assistant, and Tom Lynn is the junior. I must be off or Bill will kill me if he gets to know I've been here wasting time. Thanks for the beer, Bob. Cheerio, Richard," and Peter left.

Richard enjoyed the time he spent there talking "shop", especially to Tony Smith who had been using Nembutal as an anaesthetic in dogs and advised Richard to use it because it was safer than chloroform, but to read up the literature first. Bob was the Veterinary Officer with the Yeomanry, and when the conversation came round to the serious situation in Europe, he said that he expected to be called up at once if war broke out.

After thanking him for the beer and saying goodbye to the other two, Richard left in a very serious frame of mind asking himself hypothetical questions. He had read that the veterinary profession would be a reserved occupation, but what would happen if he were called up? He could not just leave a practice in which he was going to mortgage the future for Flora and himself for many years ahead. Again he wondered why the Parsons were so unfriendly, why other veterinary surgeons never came to see them, and why, though they drank beer and cider with their meals, they never offered a glass to Richard. He decided not to make any friendly gesture to the Parsons, but to concentrate on making more contacts with his own and Flora's relatives. With this end in view, before his next weekend off, he asked Flora if she would like to have two days away. She was enthusiastic, so Richard telephoned Uncle Dick, who immediately invited them to stay. Not having met since Annie's wedding, Alice and Flora had a lot to talk about, while Richard enjoyed walking the sheep with Dick and meeting Tom and George again. When they were alone Richard told Dick about the house. Dick was very interested, and advised Richard to remember that there was no sentiment in business and if he required a second mortgage he would lend Richard the money at the current rate of interest and under the usual conditions. Richard thanked his uncle for the offer, which would be useful next year when he had to buy the practice, but was a little sad that it was not his father who had made the offer. Since he had received a Christmas card from him, there had been no contact, so Richard decided to make no new approach to his father and sister, but with Flora's help to buy the house and then the practice, without their assistance.

Next week Joe Bolton informed them that Mrs Walker wanted £995 for her house, and when Richard asked what was the least she would take for the property, Joe replied that she would not reduce it. Flora offered to go and see Mrs Walker, to try and obtain a reduction in the price. While there Flora turned on the charm and told Mrs Walker that they had only been married two years and had very little money. She explained why they wanted to buy the house and expressed her regret that no reduction in the price could be made.

"Who said that, Mrs Holden?" asked Mrs Walker.

"Mr Bolton, he said all negotiations had to be through him and that no reduction could be made in the price," said Flora.

"It's my house and I want a quick sale. I'll take £950. You go and tell him that's your bid, but don't let on I told you to do it."

"Of course we won't, and thank you very much, Mrs Walker."

"And another thing, you come and see me just before I move. I can't take all my furniture to my sister's, you know, Mrs Holden."

"I'll do that, Mrs Walker, and thank you so much. I won't forget."

Richard was a bit hurt when he realised that Joe was not being completely truthful about the price, but, remembering his uncle's advice, told Joe that his final bid was £950. Joe scoffed at the bid but said he would inform his client and let Richard know the result. Next day he telephoned Richard and said he had talked Mrs Walker into accepting the bid. Richard thanked him and put down the phone and he and Flora collapsed onto the settee roaring with laughter. Some days later he signed the contract in Mr Duke's office and the deposit of £95 was paid. Joe Bolton arranged a 15-year mortgage through the building society and the completion date was July 16th.

It was a nice surprise to receive the invitation to dinner from Edna and Thomas Evans. When Terry and Gladys Lawson and Jean and Mary arrived it was a family get together. It was a perfect June evening when they gathered on the terrace and drank sherry before dinner. The Vicar and Edna kept a good table, so they all enjoyed a five course meal and drank choice wines. The meal finished, they went into the lounge; soon the photograph album was produced, from which "snaps" were extracted and handed round. There were the usual ones of babies lying on white blankets, Edna and Gladys carrying hockey sticks when at school, and Terry and Jean riding their ponies. While Jerry and Tom smoked their cigars, the five ladies enjoyed looking at the wedding photographs and so the evening passed very quickly and they were all sorry when it ended. Richard and Flora drove Jean and Mary past 2 Cross Street, so that they could see the new acquisition. Jean expressed the opinion that they were over-stretching themselves financially, but Flora replied that they had decided to have a large well-planned practice house no matter how difficult it might be for them in the next few years. They both said they were glad they had decided to stay in Sandhaven because they had many friends and felt at home there.

Richard wanted to move into the house and make an up-to-date operating theatre for small animals and a casting bed for large animals in the old coach house. He was frustrated because he was so limited in the amount of major operations he was allowed to do on dogs. It was all work of a minor nature: excising tumours; removing broken claws; or lancing haematomas or abscesses. On the other hand, he operated on many cats and this work continued to grow. Charles still destroyed many dogs and cats, which were then put into a sack and taken to the Council's domestic waste disposal works, locally called the "Destructor". There an employee would lift a manhole cover and the sack would be dropped into the furnace below. To circumvent Charles' obstinacy and resistance to change, Richard ordered drugs and instruments on his own account; by telephone he discussed new treatments with his veterinary friends, and bought newly published text books on medicine and surgery. On Saturday he went on from Southall to Corchester to meet Major John, and from him received instruction on the new treatment for "whites" in the cow. Using Vulsellum forceps to hold the Os. Uteri still, a single way uterine catheter was passed through the Os and a diluted solution of Lugol's iodine was injected into the uterus. In many cases this was an effective treatment, resulting in conception at a later mating. The Major took Richard to two farms, where he carried out the treatment, following the Major's instructions. Arriving home, he immediately ordered the instruments required to carry out Neilsen's treatment and also a return flow catheter for the treatment of pyometra.

Charles gave Richard a week's holiday from 11th July and the next morning he and Flora went to see Mrs Walker. She told them that her husband's condition was little changed; his left arm and leg were still paralysed, and he needed constant nursing, and said that she was moving out on the fourteenth. Then she sprang the great surprise; taking them into the lounge she told them she was leaving the carpet and curtains, also the carpet which went from the hall up the stairs to the first floor. In the second bedroom she asked Flora if she liked the walnut bedroom suite and when Flora said yes she told her that she could have it, because it would only bring five pounds in the auction rooms. She also gave them the kitchen table, the gas oven, the dustbin, lawnmower and a ladder. Flora was so moved by the old lady's generosity that she began to cry and thanked Mrs Walker and then kissed her. Richard again marvelled at the way Flora could make friends with people in a very short time and was really grateful for everything Mrs Walker had given to them.

The 16th July was a sunny day and the move into 2 Cross Street was completed without mishap and they spent the day unpacking and getting organised. The next morning Richard found a lot of garden tools in the stable and at once began to attack the overgrown garden, while Flora worked inside the house; later that morning a telephone was installed: Sandhaven 585 was the number. They decided for the moment to live in the large lounge on the left of the hall, because the kitchen was behind it. The three rooms on the right of the hall were untouched, because they would later be converted for practice use, during the next eight months. Richard spent three nights distempering the ceiling and walls of the lounge a bright cream colour and at the end of the week Flora had made a delightful lounge and said everything was great. She had one regret: that she could not see the ships on the river from the lounge window.

Richard also found time to go to the Confirmation Class which started on the last Thursday in the month and to begin painting the outside of the house, using the extension ladder which Mrs Walker had given him. It enabled him to clean out the gutters which had not been done for a long time and to repair the sash cords and make the bedroom windows open again. He cleaned out the house drains, burnt all the garden rubbish and then got George Wallace, the electrician, to install electric bells at the front and back doors and lights over both of them. It was the end of August before he finished painting the house with royal blue paint; Flora in the meantime had found a Georgian door knocker, door knob and letter box, which he fitted to the front door and they were both pleased with the smart appearance. They were planning to buy more for the house, when the statement of the balance of Richard's account came from the bank and put a stop to it. The credit balance was £104, and Richard and Flora immediately decided to reduce expenditure to the minimum, so that they would have some working capital when April arrived.The money spent on equipment, the deposit on the house, and the surgeons' fees was unavoidable, but it made Richard determined to husband his resources.

The letter from Aunty Joan had been forwarded from the flat in Ladysmith Terrace and had been written five days before. It told them that Uncle Harry had had an operation to relieve a strangulated hernia and was slowly recovering. Richard was concerned that he could not go and see him, having just had his annual week's holiday, so he telephoned Uncle Dick to see if he knew that Harry was ill. Dick said that he and Alice had also had a letter and were going to see Harry.

Richard asked him to give Harry their best wishes for a speedy recovery and an invitation to any of the family to come and stay with them now they had room. Extending the invitation spurred Richard on to decorate the bedroom which contained the walnut suite. Having finished that room, he used up the distemper he had left over by decorating the second room on the right in the hall, which he had decided to make into an operating theatre for small animals for the present.

On the east side of the railway cutting between the station and the road to Droughton were many Council owned allotments, for which there was a great demand. Potatoes and other vegetables, fruit and flowers were grown; there were some pigeon lofts, and poultry houses. On two allotments pigs were kept and many of the houses on Wyreham and Droughton roads had a pig in the sty at the bottom of the garden. In the sultry weather of that August many cases of swine erysipelas occurred which Richard treated with serum and aspirin powders. It was through treating his sow, which recovered, that Richard met Dick Hoggarth who was a first class joiner. He it was who made a wooden box with a plate glass top, for use when giving anaesthetic to cats; it was just like the one Richard had made in Holme.

They were having breakfast and Flora was looking at the newspaper, when she said to Richard:

"Listen to this, it says there was a fire early yesterday morning at the Black Bull Hotel near Oxford, in which five people lost their lives. The police say one was a member of the staff of the hotel, two were commercial travellers and the other two were a farmer and his wife from East Lancashire; and the names of the dead will be released as soon as they are positively identified."

"Here, let me read it, Flora, you don't think it's Dick and Alice do you?"

"I don't know but I don't think there will be many farmers from East Lancashire staying in Oxfordshire at the moment and it is on the way back from Uncle Harry's."

"Well there's one way we can find out. I'll phone them at Higher Hindshead," said Richard.

George Greaves told Richard that the police had been and confirmed that it was Dick and Alice who had died in the hotel fire. He said that he and Tom the shepherd did not know what to do, so Richard told him to get in touch with the bank manager and to ask him to let Uncle Dick's solicitor know. When he returned to the breakfast table Flora was crying, but suggested that Richard rang Uncle Harry who would know what had to be done. Harry had been informed and told Richard that though he was not well enough to travel yet he knew quite a lot about Dick's business and would ring George Greaves at once and advise him on what should be done, then Joan would go there by train.

On the northern edge of the area covered by the Holme practice was the village of Newchurch hidden by the great bulk of Pendle Hill. Flora said she felt she was coming home when they parked the car near the Georgian church and noticed that the blinds and curtains were drawn at the windows of many houses in the village. St. Mary's was full for this double funeral on this lovely autumn morning. His sister Jane had brought Harry by car to join his wife Joan and with Flora and Richard the five were the chief mourners. Harry made Tom and George Greaves sit with Jean, Mary and Bill Dickenson in the pew behind them. Later when they left the graveside Richard and Flora talked to Mr Brookman and then Bob Mattinson, and at the lunch to many friends and farmers from the immediate area and from Holme. Harry, Joan and Jane had to go back to Alresford, so Richard and Flora said their goodbyes to them and to Jean, Mary and Bill, and, feeling very sad, drove back to Sandhaven.

Bob Laithwaite was the rag and bone man in the town and also did light carting with his big black horse and lorry. Though he was born in the nearby village of Wyreham, no one knew his age, but he must have been very old because he could not read or write, never having been to school. He was well known in the area, having worked on many local farms since his childhood, and could do any job on a farm, so always found work at haytime and harvest. He was a mine of information about the history of all the local farming families: their successes and scandals; and of events which had taken place in the area over the years. The stable was in a yard where all the material he collected or "acquired" was sorted into heaps: of metal; bottles and jars; rags and old car tyres; by Ernie Beetham, an old ex-groom.

Both of them shaved only once a week and wore red cotton kerchiefs knotted round their necks; they were a piratical looking couple. The horse was being led round the yard by Ernie, and on examining it Richard soon diagnosed a spasmodic colic. Ernie who had seen a horse stomach tube passed before, brought a large bucket of water, poured into it the two powders Richard had given to him and stirred the water with the stomach pump. Ernie then held the horse's head while Richard passed the tube. Bob watched this take place and with astonishment his mouth fell open; he shook his head and walked to the rear of the horse, lifted its tail and looked at its anus.

"What are you doing, Bob?" asked Richard.

"Why, looking for the end of that rubber tube coming through," replied Bob.

Richard and Ernie roared with laughter. "It can't come through, Bob, it only goes into its stomach," said Richard.

"I just don't believe it, I only hope it does some good," and he lifted the horse's tail and had another look, while Ernie shouted:

"That's the daftest thing I've seen in years."

Bob dropped the horse's tail and muttering to himself walked away, shaking his head in disbelief.

His horse soon recovered after the two gallons of medicine had been pumped into it. Bob took a little longer and talked about nothing else in the taproom of the Market Hotel for days afterwards, until the worsening situation in Europe introduced another subject.

It appeared to come so suddenly to a crisis to the man in the street, when in the newspapers pictures appeared of trenches being dug in the London parks and Government buildings being protected by walls of sandbags. Gordon Hindle's brother Charles was also an engineer who worked in the new Government factory which had been built to the east of the shipyard. In the factory gas masks for the civilian population were being assembled, and a chance remark that Charles made to Richard led to Flora obtaining a position as one of the assembly inspectors. It was monotonous work examining each mask as it came off the assembly line, prior to its being packed into a cardboard box. Flora enjoyed the work and the liveliness of the girls who sang as they worked and were always cheerful in spite of the ominous threat of war which grew greater every day. Mr Chamberlain the Prime Minister had to make two journeys to Berchtesgarten to confer with Herr Hitler before the Munich agreement was signed and everybody breathed a sigh of relief. But not at the shipyard where a night shift commenced; nor at the steel works on the other side of Droughton, where continuous working began. On 30th September Herr Hitler got all the Sudetanland and it was obvious that he would annexe the rest of Czechoslovakia in the not-too-distant future.

Two weeks later gas mask assembly was transferred to another factory near Holme and Flora's employment ended. She was asked if she would go and work in the Royal Ordnance factory at Brierley. Though the wage was good and would have helped their finances, she refused because it would have meant catching the work's bus at 7.00 a.m. and not arriving home until 6.45 at night. She told Richard that she thought it was more important to be at home and look after him and Richard agreed with her. She worked hard in the house. She had painted white all the woodwork in the three rooms on the right of the hall and went to the sale rooms every fortnight looking for suitable furniture. Jean in Holme was going to Maurice Reed's and she it was who brought a steel framed table, a metal trolley and four cupboards with glass fronts, all of which had come from the casualty department of the local hospital which was being refurbished. Flora bought three rolls of linoleum at a pound a roll and, with Richard, laid it on the floors of the first two rooms and later painted the furniture white.

Though the weather was stormy, all calls were attended to and it was a particularly wild evening when Richard went to treat a cow with milk fever at Jack Booth's Intack Farm. He noticed that electricity had been laid on and an electric milking machine installed and asked Jack how he liked it.

"It's a wonderful improvement, to have electric light and power at the touch of a switch, but it cost a bit, you know, Mr Holden."

"Yes, I didn't think you'd get it for nothing," said Richard, "Has anybody else got it?"

"Oh yes, George Meadows at Boundary and Arrowsmith at Moss End and me shared the cost to have it brought from a substation, now the National Grid is finished. You know, the setting up of the Milk Marketing Board and now electricity will help to make farming pay."

While Richard was injecting the cow, the thunder crashed and the lights flickered. A few minutes later there was a very brilliant flash of lightning and the lights went out as the thunder crashed overhead, the milking machine stopping at the same moment.

"I knew this would happen, in spite of what that chap said from Droughton Corporation electricity department, so I kept my old engine," said Jack.

He and his son quickly retrieved the clusters and then went to the engine house, but it was some time before milking began again, accompanied by the steady plop, plop, plop from the engine's exhaust. In the darkness the cow had recovered, risen to her feet and was now in her stall.

The thunder and lightning were moving away, but the rain was very heavy, as he drove down the long hill from the farm. He had almost reached Sykes where the brook flows beside the road, when he drove into water and the engine stopped and would not restart. The swollen brook had flooded across the road and as he was wearing his wellingtons, he got out of the car into the water which reached the running boards. He pulled his cap well down and turned up his coat collar and was wading past the car when there was a loud splash behind him,

"Why the hell can't the damned Council stop this flooding," a voice shouted in the semi-darkness, and more cursing followed from a figure who became visible wheeling a bicycle.

"Oh, it's you, Tom," said Richard, "A bit late for a swim, isn't it?" Richard laughed heartily.

"You're bloody well right it is," said Tom, who was the pork butcher. "What a hell of a night."

"It is that, I'd just run into the flood when you arrived, so I'm going to Sykes for some help."

They waded on. "I've been up at Further Marsh cutting up a pig I killed for them on Wednesday. I'll be glad to get home, I'm soaked to the skin coming off my bike like that. Goodnight, Mr Holden," and he remounted and slowly cycled away.

"Goodnight, Tom," said Richard as he walked into the shippon at Sykes. Ted soon brought a horse and a rope to tow the car out of the flood; then by the light of a torch he dried the plugs and leads, the engine started on the first pull on the starter, so he thanked Ted and drove off home.

Dick Hoggarth had made a wooden top for the metal table. Richard bolted it on, covered it with lino and secured it by screwing right angled aluminium strip round the edges. In the sitting room Mrs Walker had left a large circular pendant electric centre light which carried four bulbs. Richard took this down, fitted it over the table and plugged in four 100-watt bulbs, which gave wonderful illumination. He and Flora spent one evening unpacking the tea chests which contained all the surgical equipment he had accumulated over the last six years. In the first cupboard was all the preoperative equipment and the second cupboard contained all the syringes, thermometers, anaesthetics and the glass-topped anaesthetic box. All the surgical instruments were put in the third cupboard and in the last all the bandages, cotton wool and surgical bowls, basins and tins of elastoplast. When they had finished they were really proud of the professional appearance of the operating theatre. Next morning Richard visited Tom Wright to come and fix a sink in one alcove and install hot and cold water, which he did a few days later. When he had finished this, he measured up the piping he would need to fit hot water radiators in the downstairs rooms. Richard hoped the system could be supplied from the anthracite stove in the kitchen which, having a back boiler, supplied all the domestic hot water. But Tom said it could not be done and brought a second-hand stove which he installed next to the one in the wide fireplace in the kitchen, and then installed the central heating. Through a box number 207 in the *Veterinary Record* Richard bought, second hand, an ophthalmoscope, a small animal mouthgag and catheters, because Charles had not got any of them.

Richard told Charles about the operating theatre and asked him to come and see it. He did not, but Richard got permission to carry out operations there when he needed better lighting and facilities. Charles must have mentioned this at The Elms because, unknown to her father, one morning

Marjorie arrived at 2 Cross Street. Flora showed her round the house and then made coffee, after which they talked. Flora soon gained Marjorie's confidence and was told how much Marjorie would like to work and have some money, so that she could get out of the cold, gas-lit old-fashioned Elms. By friendly questioning, Flora coaxed more information out of her, and discovered that she had been to the Technical School in Corporation Road; there she had enjoyed herself and obtained her certificate for typing and shorthand and had a boy friend, but when her parents discouraged this, the association ceased. Before she left, she begged Flora not to tell her parents and of course Flora agreed.

When Richard came in for lunch, Flora said:

"I've had an interesting morning talking to Marjorie."

"Really, what about?"

"Getting to know more about her. She will be a good receptionist and secretary when we want one, because she wants to get out of that house."

"What's she know about secretarial work?" asked Richard.

When Flora told him, they agreed that at first it might be a good idea to employ her part-time, because she had kept the practice accounts at home and so she knew all the clients. But Richard stressed that they would not be able to employ her full time because he had so little money in the bank and was worrying about how much money he would have to borrow to buy the practice.

In November Richard received a letter from Baker and Hodgson, Solicitors, Clitheroe, which explained that as his late Uncle Dick had been five years older than his wife Alice, in law it was presumed that he had died first in the hotel fire. He had left a will in favour of his wife and she had substantial estate. Under her will, the children of Ted, Harry and Bert Gould were to receive £200 each, and Tom and George Greaves £100 each. Richard was really delighted to receive the cheque, it eased his financial problems; and he notified the solicitors of its receipt.

When he arrived home for breakfast next morning, he found Flora in tears and his heart sank.

"Love, whatever is the matter? You're not ill again, are you?"

"No, Richard, it's just I'm upset that people can be so kind, I hardly knew Alice and look what she has left me."

Richard took the letter which was from the same solicitors and read that she had bequeathed to Flora:

One Georgian candelabra,

Two silver coasters and one silver ladle.

A Queen Anne walnut veneered bureau,

2 Chippendale upholstered chairs and a Hepplethwaite bow fronted mahogany sideboard.

"Well, how nice of her to think about you, Flora, but it's just like her."

Flora wiped her eyes and said:

"Yes, but what made me cry was the fact that she must have had a presentiment, because these are all the things I admired in June when we were there, and obviously she must have made the will soon afterwards."

"It's strange you should say that, because when I asked you to go in June, something had been bothering me for days about them," replied Richard, "and I didn't tell you but Uncle Dick offered to lend me money for a second mortgage if I needed it. It seemed strange to me for him to suggest it out of the blue."

"You never told me before that you are psychic," said Flora.

"Oh I don't think I am, but I feel things are wrong before they happen, though I couldn't tell you what was going to happen."

"Well, if that's not psychic, I don't know what is. Let's get on with breakfast and then we'll have to arrange to get these things here."

It was a week later that Maurice Reed brought the furniture, the silver and eight bentwood chairs which Richard had asked him to find for the waiting room. Flora had the furniture put in the large front bedroom, which she was planning to use as a lounge and dining room when the practice needed all the ground floor rooms. She and Maurice had a good talk and he told her to look after this lovely antique furniture and the silver. She said she would and decided to go and see Auntie Winnie and find out from her all she could about old silver and furniture. When Richard arrived home he was delighted to see what Flora had got from Alice and said though it looked great now, it would look wonderful when there was a carpet on the floor. Flora replied that as she had got the furniture, he could buy the carpet from her brother Bill. When he was twenty-one Bill had left the jeweller's where he worked and with the money he received under his grandfather's will bought a junior partnership in Moore's, the house furnishers, who had a huge shop in Holme.

Bill was very like Flora, had the same good looks; could be very charming and got on well with people. He was in his element when, immaculately dressed in a dark grey suit, he sold furniture and carpets to customers. He was very interested in furniture and went to night school studying furniture construction and design, and its history. Flora could twist him just like Richard round her little finger. But Richard was worried about spending money, because he knew that without the legacies of Uncle Ezra and now Alice he could not have paid the doctor's fees and had the deposit ready to put down on the house, and he knew he must get another car before long, definitely before he took over the practice. It had taken them four months working together to decorate the house right through and now Richard was deciding on the best use for the stable block from the practice point of view. It must produce some money and so the two-stall stable would be a hospital for small animals and a kennels; the coach house would be converted into a loose box. Flora persuaded Richard to make the upper storey into a self-contained flat for a staff member who would look after animals and also answer the telephone in the future. For the moment, with Dick Hoggarth's help, he worked two nights a week altering the stable and the coach house. It was cold working in the stable at night because the weather had become very wintry with snow and frost, but in a fortnight the stall divisions had been removed, the hospital room made ready and a door fitted at the bottom of the stairs.

Charles was now a "Panel A" inspector for the Ministry of Agriculture and Fisheries, which this year had taken over all the disease control work formerly done by the County Council. He had been doing an investigation into an outbreak of swine fever and got very wet and cold. He became ill and Richard was left to run the practice single-handed, which was almost more than he could manage.

It was easy to deal with all the daily fairly urgent work, like milk fever, calvings, acute mastitis and pneumonia in cattle; laminitis and strangles in horses, and sheep and pig troubles, but it was the chronic conditions which were difficult to resolve. Some owners were philosophical about chronic disease and sold their affected cattle in the market to any unsuspecting purchaser, or for slaughter. Others grumbled and nagged at the veterinary surgeon even when the condition was the result of overcrowding or lack of hygiene on their part. He had cleansed two cows at Vickers at Poolside, and was feeling cold when he arrived at Tom Walsh's Further Marsh Farm. He was a cattle dealer as well as having a dairy herd and began to grumble as soon as Richard got out of his car.

"Good morning, Mr Holden, I've sent for you because those calf scour powders I got last week were no good and two calves have died."

"Right," said Richard, "Let's go and look at them."

Tom led him into a single-storey building which had a brick floor. There were three pens containing calves, some of which were obviously ill, hind quarters and tails soiled with faeces. There was a sour smell, the air was very cold and discharges from the pens ran down a channel the whole length of the building.

"Yes, you've got a real dose of calf scour here," said Richard. "How did it start?"

"I think it came with those two there, they scoured slightly for a day or two after I bought them, but they kept drinking and are better now, but I've lost two out of five of these Ayrshires which I bred here."

Richard examined the calves and then some more in the top pen, all showing symptoms.

"I think you are right, Tom, but the conditions in here aren't helping either."

"Why? what's wrong? calves have done well in here before this year, but up to now I've lost five, and I can't supply my customers with ill calves," said Tom sharply.

Richard patiently explained that they needed dryness, warmth, fresh air and isolation from each other and told Tom how to achieve it. He injected the calves with serum and left him more powders. It took three more visits and some frustration for Tom and Richard before the outbreak improved, but though most calves survived, the condition continued to recur in bought-in calves. The Ayrshires bred on the farm were now suckled on the cow for three days and then kept on the path behind the cow, tied by a little halter to a ring on the wall. They did really well; but though all bought-in calves were injected with anti-scour serum on arrival at the farm, the odd one still died, in spite of much better housing.

He went on to Jack Booth at Intack, where mastitis was becoming a problem in his Friesian cows, especially chronic cases. He irrigated the udders of two cows with Acriflavine solution to try and cure their chronic mastitis. Jack said that one which had already been treated this way was not better, so Richard irrigated its udder again. Any cow showing symptoms was milked last and clusters plunged and rinsed in hot water between each cow. With these measures the condition was controlled in the herd but not cured, and more herds were beginning to be affected. Tom Hoggarth at Tithebarn still hand-milked, never had any mastitis in his cows and blamed the disease on milking machines, and Richard could not contradict him.

In the afternoon he made up packets of powders, restocked his car and was glad to leave the cold surgery and drive home, in the twilight of that bitter November afternoon. Flora made a cup of tea for him and he had just become warm, when the telephone bell rang.

"You're not going out yet," said Flora.

Richard picked up the receiver and said, "Hello, Mr Holden, veterinary surgeon here."

"Just the man I want to speak to. It's Bill Bainbridge from Duckworth Hall here. Can I bring my heeler bitch over right away, she can't whelp and my vet doesn't deal with dogs."

"Mr Bainbridge, tell me, has Mr Townsend been treating your dog?"

"No, he hasn't, Mr Holden."

"Then in that case bring her at once."

"I will, I won't be long."

Richard put down the receiver and, turning to Flora, said, "Did you hear that, it's Tom Seed's son-in-law Bill Bainbridge from Duckworth Hall, he's bringing his bitch over at once. It sounds like a Caesarian operation, so come on and let's get ready."

"How exciting," said Flora.

"It might be exciting to you, but I must make a success of it. Let's get the sterilizer filled and put on the gas. Will you wash the table with disinfectant and the trolley top." When they had done this, he put a rubber sheet over the table, and then scrubbed his hands using Neko soap. Richard had used Nembutal intravenously twice to destroy dogs and decided to use this anaesthetic if an operation was required. When the sterilizer had been boiling for five minutes he turned off the gas to allow the contents to cool, and got out the catgut tubes.

It was half an hour later that the door bell rang, and Flora led Mr and Mrs Bainbridge into the operating theatre.

"I'm sorry I've been a long time, Mr Holden, but the snow's coming down hard."

"Yes it's a bad night. Will you put her on the table, Mr Bainbridge. When did she start trying to whelp?"

"I don't really know; she was a bit wet behind at breakfast time, but we've not seen her straining."

"When was she mated? Do you know the date?"

"Yes, Mr Holden, the sixty-three days were up yesterday."

"Then she definitely is whelping. I'll just put on a muzzle on her and examine her."

"You've no need to put a muzzle on, I'll hold her."

Richard disinfected her vulva and with care examined the bitch vaginally. While he was doing this, Mr Bainbridge was talking to the bitch.

"It's all right, Emma, keep still, it's for your own good. What's wrong, Mr Holden?"

"It's what I suspected, there is a pup lying across the entrance to the passage, so it can't get out and it's blocking the way for the others. She has lost her water and is very dry and not contracting."

"Well, what are you going to do?"

"The only answer, Mr Bainbridge, is a Caesarian operation; now, it's a bit risky, first of all from the anaesthetic and then from septic infection afterwards."

"Look, Mr Holden, I want that bitch saved. She goes everywhere with me and means more to me than my whole damned herd. I don't care what it costs, but please get on with it. Can we wait for her?"

"No, there's no point. She will be some hours coming round and then wants to be kept quiet and warm. I'll look after her, you leave her here."

Mrs Bainbridge wiped tears from her eyes. Bill patted the dog's head, and said:

"Come on, May, we must get back. I want you to ring me, Mr Holden, doesn't matter what time it is."

"I'll do that. Goodbye now."

Richard injected the Nembutal solution very slowly until the eye reflex was about absent and there was no response to pinching the bitch's foot.

He operated through an incision in the mid-line of the distended abdomen and soon delivered two dead and two live pups, which he gave to Flora. He dusted sterile sulphanilamide powder into the uterus and abdomen, rapidly sewing up both. When he had finished, he was glad to find the eye reflex coming back and the bitch breathing regularly. He gave her a small dose of Pituitrin intramuscularly, wrapped her in a blanket and laid her against the radiator. Flora had cleaned up the two live pups and was holding them on top of the warm sterilizer.

"That did go well, Flora, thanks a lot. I don't know what I would have done without you."

"I've enjoyed it, really. It's far more interesting than watching father pulling teeth out years ago."

"Now I know why you didn't faint." Richard put a narrow strip of gauge onto a piece of Elastoplast, covered the wound on the bitch's abdomen and then put the two pups on to a teat each; with a little coaxing both began to suck. They washed the table and the instruments and dried them and took off their stained white overalls.

"That's that," said Flora. "Let's go and have our meal. I'm starving, do you know it's ten to seven?"

"Really? Time has flown. I'll ring Bill Bainbridge now."

The latter was relieved to hear the news and profusely thanked Richard, who then was glad to get his evening meal. He had only just finished when he went to Tithebarn Farm and delivered a cow of a live calf much to Tom Hoggarth's satisfaction. It was a weary vet who climbed into bed at eleven o'clock that night having seen Emma, fully conscious, suckling her two pups.

The telephone bell ringing woke Richard at ten to six and soon he was on his way through six inches of level snow to Tom Priestley's to a cow down with milk fever. Smith held the cow's head while Richard injected the solution. He was annoyed with himself because he could not remember which eye Smith had lost in the accident, so he covered his embarrassment by asking him how the engagement party had gone.

"It was a good do, Mr Holden, there were sixty people there and it went on till midnight. I had to carry our John to the car; he was drunk, but don't tell Dad will you?"

"No, of course I won't, Smith," said Richard as Tom came up and with his help the cow got to her feet.

"While you're here, Mr Holden, will you open a cow's teat, she calved yesterday and I can't get any milk out of it, and there is a cow with a chaff in her eye."

When Richard arrived home he was very cold and just in time to meet Bill

Bainbridge holding the pups.

"I'm glad I've just caught you. If she starts interfering with the wound put a muzzle on and let me know. Keep her quiet, with no running up and down steps and give her these tablets as directed three times a day for three days, so no infection starts up. In a week, bring her back."

"I'll do that, Mr Holden and we both thank you once again. I'll remember what you've done for us; don't you forget it," said Bill.

"Right, off you go and keep her and the pups warm, it's such a cold morning."

He turned back into the house and really enjoyed a huge breakfast.

When he arrived at Whingate Farm later, Bill Meadows was a bit fed up. "The cow's in a box, Richard. I think it's starting with John's disease like that one I lost in the spring. Is it right that Jerseys are more prone to it? I was a bit annoyed with myself the other day, I was talking to a chap and he said they are more likely to catch it. I thought, well you are a fool, to have bought trouble."

"Wait a minute, Bill, and I'll try and answer your questions. Any cow can get this disease if the germ gets into its body. We know ponds and pits harbour the germ, that it takes a long time to develop in the animal and there is no treatment." As they walked in the box, Richard asked, "Did she come from the same place as the other cow?"

"No, she didn't and the other was younger. This one has just had her second calf; but I put it on another cow."

"That's sensible, because the scour contains millions of germs. But she's not scouring today."

"No, but she was a bit yesterday, and the day after she calved last week."

"That does sometimes happen in the early stages. Have you any more scouring?"

"No, everything is quite normal."

"Good. I'll take a sample of her dung and examine it microscopically tonight. I must go. Mr Parsons is ill again and it's slow work driving in this weather. I'll let you know tomorrow. Give my regards to Elizabeth."

"Yes, I'll do that. Cheerio."

Back at the surgery, Marjorie had two more visits to be done.

"How's your father, Marjorie?"

"He's a lot better this morning, thank you, Mr Holden. The doctor says he can get up tomorrow, but he won't have to go out until the weather gets milder."

"I'm glad to hear that. I'll be off now."

As Richard drove along, he said to himself: they are a peculiar family. In freezing weather I am not even offered a cup of tea. I'm not asked into the house to see my boss and I've not seen his wife for weeks. I've got everything to do and all the decisions to take, which I suppose is good training for next year, but I'll have to discuss the buying of the practice off him because he has never mentioned it. At lunch time he and Flora talked over what they should do about the purchasing of the practice and they decided to go and see Tommy Duke the solicitor.

He was pleased to be asked to act for Richard in this matter and said he would begin to make enquiries as to the way in which Mr Parsons proposed the sale to take place.

On Advent Sunday evening, St. Luke's Church was the venue for the Confirmation service. Mary and Jean sat with Flora and watched the Reverend Evans direct the nine adolescents to stand on the left facing the Bishop of Brooksby and the four adults, who included Richard, on the right. When their time came the four knelt before the Bishop and when he laid his hands on his head Richard experienced a feeling of satisfaction that he could now join Flora when she took Communion. This act he knew would reinforce his implicit belief in the Creed and would increase his enjoyment of such of the Church services which he was able to attend. Mary and Jean could not stay after the service, so he and Flora drove them to the station to catch the train back to Holme. During the drive there it was decided that all Flora's family would come to Sandhaven at Christmas.

The thaw started on the Monday and soon the snow was gone, making driving easier. Mr Parsons, looking thinner and whiter than ever, began to work a little and did some dispensing. On Wednesday afternoon Flora went to Morton to see Aunt Winnie and Richard did the laboratory work in the surgery. Two milk samples were positive for TB bacilli and, though Bill Meadows dung sample had been negative, one from Parkside was positive. Richard felt sorry for Stan Jones who was upset when Richard told him to slaughter the cow, because he only had twelve milking and had only been farming on his own account for twelve months.

"Look, Mr Holden, isn't there a test you could do to tell if a cow has the disease?"

"There is a test, Stanley, but it is not reliable. It sometimes indicates a cow has the disease when she has not got it."

"That's not much good for farmers. Anyway, I'll get her sold to Noblett the butcher at once."

"Has she been out grazing or with your young stock?"

"No, Mr Holden, I only bought her in October."

"I'm glad to hear that because the germ lives in ponds and young stock pick it up easily."

"While you're here, would you look at a cow which has whites?"

"Yes, but did she calve to time?"

"I don't know because I bought her in the auction, but the calf is a good big bull and she only showed a bit of discharge the other day, though she has been calved three weeks."

"Stanley, I'm going to give you some advice. I don't want you to have an abortion storm, so buy every cow on the condition it passes or has passed the test for abortion. It will only cost you a few shillings but an outbreak of abortion could break you, I'll take a blood sample from this cow and then wash her out."

Richard did this and was pleased for Stanley when the laboratory report was negative.

Flora had spent a pleasant afternoon with Winnie, who had told Flora a lot about old furniture, especially to keep it away from the hot water radiators and only to use the best wax polish when cleaning it. She showed her the collection of old silver she had acquired over the years and impressed on Flora never to polish the marks or they would wear away. They had tea together, and when the maid had cleared the table, Winnie became rather sentimental and said how much she missed her family and how hurt she was because they never came to see her. This astounded Flora, because she was about the only member of the family who was allowed over the doorstep. The old lady was lonely, this fact struck Flora, but she realised there was little she could do unless Winnie changed her ways. They parted good friends, with Flora saying she would come again soon, if possible before Christmas.

It was a week later in the gloom of the early afternoon when Joe Bolton arrived with his black labrador, which had been shot. The Colonel had organised a shoot that day in the Hall Park and then the Home Farm, and the dog had been retrieving when one member of the party had accidentally fired his gun. The dog had been lightly peppered with shot, had bolted and torn the skin on its back as it ran through barbed wire.

Joe was furious. "I hope he's not invited again, he could have killed somebody in his sozzled state—I kept seeing him drinking from his hip flask."

"All right, Joe, let's have him on the table."

Richard put on a muzzle and gently washed the dog's back clean of mud and grass. A right-angled flap of skin had been torn backwards high on the chest wall and when Richard held it up to the light he could see a few holes in it made by the shot.

"Look Joe, can you see the holes the dog has? Some shot in its body, but I think it's been lucky because they've not hit anything vital, its pulse is good and its mouth is a good colour."

"Are you going to get them out, Richard?"

"No, there's no way of knowing where they are, unless the dog is X-rayed and we've not got one; anyway I don't think there's any need, I am going to stitch this flap back now under local anaesthetic."

Richard went to get Flora and together they tied the dog down. The wound was cleaned and disinfected again, then infiltrated with anaesthetic. Soon it was all stitched up, dusted with sulphanilamide and bandaged.

"Give him these tablets three times a day for three days and then bring him back, also let him have plenty of water to drink."

"Thanks, I'll do that, Richard," and a calmer, happier Joe left with his dog on a lead. As the movements of the vigorous dog caused some of the stitches to tear out, it took three weeks for the wound to heal completely, but after this, he worked well for his master and was still rock steady when shot over.

The arrival of the first Christmas cards put Flora in a panic and she and Richard decided that they should make a big effort to enjoy themselves with their families and friends, because once they had taken over the practice, it would probably be impossible to have a house party for some years. One card came from Doncaster from Ted and Mary, but did not give an address there. Richard wondered what had made them leave lovely Gloucestershire and go to a busy industrial town in Yorkshire, moving house for the second time in two years. They decided to have the party in the evening of the day before Christmas Eve. Mary brought Jean in her car and they helped to decorate the house, and to arrange the lounge, bringing the eight chairs from the waiting room. They polished the floor of the latter so that they could dance there after supper. Flora and Betty Heyes prepared the food and Richard was in his element getting the drinks and glasses ready. They had invited the Vicar, the Reverend Evans and Edna; Tom, Nellie and Frank Bradshaw; and Jack and Margaret Lawson; in addition to all the friends they had invited the year before. With the arrival of Bill Dickenson and Dr McConnell, Richard and Frank found it a busy struggle to keep everybody supplied with drinks until nine o'clock, when supper was served in the big kitchen. At ten they began dancing to the music on the wireless in the waiting room, and quickly Flora had everybody on the dance floor to win the spot prizes.

Later two party games were played by all present, who had been divided into two teams each having a captain. The first was a treasure hunt with clues hidden all over the house, and soon they were all chasing each other up and down the stairs and even into the garage. The second was the lions and the lambs game. In this every member of both teams had an empty jam jar, into which they put the dried peas, again distributed around the house in the most unlikely places. When peas were found the members of each team roared like lions or bleated like lambs respectively, until the captain collected the peas. The captain with the most peas at the end was the leader of the winning team. The fun was fast and furious and the uproar terrific, until the silly prizes were presented to the winning team. And so the happy memorable evening ended with the singing of Auld Lang Syne at midnight. During the grim years to come, Richard and Flora often thought about that lovely care-free party and longed for the time when they could all be together again.

This night was the first time that Flora and Richard entertained Jean, Mary and Bill at 2 Cross Street. Mary and Frank Bradshaw had been very attracted to each other at the party and so they invited him, and Jim and Isabel Lord, to lunch on Christmas Day. The sea air had worked wonders for Isabel Lord's health; she and Flora saw each other regularly and had become good friends. After the lunch was finished, Flora gave everyone a small present from the Christmas tree and the guests produced theirs for Flora and Richard. The guests left on Boxing Day and the house was quiet for the first time in days, as Flora put the presents away and collected all the sheets and pillowcases for the wash. Richard took the centre section out of the top of the mahogany table, carried the chairs back into the waiting room and then put all the crockery away in the kitchen cupboards.

They had been invited to a party at the Heyes' and so, on New Years Eve, Richard asked the operator at the telephone exchange to transfer all calls from 585 to their number.

They had a jolly night and having seen in the New Year had just arrived home at 1.00 a.m. when the telephone rang. Richard set off at once to Brook Farm to treat a cow with a prolapsed uterus. Walter Scott Black and his son Duncan had both been well and truly celebrating Hogmanay and were singing at the top of their voices when Richard walked into the shippon. They hoisted the rear end of the cow and rested it on a bale of straw. Richard soon replaced the uterus and put on the strappings. After he had washed and dressed, Walter in his most persuasive Scottish manner invited Richard into the house, where he was introduced to all the family and a large glass of whisky put into his hand. After many toasts had been drunk, Richard excused himself, then drove home slowly because the whisky had had a great effect on him. He was very pleased the New Year had begun so well and made a resolution to have everything ready for the 5th April; the two years of waiting would soon be over.

There was little work to do that day, so in the afternoon, true to his 2.30 a.m. resolution, he began to review the preparations they had made. They decided the waiting room was satisfactory, but realised they would have to have opaque glass fitted to the lower half of the windows in the consulting room. Flora made a list of the jobs to be done and suggested that they had the fireplace bricked up in the consulting room, but Richard decided to have the grate removed and the recess tiled. The chimney would be shut off except for a small hatch through which steam could escape from the sterilizer, which would stand on a table in the recess. On a bitter, snowy day before Christmas, Flora went to a house contents sale, and bought a well made double oak wardrobe, a kitchen table and two stand chairs for £2 15s. 0d. Richard had fitted shelves inside the wardrobe and this, the kitchen table and the chairs, went into the dispensary, which had been made by Dick Hoggarth fitting a second-hand glazed room divider in the last room on the right of the hall, so dividing it into two. The other half would be the office. Further jobs to be done were shelves to be made and fitted to the walls in the dispensary; for the office a converted wardrobe, a second-hand flat top desk and a chair would have to do. It was three weeks before these things had been accomplished, most of the work being done in the afternoons, when often there were no cases to visit. This worried Richard, who wanted the practice to grow so that he could the sooner pay back the money he had borrowed. He spent two nights fitting a second door in the kennel room and one in the hospital room to try and prevent animals escaping. He had learnt that Ted Roberts at Sykes was a fully qualified builder as well as a farmer and with his help in two weekends they built a wall across the open end of the cart shed, converting it into a room big enough to act as a large animal operating theatre. A wide door and a large window had been built into the wall and when hot and cold water and electric light had been fitted, Richard was pleased with the result.

With all this work at home and the treatment of all the winter ills of horses cattle and sheep it was February before he had an appointment to see Tommy Duke, the solicitor. As he was ushered into his office, Rusty the red setter met him, wagging his tail.

"Good morning, Richard," said Tom, "It must be nice to be met by a satisfied client."

"It does one's morale a lot of good," he replied, patting Rusty on the head. "And I must add that Mr Parsons is also satisfied with your integrity, because I have heard from Avenham and George, his solicitors, to say that payment for the practice good will, stock of instruments, and drugs will be by a promissory note."

"And what is that, Tom?"

"It's a document which has to be signed which contains a written promise that you will pay to Charlie Parsons, or to the bearer of the note, a stated sum either on demand or on a date specified. Also he is not charging you the current rate of interest on the capital sum, only 2%, which will be a good saving for you."

"Well, that is nice of him. I didn't think he thought much of me, he never invites Flora or me into the house."

"Richard, I don't know anybody in Sandhaven who has been in the house; they don't seem to want friends."

"Still, I am pleased, but I really don't know much about business, except what I picked up running the practice in Holme, so I'd like your advice."

"You must get a good accountant."

"Who do you recommend, Tom, and is it a good idea to have one in

Sandhaven? because I don't want my business discussed in Miss Bishop's café."

"I am certain they will not talk about your affairs. There's Fortune in Droughton who I have, but he is expensive and there is my brother George in Church Street."

"I'll have him then, it will be handy having him fairly near. Shall I go and see him, or will you introduce me?"

"I'll let him know you will be going to see him. As for what you want to do on the business side, I'll think it over and make a list for you."

"Thanks very much, Tom. I must be on my way but I'll ring you later in the week."

"Yes, you do that. Goodbye now."

The next morning in the surgery Richard thanked Charles for proposing payment by a promissory note.

"I did it, Richard, because it will rule out you having to get another mortgage. The valuer and the accountant have come up with a figure of £1,250 for the practice, and the instruments and drugs I am selling."

"How did they arrive at the purchase price of the practice?" asked Richard.

"They did it by taking the average of three years' turnover, which since you came has gone up from £950 to £1,250. They will send the relevant statements of the accounts and the valuation to Tom Duke."

"Thank you very much, Charles. I am really grateful, because I have little capital."

"I realised that," replied Charles, "but don't worry, I know you will do well."

After seeing George Duke, who was pleased to have Richard as a client, he went on to Tom Duke's office.

Tom talked long and earnestly to Richard and the main points he outlined were that he should:

1) Make a list of all projected expenditure—mortgage and promissory note payments; salary for Flora and himself; rates; subscriptions and any other outgoings including car expenses, divide it by 52 and that would give him a minimum amount each week he would have to earn.

2) With George, to draw up a price list for all professional work and a mileage rate to be charged for visits. Also, not to overlook discounts which could be claimed for early settlement of bills.

3) To have third party insurance and a life assurance. He stressed that professional insurance through the NVB and MDS was essential, and that a consent form to be signed by the owner before operations were performed would be an added safeguard.

4) To buy a fireproof safe in which to keep all ledgers and cash books, and a fire proof filing cabinet.

5) Not to try to fiddle the Inland Revenue, and to be careful not to put financial temptation in front of staff; one trustworthy person to be in charge of all money and have the key to the cash box and safe.

Richard left the office with his head in a whirl, there was so much to do. He wrote to the Divisional Veterinary Officer of the Ministry of Agriculture and Fisheries in Droughton and asked to be put on the Panel A of Local Veterinary Inspectors as from 5th April.

On his half day he went with Flora to Droughton and ordered a professional plate 12 inches by 8 inches in bronze with white lettering to be mounted on a wooden wall board. They then went on to the printers and ordered professional stationery and envelopes. Each day they tried to do something to make ready for the takeover and on the day in March when they went to see Jean in Holme, Hitler, in flat defiance of the Munich agreement, proclaimed the annexation of the remainder of Czechoslovakia and then his army occupied it. Richard was depressed; all the newspapers said war was coming soon and he was beset with doubts as to whether he should buy the practice after all. In the end Flora and her family were instrumental in rekindling his enthusiasm and so he signed the documents and the contract and bought the practice. The three days before the fifth, he spent all his spare moments bringing everything he had bought from The Elms and putting it away in the dispensary and the office. All the large animal equipment and instruments he put temporarily in the large animal operating theatre, and on Tuesday night, 4th April 1939, Flora and he drank a toast to their future and then waited for Marjorie to come.

It was decided that she came to do office work on Tuesday, Thursday and Saturday mornings from 9.00 a.m. till 1.00 p.m. She thanked them for giving her the part-time job and expressed her admiration of the bright, warm and well decorated rooms, especially the office whose windows looked on to Victoria Street. It was almost dark when with Flora's help he put up his plate on the wall to the right of the front door They stood back and looked at it and read:

R.B. HOLDEN BVSc, MRCVS

Veterinary Surgeon

Surgery hour 6-7 p.m. Monday to Saturday.

They walked into the house and closed the door, both realising that the die was cast and that there could be no turning back. Richard took Flora in his arms and kissed her and said:

"Thanks, darling, for all your help. I'm sorry it's been so hectic that I've not had time to talk to you, but just remember that I love you."

Flora kissed Richard and with tears running down her cheeks said, "Love, that's all I wanted to know."

He released her and asked, "Did you finish the envelopes?"

"No, but there are only twenty or so left to address."

VII

Richard had had a letter printed which gave the news that the practice as from April 5th would be run from 2 Cross Street, Sandhaven; Tel. 585 and 264. Flora, with all the clients' names and addresses from the ledgers, had spent most afternoons recently addressing the envelopes. They finished the last few now and, having put stamps on them all, packed them in an empty shoe box and took them up to the post office. They were glad when they had all been posted and, very tired, they drove home and went to bed at once.

It was just before 6.00 a.m. when Richard answered the phone and Charles said, "Jack Booth at Intack has a cow down with milk fever. I'd like to remind you that the telephone men will be taking out my phone today and, I expect, installing it in your house."

"Thank you, Charles. I'll get onto Intack straight away; and thanks for reminding me about the phone. I'll tell Flora to look out for them."

Richard kept beside the bed a thick knitted blue fisherman's pullover, a pair of blue Melton cloth trousers and a pair of white wool long stockings so that he could dress quickly to go to emergencies. He dressed, and ran downstairs and into the kitchen where he put on his jacket and cap and wellingtons. They were all warm and dry, having been near the stove all night. In less than five minutes after the phone rang he drove away. He arrived back an hour or so later, and quickly ate the breakfast Flora had ready for him.

"How did you get on?" she asked.

"Very well. She is a good milker, and I had to give her two injections, after which she got up. He also wanted some powders."

"I've taken three messages while you've been out. By the way, will you put a Yale lock on the back door, because when you go out in a morning anybody could walk in, and at night as well."

"Yes I will, and we must also take precautions against burglars."

He had finished the visits by lunch time. In the afternoon he discussed with Flora ways of keeping down costs and increasing income. They decided to ask Marjorie to come on Tuesday and Saturday mornings from 9.00 a.m. till 1.00 p.m., for two shillings and sixpence each morning. Richard also decided to strip dogs, and board cats, and so put the hospital room to good use. The next thing would be to make cages to house cats; this he decided to do himself.

He was very pleased two weeks later to receive a large, buff-coloured envelope marked On His Majesty's Service. It contained a letter, which informed him that he had been appointed to Panel A of Local Veterinary Inspectors; there was also a folder which contained instructions for carrying out the various duties and a list of herds to be examined under the Milk and Dairies Acts and Orders.

Miss Bishop rang quite early one morning, and asked Richard to visit one of her cats. It proved to be Hector, a ginger and white cat which Richard had castrated as a kitten soon after arriving in Sandhaven.

"What's wrong with him, Mr Holden?" she asked as she held the cat, while Richard took its temperature, and then gently touched the swelling below its right ear.

"It is an abscess developing, he has a temperature of 104°F."

"What can you do for him?"

"I'm going to inject him with Omnadin, and you are going to bathe that swelling every six hours with hot water. The abscess has got to come to a head and then I will lance it."

"Very well, I'll do that and you will come tomorrow?"

"Oh yes, Miss Bishop, I will, probably just after lunch."

When he arrived next day, there were three dustbins outside the shop and four tea chests. The cat's abscess was coming to a head.

"Miss Bishop, I'll take him to the surgery and lance the abscess, and keep him overnight. I'll bring him back tomorrow, when I am sure he will be a lot better."

Richard put him into a basket and secured the lid, and then asked:

"Miss Bishop, what do you do with those empty tea chests you have outside the shop?"

"Sometimes a man comes from Droughton and collects them, otherwise the bin men collect them."

"Could I buy four off you, then?"

"Don't be silly," she replied, "Mr Holden, you can have them now, take them out of the way."

He did. At the surgery he wrapped Hector up in a blanket and Flora, wearing gloves, held him firmly. With the point of the scalpel he quickly slit open the abscess and yellow, foul-smelling pus ran into the kidney dish. He syringed weak warm Dettol and water into the cavity, put Hector back in the basket and took him up into the hospital room in the stable block.

During two evenings he made doors to fit the tea chests. The doors were really a hard wood frame onto which was securely nailed fine mesh chicken wire. He drilled holes in the bottom of the chests, fitted the doors and took the four complete cages to the garage where Gordon Hindle sprayed them pure white. From the day he put them in the hospital room they were rarely empty. Hector made a complete recovery, and then Miss Bishop had all three

"I agree with him," said Flora, "You know, you were nearly twenty minutes with his dog."

"Yes. George Duke's figures are nearer the mark, his pricing adds up to £1 1s. 6d."

"You had better use his figures in future."

"Maybe, but that's half an ordinary chap's wage for the week," said Richard. "They could not afford that. Where does Mr Twining live?"

"Worsthorne, The Crescent."

"He must be wealthy to live up there, and they are the sort of client we could do with."

"We could do with an appointments book for operations," said Flora, "and even for surgery consultations except for emergencies." And so in a few weeks, surgeries were going smoothly, with the surgery card, the pricing book and the appointments book all in use, and all clients paid cash.

But Richard's day was not finished. Now, at half past seven, he began to examine the milk samples he had taken that morning. When he had prepared the three films of the milk sediments he patiently examined them, but found it difficult to move the slide so slowly that no part was missed. He decided that he must have a mechanical stage, and wondered how Charles had managed without one. He ordered one from a firm in London.

With so many things to do the spring days were passing quickly, and it was a good lambing time. Richard lambed some ewes; he now asked the farmers to bring them to Cross St. and he delivered the lambs in the new large animal operating room. He did this because the conditions were better, and also because he could lamb three ewes at Cross Street in the time it would have taken him to go to one farm.

When the cows were turned out, cases of staggers or hypomagnesaemia began to occur. With increasing milk yields from cows, more cases were seen each year. Richard made up 25% solutions of magnesium sulphate in 200 cc. of water for injection; but though he always rushed to these cases, even driving in the car right up to the cow in the field, only about one in four recovered. He began to use Willows' Glucomag injection, and found he had better results in mild cases, but the advanced cases still died. One May morning when he was relieving a blown cow using a trocar and canula, he thought of Ezra and John on that spring morning long ago.

There were not many colts to be castrated that spring. He operated on four on the farms, but two well grown Shires were brought into Cross Street and he operated on them in the big theatre. But there were many foals to dock and he did them all before flies became numerous.

He saw more of Bob Whiteside that spring than he wanted to, because he collected the cows which had died of staggers, and also because Richard had to go to his yard at Southall and make a post mortem examination of two cows which had been slaughtered under the Tuberculosis Order of 1937. Then there was Tom Collinson's show-winning cow which was new-calved, down and unconscious. Richard examined it and injected it for milk fever but it died half an hour later. Tom quietened down when the post mortem examination showed an enlarged pale heart, a large yellow fatty liver, and an enteritis. In the Friesian herds where there were high-yielding cows, he advised the farmers to feed Boots iodised mineral salts.

All the Shire mares foaled easily, except two. A different black stallion travelled this district, and few cases of deformed foals were seen. Richard took Charles with him as a second opinion in both his cases, but both could not be foaled and were shot. Bob Whiteside commented that he had never known it so busy and now he was employing four butchers.

Then the large animal side of the practice went quiet, just as it had at Fernhall seven years before. He began to wish the 'phone would ring, but began to be a bit depressed by events. A ewe he lambed developed gas gangrene and, though the farmer had tried to lamb it before he sent for assistance, Richard blamed himself. He operated on two bitches which were suffering from pyometra but both died and then there was the cat belonging to Frank Madden, the verger at St. Luke's. He brought it to evening surgery and asked for it to be castrated. It was a full-grown ginger tom cat, which was the apple of the widower's eye. Richard asked him if it had been fed; Frank replied "No", and went and sat in the waiting room. Richard and Flora put the cat in the anaesthetic box and closed the glass lid. Richard turned on the ether-oxygen anaesthetic and after a few moments saw to his horror that the cat had stopped breathing. In spite of artificial respiration, oxygen, and smelling salts the cat died. Richard went into the waiting room and said,

"Frank, I am sorry to tell you your cat died as it was going under the anaesthetic."

"Oh no, it can't have; it has been my pal since my wife died and you've killed it."

"No I haven't, Frank. I examined its heart and it was perfectly well; to me it is a mystery, so I would like to do a post mortem, seeing you said it had not been fed."

"It hadn't, and I want to see it opened."

When Richard opened the abdomen, a distended stomach could be seen, which he cut open and out came at least half a pound of fish.

"Well, I'll be damned," said Frank, "It must have got in through the larder window and eaten it and gone out the same way; that was for my tea."

"I am sorry it died, Frank, but a full stomach pressing on its heart and lungs just stopped everything."

"I can see that; I am sorry I was rude and upset Mr Holden."

"Forget it, Frank. I'll try and find you another."

"Yes, do please. I love cats; they are such company." Flora showed him out. Richard was a bit numb, yet thankful he had had a consent form signed.

Later that evening he added up the cash and cheques which had come in during the week and realised that April and May accounts were being paid very slowly. He thought that not many things seem to be going right at the moment. Flora made him go to the pictures on the Saturday night. Gracie Fields in *Shipyard Sally* cheered him up, though the news was ominous. Richard, like millions of others in Great Britain, realised at last that war was coming. Events in Czechoslovakia and Albania that spring meant very little; but now Mr Chamberlain the Prime Minister, addressing Parliament, said that it was his intention to stand by Poland if her independence was threatened by Germany, and Hitler was boasting that he would settle the Danzig problem once and for all. When he and Mussolini signed their Pact of Steel in May that year, everyone realised that war was not far away, but chose to forget it.

Though he had only had the practice for three months, Richard could see that some of his arrangements were inconvenient. The office was too small, and in the wrong place to hear the telephone plainly. When he had taken over Charles' number, 264, he had had the telephone put in the front room to the left of the front door–the room they used as a lounge-dining room. The other 'phone, 585, was in the office at the bottom of the hall and could not be heard.

Flora and he decided to make the lounge into the office and to move the phone 585 to be with 264, which would allow the dispensary to be increased in size, and increase the working space. Also, from the lounge window the secretary could see everybody who came into the building, because the sign by the bell push said, "Please ring and enter". So on two evenings he and Flora worked together, taking up the carpet where they had the furniture which came from Auntie Alice. They decided to eat in the kitchen in future, so the dining table and chairs and the two big easy chairs were taken upstairs. They had soon moved everything across from the office, but did not put anything on the floor, deciding to buy either a carpet or linoleum at the sale at Joe Bolton's. Richard took his building society book with him when he went to ask Joe when he would have his next sale. He collected it two days later, and was surprised and shocked to see that he owed the building society more than he had done a year ago when he took out his mortgage. When he arrived home he showed the book to Flora who immediately said:

"I'm not surprised, Richard, because we have not had any spare money to save this year; we have spent it all on getting the house ready for the practice."

"So, you are not disappointed, because I am."

"Don't be silly," replied Flora, "It's our practice and in three months we have paid everybody, kept ourselves, and paid a little bit off–things can only get better."

"What, with a war coming?"

"Yes, even with a war coming, and this is always a quiet two months in the practice. We have just to try and make everything pay and pay off that mortgage as soon as we can."

"I'm glad you feel like that about it, Flora, because I was a bit despondent."

"Don't be, we will be OK. When is the next sale?"

"It's in ten days time and Joe said there will be some good stuff on sale."

Flora was pleased when she got a good carpet to cover the office floor for £4 17s.6d. Bradshaw brought it on his cart the next day, carried it into the office and unrolled it.

"That's a good fit, Mrs Holden and a nice carpet."

"Yes, I'm pleased with it. Joe Bolton said there would be some good stuff there and it is a good carpet."

"Did you hear that he's been taken ill and rushed into the Memorial Hospital?"

"No, I hadn't, but thank you for telling me." She paid him and immediately phoned Mary, but there was no reply. After evening surgery was finished she rang again. Mary's mother answered the 'phone and told Flora that Joe had died; it had been a severe heart attack and he had never recovered consciousness. Richard and Flora were both very sad that suddenly one of their small circle of friends had died. Flora went with Edna Evans next morning to comfort Mary, who was in a state of collapse after her husband's sudden death. Four days later the people of Sandhaven showed their respect for Joe by crowding St. Luke's for the funeral.

Richard noticed with some apprehension how war preparations were being made which directly or indirectly would affect him and the practice. Tom Priestley told him that he had been proposed to serve on the War Agricultural Committee for the area. When Richard asked what the Committee would do, he was surprised at Tom's answer.

"Well, we will inspect farms to see if the land is being put to the best use."

"And what happens if it isn't?"

"In that case, Richard, an order will be made compelling the farmer to carry out the recommendation."

"What will be advised?"

"Mainly producing as much potatoes, wheat and milk as possible, which means quite a lot of pasture will have to be ploughed up."

"But Tom," said Richard, "you know a lot of farmers round here are milk producers, they don't plough up good pastures. If they did, would they have to reduce the number of stock carried?"

"In some cases, yes, and especially if the feed stuffs position got bad."

"Well I hope it goes off OK but I wouldn't like to face some chaps round here and give them orders like that."

"Look, Richard, we will have the law behind us. More than that, if a farmer produces as much as he can, we won't interfere and he will make a good profit."

The fact that farmers would have to produce as much as possible made Richard happier. It meant more horses, cattle, sheep and pigs; also he had read that veterinary surgeons would be in the list of Reserved Occupations; so though he had Certificates A and B from his OTC days he would not be called up. Nevertheless, he had to complete a postcard giving personal details and return it to the organising veterinary surgeon for the area. This was necessary so that a veterinary first aid force would be ready to deal with animal casualties in the event of bombing from the air.

When the Ford went in for service Gordon Hindle told Richard that it was time he thought of getting another car. Richard said he knew his car was old, but he could not afford a new one at the moment.

"Oh, I don't mean buy one straight away. I'd hang on a bit because if war comes a lot of people won't get enough petrol to be able to use them and so they will sell them for what they can make."

"Like me, you think war is getting near."

"Yes, we are getting all sorts of information about petrol rationing and coupons and how the system will be administered. Also we will have to assist the Auxilary Fire Service, by having fire fighting appliances handy and things like that. Tyres will soon be in short supply so I'd have a few in store if I were you."

"Thanks, Gordon, for your advice, I'll do that."

The next time Richard saw Dick Hoggarth he asked him to come and take the partition down which divided the office from the dispensary. Flora and Richard discussed what to do with it and finally it was put in the loft over the kennels. Dick told Richard that there was a waiting list now for the allotments and that he had sold some of his pigs to other people who were beginning to keep them, having built pig sties; so he would have more work there. This was soon the case because he had to treat a lot of cases of swine erysipelas, brought on by the hot weather. Looking back in later years Richard saw how July-August 1939 was the time when his fortune suddenly changed for the better. He was treating a horse at Uncle Tom's in Droughton and when he had finished Frank said,

"Richard, me Dad wants to see yer."

"What about, Frank?"

"Ee I don't know, but he's in t'office."

Richard walked in and his uncle asked:

"Is everything OK?"

"Yes, I wouldn't work Number Four for a few days; he's got a greasy impetigo on his neck probably caused by the collar rubbing. You should get it restuffed. I've given Frank some dressing for it. Also I've rasped Number Eleven's teeth, he had some sharp points which were making him quid a bit."

"That's good. Now why I wanted to see you, was because I bought a really big Shire in the spring and I've just sold it to the steel works, to haul loads round the yard. I saw the manager, he asked me who was my vet, so I've given him your name."

"Thanks a lot, Uncle, I can do with all the work I can get, what with the mortgage on the house, and I want another car."

"Don't worry, Richard, you've got a good name, you'll do well. Come on and have a cup of tea with Nellie before you go."

He went in the house with his uncle, and two brown and white puppies ran to meet them.

"Has your Jack Russell bitch had pups, Uncle?"

"Yes, she got out to a wire-haired fox terrier belonging to John Whalley, one of the drivers."

"What are they?"

"A bitch and a dog, but the bitch is spoken for already."

"Well, could I have the dog for company for Flora?"

"Yes, of course you can, Richard, but you'll have to wait a bit, they are just five weeks old."

While drinking his tea he chatted to Nellie and Tom about the international situation. Tom said he was convinced war was coming, because one of his young drivers had been called up and because he had received an information sheet from the Government about fuel supplies. On his way out of Droughton Richard stopped at the scrap yard to see if they had any metal containers the size of a tea chest. He wanted to replace his wooden cat cages soon, because they were difficult to clean and because the three-ply wood absorbed urine, buckled and smelt badly. There was nothing suitable, but the owner told Richard to call in a month's time, because they were soon to bring a lot of scrap from the Government factory and if there were any metal boxes he would save them for him.

He called in at the surgery and went at once to George Collinson at Church Farm to see a cow off colour.

George, the elder son of Tom Collinson of Park Hall, had married Mary Booth from Intack a year ago and at once took over Church Farm and was working hard to get it straight, because it had been neglected by the previous tenant.

"Hello, George, where's the cow?"

"In the small shippon; since Dad rang you she's got a bad quarter."

"So that's the trouble, is it? I'll just examine her. Did she eat this morning?"

"No, Mr Holden, she was quiet and gave very little milk, though she's been giving over five a day."

"I'm not surprised she gave very little milk, her temperature is 105.5°F."

The cow's heart rate was fast and the pulse full and hard. Richard examined the quarter, which was hot, and the milk was watery, but somehow it was not bad enough to make the cow as ill as she was.

"Very well, George, give her two powders now, then one at four and one last thing. Strip out that quarter and rub in this lotion now and each time you drench her. I'll see her again in the morning."

"Shall I turn her out?"

"Yes, it's a lovely day; it won't harm her and she'll probably pick a bit. I'll see you tomorrow."

Richard was finishing his lunch when the phone rang.

"Tom Collinson here, Mr Holden. Will you go back to our George's; that cow's been badly hiked and is bleeding. I'll meet you there."

"Right, Tom, I won't be ten minutes."

The cow was standing in the yard, blood trickling from her vulva and running down her tail.

"Let's have a bucket of hot water, soap and a towel, quick, George."

Richard took off his jacket, rolled up his sleeves and put on his calving overall. He poured disinfectant into the water George had brought and then soaped his arm.

"Nose her, George, please."

When she was securely held, Richard pushed his hand into the cow's vagina and found it full of faeces; there was a tear a foot long in the top of the vagina and the torn rectum was hanging into it. As he explored further he felt hot blood spraying onto his hand, but he could not find the artery in all the torn tissue.

"I'm sorry George, it's a fatal wound; it goes the length of her passage and has ripped her rectum open as well and she's bleeding internally."

"I'll take her up to the abattoir at once," said Tom, "The cattle truck is here behind the barn."

"Do that, but I don't know if she'll pass."

"Oh I think the forequarters should, at least we'll get something back."

While he was fetching the truck, Richard washed himself well and his overall.

"Do you know which one did it, George?"

"Yes, it's a crossbred Ayrshire-Friesian; she is a bad devil, and she had blood on one horn, I heard some bellowing and looked and could see some fighting, so I went and found it was this one, so I brought her up."

"Bad luck, George. I must be off. Cheerio."

It was three o'clock when the manager of the abattoir rang.

"Is that you, Mr Holden?"

"Yes, what's the matter?"

"It's Dick Williams from the abattoir. You sent in a cow from George Collinson's, didn't you?"

"Yes, I did."

"Well, can you come and see her. The butcher has partly dressed her and thinks she's got anthrax."

"Good God, I hope not, I'll be there as quick as I can."

He got an anthrax specimen box from the dispensary and a little bag which contained a scalpel, some microscope glass slides and a spirit lamp; then he drove to the abattoir at high speed.

Dick Williams led Richard into the main slaughtering hall where the carcase was hanging from an overhead rail. The skin had been cut from the belly and turned back and the belly slit open. The stomach and intestines were hanging out, and a huge blue-black spleen.

"Yes that's anthrax all right. I'll take a swab of the blood and a couple of slides. Will you block that drain with a brick or something. Get a bucket of hot water and put this disinfectant into it and get the butcher to wash his hands and arms, and his apron, wellingtons and knives as well. Did the blood run into that bucket?"

"Yes, it did."

"Right, leave it there; don't pour it away. Fill another bucket with water and disinfectant, put it at the door and we can clean our wellingtons with it."

While this was being done Richard took his swab and made his slides, then he disinfected himself and drove off at high speed. He was going along the main road, when a car roared past and the driver signalled him to pull into the side of the road. The driver was the inspector of police. Richard wound down the car window.

"Good afternoon, Mr Holden. Do you know you were doing over 50 miles an hour?"

"Yes, Inspector, but I'm in a hell of a hurry. A cow has just been killed in the abattoir. It has anthrax and I've got the blood samples here which I must examine at once, and then report it to the Ministry of Agriculture and Fisheries in Droughton. Also, the slaughterman has been splashed with blood."

"Off you go then, but keep to the speed limit in future."

"Yes, Inspector, I will."

The microscopic examination of the smear showed the fat black bacilli of anthrax in a pale pink background. Richard reported the case of suspect anthrax at once to Droughton and was told to send the swab and diagnostic smear immediately to the Central Veterinary Laboratory.

Two weeks later a cow was being unloaded at Leach Farm, when it sprang off the back board and broke a leg. Richard told Jack Clough to send it to the abattoir. He would meet it there and give Dick Williams a certificate and then examine it post mortem.

When he walked into the abattoir, there was a shout: "The devil's here, get him, boys," and Richard was immediately surrounded by two butchers and three other workers holding choppers and knives. Richard was scared for a moment until Dick Williams burst out laughing and told him the reason for the demonstration.

Immediately Richard had informed Droughton, they had ordered Dick to detain all employees on the premises and two veterinary officers had gone straight to the abattoir. Cleansing and disinfection had been carried out and the carcase burnt. Then all who had been in contact had been taken to the hospital, had been injected with serum and given tablets to take for three days. Because the site of the injection had been very painful, the employees had decided to let Richard know their feelings in a good-humoured way.

The case was confirmed by the Ministry of Agriculture and Fisheries as one of anthrax.

Richard never told Flora about his brush with death in the form of anthrax, but she soon got to recognise swine fever by a certain smell. To get to Poolside Farm, one went into the centre of Shipton village and turned to the right into a country lane which led down to the farm a mile and a half away. Bill Parkinson was the tenant and kept a mixed bag of livestock: ten milking cows; some bullocks; thirty breeding ewes; and many pigs. He was as happy-go-lucky as his Irish wife and they had six children, four boys and two girls. He was a swill feeder, that is, he fed his pigs on boiled waste food from hotels, factory canteens and bakeries. His buildings were poorly maintained and he always gave the impression of being hard-up, though the contrary was true. Richard had been sent to the farm by the Ministry of Agriculture and Fisheries to conduct a suspect swine fever inquiry. It was a hot summer morning when he arrived at the farm and was met by Bill who took him into one of the pig houses. The sickly smell of boiling swill was everywhere and flies were numerous.

"This is the pen, Mr Holden, they're ten-week-old stores I bought at Droughton. They did well for the first few days and then went sickly and then two died yesterday. I didn't like the look of it, so I reported it to Hibbert, the bobby in the village."

"Yes, they look in a poor way, Bill, I must say. Anyway I have got to post mortem these two and then there are forms to fill in. So let's have a bucket of water."

Bill brought the water. Richard poured in disinfectant and soaked his hands in the fluid, then he proceeded to open the pigs. The lungs showed pneumonia; there were little haemorrhages in the kidneys; the stomach was empty but inflamed and bile stained. After he cut open the bowels, he washed them in the disinfectant and found the mucous membrane ulcerated. He put all his specimens onto a big sheet of grease-proof paper and then wrapped them up.

"You won't be having them for your tea, Mr Holden?"

"You're right, Bill. I've got to send these to the Veterinary Laboratory at Addlestone near London, because they do the diagnosis."

"But can't you tell me if they've got it or they haven't?"

"No, I can't, but to me it looks suspicious. Let's go outside and I'll disinfect my rubber coat and boots and then we can go in the house and fill up the forms; and I must check your Movements Book."

It was very pleasant to get outside into the fresh air blowing in from the river and to drink the tea Mrs Parkinson had made.

"Well, Bill, that completes it. You've got more pigs on than I thought."

"Aye, they are all ready for killing. I work it so that I have a lot of young pigs just bought at this time of year, to go onto all the extra food I get from the hotels and boarding houses now that the Wakes are on and they do do well. Now, Mr Holden, what would you do in my shoes?"

"Get every pig off for killing first thing tomorrow morning except the ill ones; but if any more die you must tell PC Hibbert in the village."

"Thanks a lot. I'll do that."

Richard carried his specimens in the cardboard box to the car and drove back to the surgery. He filled in the two labels, put one inside the cardboard box, wrapped it in strong brown paper, tied it with string attaching the other labels and sealed the knots with sealing wax. Flora said as she came into the office:

"What a dreadful stink, what on earth is it?"

"Pig guts for the Ministry. I must fly to get them on the first train."

Arriving at the station he took the box into the parcels office and the clerk said he would see that the guard on the 11.10 a.m. express got the box.

"I don't think he'll like it though; it smells pretty rotten already."

"Yes, it does. I'm glad I haven't to open it in London."

Richard's Ministry work increased. He had got another list of herds to inspect, and found two TB cows in the first week, one with chronic cough and emaciation and the other with an indurated udder. He did two visits on his way to the yard at Southall and Bob Whiteside opened the cows for him. They were both rotten with bovine tuberculosis.

"I can't understand these farmers, keeping cows till they get in this state," said Bob, "can you?"

"No, if only they slaughtered them at the first signs they would probably salvage something, but these are only worth thirty bob."

"If that. By the way, have you been to our George's at Seedhill?"

"No I haven't, Bob. I didn't know he was your brother."

"He isn't, he's my cousin. He's fed up with that Droughton chap, he seems to be a funny sort of vet, forgets to come to your farm when you've rung him. Anyway, I told George to ring you."

"Thanks, Bob. Is he milking?"

"Aye about forty, and he rears pigs as well, and fattens for the Loxhams, the butchers in Droughton and Brooksby and here in Southall. He never buys owt on and he meal feeds with skim milk from the milk factory."

"I'll look after him, Bob, when he rings me."

His last call that morning was to the stables on the docks, where stable cough had broken out. The four affected horses were tied up in an old stable.

He injected each one with equine catarrh vaccine and gave the foreman a large tin of cough electuary and a bottle of inhalant. To use the latter the horse was tied up short to the manger and a bucket, with hay in the bottom, was put into the manger and some inhalant poured in the bucket. Then a horse rug was thrown over the horse's head and the bucket. Now boiling water was poured into the bucket and the horse inhaled the steam, which was medicated with the creosote, eucalyptus and camphor of the inhalant.

When he arrived home, the order from the wholesale chemists Willows Francis, Butler and Thompson Ltd. had arrived. He had ordered double the amount of the drugs he needed so that he would have a stock in hand if war came. There were nearly fifty items. About half went into the dispensary and the rest into the second bedroom, being put into the wardrobe, with the big cans and jars ranged along the wall, along with tins of treacle, soft soap and paraffin. When he read in the daily paper that Parliament had risen for the summer recess, he wondered if his stockpiling was necessary and that the war scare would blow over as it had the year before. On August Bank Holiday weekend the coaches and cars poured through Sandhaven on their way to the resorts up the coast; and the railway was very busy with day excursions on the Monday, a lot of people going to the station quite early.

Marjorie had gone home when Flora came back from shopping on the Saturday morning and told Richard that she had been talking to Betty Heyes, who told her to buy some blackout material, as it was selling fast.

"But Flora, there are eighteen windows in this house and then there is the stable block; it will take days to make curtains for that lot," said Richard. "Don't do anything yet, I'll ask Jim Lord and Bishop what they are going to do."

"Well, hurry up; we will have to do something and we can't do much if the practice gets really busy," replied Flora. "And another thing, people keep asking me to board their dogs; don't you think we could put the cats upstairs and board dogs downstairs?"

"It had never crossed my mind, but now you mention it, I think it's a good idea. We could put a small dog in each room until I have time to make kennels."

Flora laughed. "You know you won't have time. I'll see that Dick does it."

That afternoon the cats were taken upstairs and by Monday there was a Pekinese dog in the far room and a dachshund in the hospital room. There was also a pony in the loose box, which had shied and backed into a shop window in Broad Street and had a lump of glass embedded in its buttock. With Flora helping him, he extracted it under local anaesthetic and then injected the pony against tetanus. With emergencies and surgeries it was a busy weekend.

Richard, thinking it was an emergency, rushed to The Boltons, a big house on the Crescent. He was admitted by the maid and then Mrs Nathan came in, a beautifully groomed elderly Jewish woman.

"Good morning, you are Mr Holden, I hope," she said.

"Yes," replied Richard, "Where is the cat?"

"Upstairs in my daughter's room; she has gone to London on war work and has given it to me, but it howls in agony all the time; it kept me awake all last night."

They walked into the room and there was a lovely seal-point Siamese cat, howling as only they can when they want a mate, standing on the end of the bed.

"That's the noise, Mr Holden. I can't stand it, take her away and destroy her."

"Mrs Nathan, the cat is not in agony. It is a female which is in season. She is calling for a male."

"But I can't keep her, please take her."

"I will, Mrs Nathan, but would you agree to me giving her to a person who has just lost his cat and wants another? It will go to a good home. I can't destroy her."

"Yes, I agree," so Richard put the cat into the basket; she was quite docile.

"By the way, what is her name?"

"Mekong after the river in Siam."

Frank Madden welcomed the cat, picked her up and stroked her.

"Will you have her? She is in season, but it will go off in a few days."

"Oh, of course I'll have her, she's beautiful and I'll breed from her. Tom Billsborough at St. George's in Droughton, breeds them. So I'll take her straight away."

"I'm glad you like her and will have her. She has a full pedigree; I'll get it from Mrs Nathan for you. I hope she has kittens. I'd like one if you are lucky."

"I'll see you get one, Mr Holden, and thanks again for Mekong."

The voice on the 'phone said, "This is Mr Croft. Could you tell me if there is distemper in Sandhaven at the moment?"

"Yes there is. This is Mr Holden the vet speaking. We always get more in summer and this year I have seen quite a lot of cases."

"Thank you, I'll bring my dog to surgery tonight for an injection."

"Yes, between 6 and 7."

Ted Croft was a black-haired, big man of middle age, who brought a big Airedale dog into the room.

"I'm Ted Croft. I rang up about distemper."

"Yes, so you did. I am Richard Holden, now what do you want?"

"Well, he's been injected once when he was a pup. Should he have another now he's here in Sandhaven, because I've taken over Joe Bolton's business."

"Yes, I advise that he has another injection, and then keep him in for a week before you take him walks round the town."

"That's no difficulty because he's the guard dog at my house I've bought on Woodfield Road."

Richard filled the syringe and said, "I'll just muzzle him."

"You won't; he won't let you, I'll do it." He pulled a leather muzzle out of his pocket and put it on the dog, which never moved when Richard gave him the injection.

"He's a funny dog, I can do anything with him but if anybody else goes near him or lays a hand on him he bites in a flash. He is called Reeth, by the way."

"Thanks for telling me, Ted, my wife will make a note on his surgery card. I will be seeing you then in the course of business. Nice to have met you," and Flora showed him out.

"Have you seen Mary Bolton, Flora? or do you know what she is going to do?"

"No I called once and the house was locked up. She has probably gone off for a holiday; she has kept herself to herself since Joe died."

"You know, I do miss Joe, but this new chap seems very nice."

"Yes, I think we can do business with him."

When he added up the cash and the cheques at the weekend, he was pleasantly surprised at the amount, much increased by the cheque from the Ministry of Agriculture and Fisheries. He made it a rule after he had had dinner on Saturday or Sunday night to fill in the paying-in book for the bank, no matter how late it was, and this night it was almost eleven o'clock.

When Flora rang her mother on Sunday, Jean asked if she could come over on the Monday and stay for a few days, with Mary coming as well because she was on holiday. Flora was thrilled and told them to come over in time for lunch on the Monday. When they arrived Jean used the back bedroom and Mary the second bedroom which had a single bed and, laughing, said it would be the first time she had slept in a wholesale chemists. Flora was glad to have them and soon found them both work to do, Jean in the kitchen and Mary working with Flora in the dispensary making up powders and medicines.

When Marjorie came on Tuesday morning, the house was a hive of industry, which surprised the billeting officer, who arrived at lunch time much to Jean's annoyance. Still, he soon saw all the rooms were in use and Flora kept excusing herself to answer the door bell and Marjorie kept talking loudly on the 'phone. In the end he said he could see that they had no spare accommodation for children and Flora said there were too many dangerous drugs in the house, especially dangerous for children. She was glad to see him go, and they ate a slightly overcooked meal.

Richard was late because he had been in to Jim Lord's to get some tins of Elastoplast and was looking at his blackout arrangements. He had had made sheets of three ply to fit over the windows and they were held in place by turn catches. Jim said he had decided on wood because it would last longer than curtains and it would protect against flying glass. He had called at Tommy Bishop's as well and seen that he had blinds fitted to the windows because they started baking at 3.00 a.m. He was also having blinds fitted to the sky lights and all doors doubled, so that you had to shut the outside one before you could open the inner one, because, as he said, I don't want a bomb through the blooming roof. But he astonished Richard by telling him that some of the windows in Cross Street had internal shutters.

Richard, on arriving home, had gone into the office and looking at the long wooden painted panels each side of the window realised that Tom was right, though the handles had been removed and the panels made fast with screws. It took him two nights to get all the screws out, and fit new knobs to the shutters of the five windows which faced onto Victoria Street and Cross Street, and when closed they were most effective. For the other windows he had plywood panels made, held in place by catches, while upstairs the three women made the thick curtains fit so that no lights showed outside. The shutters when open were a dirty brown colour and, though he grumbled because he had to paint them white, he was grateful in his heart to the Walkers because they had not disposed of them.

The swine fever investigation Richard had carried out was confirmed as a positive case; he was glad his diagnosis had been correct and that he had advised Bill Chapman on the best course of action to adopt. While he was reading the morning mail, the phone rang and a voice said:

"Is that you, Richard?"

"Speaking, who's that?"

"Bob Townsend from Wilton. I was hoping to catch you. I am the vet to the Yeomanry and we are being mobilised, so it looks as if war is not far away. Really, I want to ask you if you will help the new graduate I have got here. His name is Tommy Knowles and he'll be running the practice from now on."

"Of course I'll help him, Bob. Tell him just to ring me if he's in need of assistance."

"Thanks a lot, Richard. I'll say goodbye. I don't know when I will see you again."

"Good luck, Bob, and if you get leave come and see me, all the best."

As he put the 'phone down, he almost hit the roof because the air raid siren sounded. It was a dummy run, a test, but the noise was very loud because the siren was on the roof of the police station lower down Victoria Street. The next envelope he opened contained the pedigree of Mekong, the Siamese cat he had taken to Frank Madden.

It was early evening when he went to Moss End at Ryton to a cow down with milk fever. It was only a few miles from Droughton and Richard had never been there before. Mr Birtwell was standing in the yard, and immediately walked over to the car when Richard drove in.

"Good evening, you are Mr Birtwell?"

"Yes, I am Tommy Birtwell."

"I'm Richard Holden. Now I just want to get this straight–you haven't had another vet to this cow."

"No, I've had enough of Wilson in Droughton; he's lost me two cows this year, so I've come to you; Walter Black at Brook Farm told me to."

"Good enough, where's the cow?"

"Down the field, we'll have to ride down to her."

They drove down the lane and across the field, and Tommy stopped Richard beside an overgrown hedge.

"It's awkward to get to her, she's rolled into the ditch under the hedge. I know it's overgrown, but it's a good windbreak."

Bending down, they scrambled through the brambles and into the ditch, which was dry, and clouds of flies descended on them. Richard gave the cow two 200 cc. injections intravenously, and the flies were biting all the time, but when they pulled the cow's head round she sat up.

"Hell, that's quick," said Tommy.

"Yes, it works quicker if you inject it in a vein."

Richard gave her a clout across her back with his rope and she got to her feet and after a minute crashed her way through the brambles and thorns into the field.

"I'm glad she's out of there, and so am I; I'm bitten all over with these flies."

"Aye, these clegs are a damned nuisance in August. One stung me on my eyelid last week and I had my eye shut for two days."

They scrambled back into the car to get away from the flies.

"Just ease her bag for twenty-four hours, Tom; don't milk her out and she'll be fine."

"I'll do that, thank you, Mr Holden"

He was in high spirits as he drove away, another new client, but his face was sore. When he walked into the lounge Flora turned round and said:

"Heavens, what's happened to your face, Richard, have you been in a fight?"

"No, they are cleg bites, there were clouds of them at Moss End."

Flora liberally plastered his face with Pond's cold cream, and started to laugh.

"You know, you look like a circus clown with your white face," Mary and Jean joined in the banter.

Richard took the pedigree round to Frank Madden, who told him that Mekong had mated with Billsborough's stud cat, and he was now hoping for some kittens.

"And don't forget to keep me one, Frank"

"I won't forget, and you look after your face, you have been badly bitten."

His face was a lot better next morning, but the lumps took a few days to disappear. Among the animals the effects were more serious, and John Huddlestone at Red Barn, asked him to go to treat some sheep as soon as he could because they "had been struck by flies". Richard put plenty of antiseptic dusting powder, and a Winchester bottle of anti-fly dressing into the car. The dressing was a recipe he had got from Major Gillmour in Corchester. It read:

Iodoformi Pulv. 2 drachms

Ol. Eucalypti 2 drachms

Ol. Citronelli 2 ounces

Creosoti 2 drachms

Ol. Colza ad 20 ounces

John had some sheep in a small pen, and one or two were looking ill.

"Morning, John, now what's happened?"

"I don't know. It could be that shower of rain about five days ago, but being shorn in June they haven't a good fleece yet to get wet round the crotch and tail. Anyway last night it was obvious some were bothered, so we gathered them, and sorted these out"

With the ewe held Richard parted the brown-stained fleece above the tail, and the smell of rotting flesh was awful. There was a hole in the skin two inches across, and he could see maggots moving in the pus and liquified flesh.

"John, clip this area short."

When he had done so, Richard washed the area with Eusol, removing the stinking discharge and some maggots; the rest he picked out with forceps, and then poured acriflavine emulsion over the wound.

"She'll soon recover, John. Let's have that ill-looking one over there."

This ewe proved to have an area the size of one's hand under-run with maggots. He cut the skin away, and treated her like the first one, then covered the wound.

"Mark her with a paint stick, and I'll give you some medicine for her."

He treated five cases, and then left John to continue the treatment on the others.

"Do the same tomorrow, because you may find more maggots, then dust the flesh with this sulphanilamide powder, and paint the fly dressing round the wounds. As soon as the wounds are dry use the dusting powder, and the dressing."

"I'll do that, Mr Holden, and I'll go through all the flock once a day while the flies are so bad. Have you been bitten on your face?"

"Yes, at Moss End at Ryton the other night, the clegs were dreadful."

"They're bad enough up here. I wouldn't like to farm on the marsh. Thanks for coming so soon. I'll let you know if they are not doing."

The dry cows were also suffering from summer garget, an acute inflammation of the udder called by some farmers "felon". The infection seemed to be carried by flies, which nibbled at the end of the teat, which was often raw. In a day or two the affected quarter of the udder was full of yellow stinking pus and the cow was very ill. When he had treated one of these cases at Harold Briggs, Brookhouse Farm, which was only four miles from Droughton, he went on to Uncle Tom's stable to deliver some alterative powders, bottles of colic medicine and a tin of horse electuary.

"Richard, you can take your pup, it's nearly nine week old. If tha' goes to th' house Nellie 'ull give it to yer."

"Thanks, Uncle, Flora will be pleased. She does want a dog for company and to bark if there is anybody at the back of the house."

The puppy was white in colour with brown patches, a white head, and one brown and one white ear. Flora fell for him at once. He would be company for her now that Jean and Mary had gone home, and at night when Richard was out.

"Well, what are you going to call him, Flora?"

"What do you think, Tommy, of course."

On his way back from Droughton he had called at Howard's scrapyard. They had kept six metal boxes which were 20 inches square with no lids. Richard was pleased; they would make substantial cat cages, once they had drainage holes made and wire mesh doors fitted. He arranged for them to be delivered to Gordon Hindle's garage.

That night he injected Tommy against distemper and, in spite of Flora's protests, he was kept in the recovery room in the stable block for a week in isolation.

The next morning, it was announced on the eight o'clock news that Germany and Russia had signed a non-aggression pact. When Richard arrived at the garage, Gordon was reading the paper and asked Richard if he had read it. Richard replied that he had not, but had heard the news on the wireless. "To my way of thinking that Hitler knows he can fight anybody in the West without Russia interfering, so it could be Poland or France any day now."

"Yes, I think the same, but we said we'll fight if he has a go at Poland."

"I know, we could be at war in a month or two, with bombs and rationing and blackout."

"Gordon, would you get me a car before Christmas because I am really flogging the old Ford to death by doing so much driving."

"I'll do that, Richard, and have you got any petrol coupons yet?"

"No, but they should come any time now, because it's been confirmed that vets are a reserved occupation and I've filled up the form and sent it off. Now, with regard to those boxes, could your George make secure wire mesh doors for them and drill drainage holes in them and when he's finished will you paint them white?"

"Yes, I'll do that. Shall I fill her up?"

"Yes, Gordon, I'll keep her full to the top every day now. By the way, could you sell me a couple of petrol cans, so I have a little petrol by me in case of emergencies."

"Yes, I'll do that, and put it on your account. You'll see the name has altered to G. & G. Hindle Ltd."

"Oh, why?"

"Well, I've a decent workshop at the back here and George has got a Government contract to make phosphor-bronze bearings, so we've made it a company. You know, each of us has put in five hundred quid and the factory is in production now. We have two turners working already."

"I'm glad you've got off to a good start. Cheerio for now. Oh, Gordon, I've almost forgotten; will you put the regulation head lamp covers on now while I wait, because there is going to be a practice black-out some night now." These were soon fitted, but on the night of the practice he did not go out in the car in the blackout, but walked round to the GPO in High Street using his shaded torch. He thought he could walk round the back of his own house without using his torch and Flora laughed her head off when he fell over the dustbin; and Tommy, alerted by the noise, growled at him when he opened the back door.

"Really, it's come to something when your wife laughs at you hurting yourself and then your own dog won't let you into your own house! You wait till

you go out in the blackout, it's not funny. You can't judge how near you are
to things."

"All right, love, I'm sorry. Come on and have your supper."

Next morning Flora asked Richard to get some bananas and oranges.
When he went to the shop Dick, Betty and the girl were serving customers
and he noticed a tall grey-haired man who walked with a limp carrying in
boxes.

"Have you got another helper, Dick?"

"Who him? No, he's not new, he's worked for me for a year in the store
room at the back on a part-time basis. He's a good worker and will do
anything."

"I could do with someone like that to help me. Would you ask him when
you've a minute to come and see me."

"Yes, Richard, I'll tell him."

When the man came to the surgery that evening a friendship began which
was to last for years. John Lamb's father had been killed in the 1914-1918 war
and his mother had endured hardship to bring up him, his brother and his
sister. She took in other people's washing and toiled day in and day out in a
lean-to at the back of the house where there were the boiler, the tubs, the
scrubbing boards and the mangle. Two clothes lines stretched across the little
back yard, while in winter clothes dried on maidens round the fire. John,
when not at school, turned the mangle or collected or delivered the laundry,
carrying it in a large white wicker laundry basket which had handles at each
end. His sister Margaret who was four years older than John did most of the
ironing in the evenings, after working all day in Miss Bishop's Market Café.
Marjorie Bishop often gave the thin white-faced girl a loaf of bread and some
cakes when she was going home at half past six. John left school at fourteen
and got a job in the ship yard. He did general labouring work and over the
years developed a powerful physique. Because he would do any work to the
best of his ability he became a painter, and life became a little easier. He
helped his mother, whom he worshipped, as much as he could because
Margaret got married and she and her husband moved into a little terraced
house on Station Road North. When John got married, he and Ruth lived in
his mother's house. Now she had given up laundry work. The British Legion
had got her a job cleaning at the Town Hall five mornings and evenings a
week. Just as life was becoming more pleasant for them, tragedy struck.
Ruth died having their first child, and though John showed very little
emotion, he began to chain-smoke cigarettes and did so for the rest of his
life. Wilfred his brother had also married, and lived in Birkenhead

It was two years later that he and another workman were standing in a
cradle which hung over the side of the ship which was being fitted out. They
were painting, when suddenly a rope snapped and the two men were hurled

into the dry dock below. John fell on top of his companion who was killed. John sustained a broken hip, which kept him in the Memorial Hospital for months. Though the compensation paid to him was very little, he didn't complain, but just got on making the best of a bad job. When he was well enough, he did part-time jobs in many trades in Sandhaven and continued to live at his mother's.

She died of a stroke suddenly in 1937, leaving the house to John and the contents to Margaret. The two decided to combine forces and Margaret and her family moved back to the family home, and she looked after John.

The hardships and tragedies of his life had left their indelible mark on John, yet he was brisk and cheerful, as he sat in the office that evening opposite Richard.

"Well John, thanks for coming round. I'll tell you what the job is. Say two nights a week come and mop the front doorstep, the lino in the waiting room, consulting room and the dispensary. Then clean my car inside and wash and polish it as well. Can you answer the telephone and take messages?"

"Oh, I can do that, Mr Holden. I learnt to use one when I was a lad doing odd jobs in the office at the shipyard. I often used to pick it up and take a message for Mr Kennedy and then go into the yard and find him and tell him, and I used to polish his car."

"Who was Mr Kennedy?"

"The manager; actually he was a Major, we always had to call him that."

"Right, John, come on Saturday about four o'clock and do three hours work and I'll pay you three shillings."

"Thanks very much, Mr Holden. I'll be here at four."

He was, and he worked hard. When he was not whistling he was smoking, and Richard's car had not been so clean for months. Richard often teased John in later years saying:

"I don't know what you did, but the day after you started working for me war broke out."

Richard and Flora sat very still on the settee in the lounge on that Sunday morning and listened to the Prime Minister on the wireless saying that "a state of war now existed between Great Britain and Germany". Flora was very tense and, holding Richard's hand, asked:

"Do you think they will bomb us right away like they are doing in Poland?"

"I don't know, love, what will happen, but I hope it doesn't come to that. Really, now I think we will have to live one day at a time, and not make any plans." He kissed her, and she rose to her feet and said loudly:

"I'm going to make a pot of tea."

As she left the room Richard was very proud of her. He thought, that's the bloody spirit; it will take more than Hitler to stop her making tea.

When he went to the GPO in the afternoon, the streets were quiet, but men carrying suitcases were coming out of the drill hall and going into the bus station, and he realised that as they were all young they had been called up. The windows of the Market Hotel looked like lattice work, being criss-crossed with white sticking paper. The windows of the police station and the GPO were similar, but both now were protected by high walls of sand bags. It was late in the evening when he was locking up, and having put out the light opened the back door to go across to the stable block, that he realised how intense the blackness of the black-out was; it took him a few moments to get his bearings.

On Monday Richard took an empty drugs hamper to the goods office at the railway station, and as he was coming out met Dr Bill McConnell who had a child holding each of his hands, and who was followed by a goodlook-ing woman who was also leading a child.

"Hello, Bill, you look busy," said Richard.

"I am that; this is my sister Fiona and these are her three children; they have come from Birmingham in case the Germans come over and bomb the city, so now I have a full house."

"How do you do, Fiona, nice to meet you," said Richard. "Bill, you must bring her round to meet Flora when you have time."

"Yes, I'll do that, thanks Richard."

As he walked away, the latter wondered how the 37-year-old bachelor and his old housekeeper would adapt to having three young children in the house. More evacuees arrived and Frank Wood the butcher met two of his brother's children from Liverpool. The organised parties of children waiting for transport had come from Manchester and, standing outside the station, looked very bewildered. Each child had a card round its neck, and carried a gas mask and a small case, or bag. Richard got into his car, felt vaguely upset, and couldn't understand this, until it dawned on him that he hadn't a child to worry about. Thoughts flooded through his mind. Why haven't we any children? Why haven't I got a son? He resolved to do something about this as he drove back to the surgery, but when he arrived there, the cares of the day banished it from his mind. Two people were waiting to have their dogs destroyed, and when later he put the bodies into the metal box, he hoped not everybody would panic like this and have healthy animals destroyed.

But the large animal side of the practice was busy, keeping Richard fully occupied most days, and this continued in October, when the cows were housed for the winter. He did the six-monthly private Tuberculin Test at the Home Farm, but the Attested Herds scheme of the Ministry of Agriculture and Fisheries was stopped; nevertheless he still had plenty of herds to examine for tuberculosis. The sudden increase in the number of dogs and cats to be destroyed had stopped, and though there was the black-out and rationing, the war was not really affecting his life, until the placard outside the newsagents one evening stopped him dead in his tracks. It said "ROYAL OAK SUNK". He was listening to the news on the wireless, when John Lamb came noisily up the stairs.

"Hello, Mr Holden, are you listening to the news?"

"Yes, John, it's a bad do about the *Royal Oak*".

"Aye it is. My nephew Frank is on her, my brother's eldest lad. I hope he's all right."

He was not, he was drowned, and John was very quiet on Saturday night, after telling Richard the news. Frank had had a hard life on the trawlers sailing out of Sandhaven and had joined the Royal Navy in 1936. He left a two-year-old boy and a lovely thirty-year-old wife called Mavis who had very dark curly hair and blue eyes.

It was a very dark rainy night when Richard turned onto the main Brookham road, and the headlights were not much use. But he knew his way to Wood End Farm and found the entrance easily. With Will Pickles' help he soon calved the cow and after downing a mug of tea set off for Sandhaven. He had driven about a mile, when he could see the road ahead was lit up. He slowed down as soon as he saw a figure in the road waving a red lamp and then stopped. He lowered the window and the policeman said:

"Will you please keep to the right of the road and go slowly, because there has been an accident. It is Mr Holden, isn't it?"

"Yes, that's right, constable, is anybody hurt?"

"Yes, the car driver is very badly injured, and he's been taken to the Royal in Droughton. Bob Whiteside has just shot the cow."

"Whatever happened?"

"Well, it looks as though the driver was going very fast and ran into a big Friesian cow standing in the middle of the road. It must have got out somehow and, being all black round its back end, the driver wouldn't see it. It was sitting on its belly in the middle of the road, when I arrived, but its back legs were all smashed up."

"How dreadful. Do you know who it was?"

"Not yet, but he must be from somewhere around here."

He was; it was Tom Seed, the traveller for cattle food, who was well known and highly respected in the district. Richard was very despondent, having lost a true friend to whom he owed a great deal, because it was Tom who had sent him to Major Johnny all those years ago. St. George's Church in Droughton was packed for the funeral and during the service Richard and many others were reduced to tears. After leaving the church he found a telephone box and rang the surgery and Flora gave him two cases to visit, which helped to lift his spirits and take his mind off Tom's death.

Frank Madden brought the Siamese kitten for Flora, but would not take any payment from Richard who immediately vaccinated it against feline enteritis. Though Flora idolised it, it soon showed that it considered Richard its master. For the first night the kitten sat under a chair, and cautiously played with Tommy, but soon they were romping together in the kitchen. One cold evening, Flora took them upstairs into the lounge, where they played happily for a little time. Suddenly there was a prolonged ringing of the front door bell. Richard rushed down, turned off the hall light and opened the door, thinking it was an emergency case.

"Mr Holden, I am the Air Raid Warden. You have a light showing upstairs. Will you put it out at once. I must tell you that further contravention of the Order will lead to prosecution."

Richard was a bit taken back and said, "I am sorry, I didn't know. I've been very careful with the blackout, where is the light?"

"It's showing from the first floor window of the room on the corner."

"That's the lounge. I'll go and put it right at once."

"You do, Sir. Goodnight."

The cat and the puppy had been playing behind Flora's armchair and, dashing under the curtains, had opened them slightly. Richard told Flora that the warden was most officious, so the puppy was banished to the kitchen, and loops and buttons were sewn on the curtains, so that they could not be accidentally opened. They called the kitten Ming.

Various conditions appeared with the onset of autumn weather. Richard vaccinated all the beef cattle at Hill Crest, where there was an outbreak of black leg and two sheep farmers over Ridgetown way came in for braxy vaccine. He got another farmer to inject all his ewes, just before the tups were put in, with lamb dysentery vaccine, showing him how to inject them at the base of the tail and providing him with syringes, needles and antiseptic. When an outbreak of coughing began in one stable on the docks, it soon spread among the equine population of Sandhaven and Richard was very busy dispensing electuary to which he had added extract of belladonna for use on mild cases. He dosed the worst cases however with sulphanilamide and used the new drug M & B 693 on two very ill cases. One recovered but the other died. When clients grumbled about coming to the surgery at 6 o'clock in the blackout Richard changed the time to between 2 o'clock and half past each afternoon except Sunday and the numbers attending increased again. The blackout did not completely stop social life, but Fiona and her children always came on a Saturday afternoon, while others of their friends came on a Sunday afternoon.

George Duke came to the office in the first week of November and went through the books. They showed that the practice was making a good profit and that the mortgage was being reduced. Richard was quietly pleased that he had lived up to the confidence which Flora had in him, and they had done the right thing in buying the practice. So when Gordon Hindle told Richard that he had got a car for him, he immediately agreed to buy it, Gordon taking the Ford Eight in part exchange. The car was a second-hand 1938 Austin Cambridge, colour black, with grey leather upholstery and a square glass ventilator in the roof. It had only done seven and a half thousand miles and was like new and the price was £135. They were both sad to see the old car go, Richard because it had been his first car, and Flora because it had been part of their lives since the day they got married; but she was secretly pleased to see TJ 2438 standing at the door, a shining symbol of their progress.

"When I was getting some cakes this morning, Marjorie Bishop asked me to tell you to go and see the cat at the bakery, Richard."

"Did she say what was wrong?"

"No, not really, just that Tommy had said it had not been well."

"I'll go and see it at lunch time," promised Richard. When he arrived at the bakery he went straight to the office, but Tommy's secretary said he was in the works. Richard found him in the mixing room, where the dough was being made in large vessels as tall as a man. Tommy was his usual cheerful self.

"Hello, Richard, come to see how the other half live?"

"No, just to see the cat and not waste your time."

"Right. I shut him in my car, so he wouldn't wander off," said Tommy, and led Richard into the garage. He opened the back door of the car and a black tom cat was sitting on the back seat. Its nose was soiled with yellow mucus and Richard noticed that it was breathing rapidly through its mouth. He picked it up and put it on the bench and he felt that it was just skin and bone under its fur. When he listened to its breathing through his stethoscope he heard many sounds and then the cat coughed–a soft cough.

"He seemed to get a really bad cold last week and began to lie about and go downhill quickly," said Tommy, "What's wrong with him?"

"A peculiar lung infection that I don't like, so I'm going to take a sample of that mucus and examine it."

In the stained preparation of the mucus Richard soon found TB germs, so he went and collected the cat and destroyed it. It had never been allowed in the bakery, being a warehouse cat, so there was no risk to Tommy or his staff, but Richard insisted that its box and bedding be burnt and its food bowl disposed of. This was the first case of TB he had diagnosed in the cat, and, being on the alert for the condition, found about one case a year for a few years. Apart from cases of TB he diagnosed doing the herd inspections, one of the most worrying conditions was calf scour, which was often combined with pneumonia. Where pedigree stock was concerned, some farmers were injecting each new-born calf with anti-calf scour serum, which Richard sold to them. He also supplied M & B 693 tablets and either powders or a medicine containing *Pulv opii* and kaolin. Most farmers kept these ready for use in any cases of scour. Flora often had to help Richard with the dispensing in the evenings and when John arrived he stuck on the labels.

During these autumn weeks it was all bed and work. Richard's only relaxation was listening to the news, and especially the ITMA show on the wireless and an occasional visit to the Palace Cinema. Though there was the blackout and everybody carried their gas mask, life continued much as usual in the pubs, clubs and cinemas, but times of opening were often shortened. The Vicar now held evensong at 3.00 p.m. because it was impossible to black out St. Lukes with its great East and West Windows, and those in the clerestory. But the smaller Methodist church had blackout curtains made and did not alter the times of its services, even though some parishioners were hurt by colliding with lamp posts and trees or falling over steps and kerb stones in the dark. As Christmas approached the shops put on a festive appearance and displayed beers and spirits; chocolate, toffee, and toys for the children, but a lot of evacuees went home.

On the Friday before Christmas, Jean and Mary came by train and brought with them a plum pudding and a loin of pork. There would be plenty for Christmas lunch, because Richard had ordered a turkey from Frank Wood. Because they had decided to have a get-together of their friends on Saturday evening 23rd December, the girls decorated the house. It had to be held in the evening because Fiona took her children to the pantomime and some of the men were going to the football match in Droughton. On that mild and fine evening all their friends came except Mary Bolton, and there was plenty of room for all, including Tommy Bishop, Jean, Fiona and her children, Gordon Hindle and Pat. The Vicar and Edna stayed only for a short time, because they had many calls to make that night, but dived into the sandwiches and mince pies along with the rest. It was a jolly, cheerful party which they all enjoyed because they had doubted whether they would be able to have one. Fiona gave the children a small box of chocolates, a toy and an orange each. The carol singers could be heard when they all left about 10.30 and drove away in the blackout. On Christmas Eve Richard missed the sound of the church bells being rung and was a little sad when he remembered how as a boy he listened to them while pretending to be asleep when his father and mother filled his stocking. He presumed Ted and Mary were both doing well in East Anglia though no information was given on their Christmas card; the message was "To Richard from Ted and Mary", in the latter's handwriting. He was annoyed that Flora had been ignored, tore the card into pieces and threw them on the fire.

On Christmas Day Richard was writing out an order for drugs, when Jean called that everything would be ready for lunch in ten minutes. Seconds later, when the 'phone rang, it was old Robert Parkinson who lived in Seaton and kept two cows on his smallholding. One of which was having difficulty in calving. Richard told the three women to have their lunch and not to wait for him. It was just as well he did, because as he delivered the live calf, the uterus prolapsed. This was replaced and the strappings put on the cow and he then injected her for milk fever. When he had washed and dressed he had a quick Christmas drink with the Parkinsons and was ravenously hungry when he arrived home. When he had eaten, he joined them in the lounge and Flora gave out the presents which were under the Christmas tree. She had bought him a Waterman fountain pen and for Flora Richard's present was a powder blue two-piece suit. Jean and Mary had bought the matching accessories for this and the three women spent the afternoon comparing notes about their respective wardrobes.

January began with some bitter weather and Richard bought a pair of leather gauntlet gloves and a Melton overcoat, even though the Austin was warmer than the Ford had been. He got very cold on farms where he had to wear his rubber parturition gown, which took a long time to dry, and his hands and arms became sore from slight frostbite. These became worse when he had to deal with an outbreak of what was locally known as Skipton disease. It was an infectious vulvo-vaginitis, which appeared in a small herd in Shipton village. The cows had a grey-coloured discharge from the vulva and were not holding to service. He examined each one, syringed the vagina with a solution of glycerol, thymol co., and showed the farmer how to use the Higginson syringe, advising him to treat each animal twice a day. Richard was glad to get fully dressed again and get back into the car. He drove a short distance down the lane, got out his Thermos flask, had a hot drink and felt better.

The next day he went to Bill Parkinson at Poolside and found some of his cows with the same infectious condition he had seen at Rose Farm the day before. Richard had presumed that the outbreak had been started by a cow which Harold Marsden had bought in Droughton some weeks before.

"Now then, what's wrong with them, Mr Holden?" asked Bill.

"It's an infectious condition which goes from cow to cow and is often brought in through a cow which has been bought."

"But I've not bought any."

"I thought you didn't, Bill. By the way, do you keep a bull?"

"Not me, I take my cows up to the bull at Eric Vickers. He's a good bull but he hasn't stopped these two cows and they calved in October."

Richard carried out the same treatment, and showed Bill how to continue it. He went back to Rose Farm and asked Harold if he took his cows to the bull at Pleasant View. Harold said that he did, but it was no good and he would have to find another bull in the area. Richard told him not to have any cows served until he came to examine them again. He went straight to Eric Vickers at Pleasant View who, though he was surprised to see Richard, asked him into the house out of earshot of the men.

"Well, Richard, what do you want?"

"Confidentially to ask you a few questions about your herd."

"Oh, what do you want to know?"

Richard explained the position in two herds he had examined without giving names and said that the common factor seemed to be Eric's bull.

"Now, what I want to know is, have you had any cows with a discharge and have any come over?"

"Well it's strange you should come today because I began to think something was wrong. You know, to avoid pick I buy new-calved Irish heifers, milk them once, get them in calf and sell them dry. Two have come over twice and I was going to ask you to come and wash them out tomorrow. The bull seems to be working as well as ever; I think most of them are in calf."

"Right, can I have a look at the bull?"

"Yes, of course," and they went across the yard and into the bull box. The big Shorthorn was securely tied up with two chains and Richard asked Eric to hold his ring while he examined him. He found no abnormality with his testicles and his tazzle was clean and almost dry.

"Right, let him go, Eric. What do you do when someone brings a cow for service?"

"I have a good look at the cow and then I bring a lading can out full of warm water with disinfectant in it. As he comes off the cow I give his pizzle a good splashing."

"You can't do more than that. Let's have a look at these two cows."

Richard found no signs of the infectious condition. One heifer had calved twins and held her cleansing for two days, the other appeared normal, so he irrigated the uterus in both cases with Lugol's solution diluted with water.

"Right, Eric, that's it. I'd be careful with your bull; don't let him serve any cows with a discharge, and disinfect him as carefully as you can."

"I will, Richard. That bull is one from Tim Tunstall, I've a lot of money at stake there."

Richard never did trace the source of the outbreak, and his hand and arms healed after liberal applications of Germoline ointment. The cows got better and a few were got in calf; the rest were fattened off for slaughter.

The last Saturday in January was a grey day with a bitter wind and light snow showers. In the afternoon after the surgery he went to Chapel House at Rushworth, twelve miles away, to treat two cows; one had a bad mastitis and the other was not eating. When they came out of the shippon John Priestley said:

"I don't like the look of it, the snow is beginning to stick, you'd better be off while I get everybody out and bring the sheep down to the in-by and the Dutch barn."

"Do you think it will be as bad as that?"

"I do, there has been snow about all day. I've lived here so long I know when it's coming."

"In that case here is another packet of sulphanilamide powders for that cow. Use them until she is better. Cheerio."

As he drove down the track to the main road, the snow was dusting everything white and the further he went the heavier it became. He was very cold, and as he had not got his flask with him, he stopped at the Cock Inn in Middleton and walked to the door through snow at least six inches deep, which the wind was blowing into drifts.

"Good afternoon, Mrs Sharples, can I have a hot toddy please?" asked Richard, as he walked across the room to warm himself at the fire.

"Of course you can, I'll just go and get the hot water."

Richard felt the hot drink bringing warmth back into his arms and legs.

"Are you off home now, Mr Holden?"

"Yes, I hope I've done my last call for today."

"Then I'd be off if I were you, the snow is getting heavier and you might not get up Beech Hill."

"I will; thank you, Mrs Sharples."

The snow was beginning to stick to the windscreen, so he wiped most of it off, turned the wipers on and set off on the last five miles to Sandhaven. Going up Beech Hill the back wheels began to spin, but the car kept going through the odd drift, which caused snow to blow over the radiator and onto the windscreen. He had met no other traffic and was worried as to what he should do if he got stuck. The car just made it over the brow of the hill and then Richard was cheered to see a cattle waggon turn out of Beech Tree Farm in the direction of Sandhaven. He followed close behind in its tracks, and after it turned left at Boundary Farm Richard drove on as fast as he dared through the howling whiteness as it became dark. When he turned into the yard at the surgery the snow was deep, and with a struggle he opened the garage doors, drove the car in, covered the engine with an old horserug and put the little paraffin heater under the radiator; then he carefully locked up. When he walked into the kitchen Flora was standing by the table.

"Oh Richard, am I glad to see you, I was getting dreadfully worried; it's become a real snowstorm this last half hour."

"Don't I know it, and the head lamp covers were blocking with snow, I could scarcely see where I was going. I know one thing, I'm not going out again today."

On the Sunday morning when Richard awoke it was still dark in the bedroom though the clock showed the time as 7.30 a.m. The reason for this was obvious when he drew back the curtain. The window was thickly covered with frozen snow. The fire in the kitchen stove was very low so, picking up the coal bucket and the shovel, he opened the door with Tommy at his heels. Neither he nor the dog however were prepared for the wall of snow which collapsed into the doorway. Looking out, Richard could see that the snow was at least a yard deep and had drifted up against the stable block to the height of the first floor windows, completely burying the garage doors; also it was strangely quiet. He shovelled out the snow and closed the door, and called to Flora to bring down the coal in the bucket in the lounge. When she came into the room Richard said:

"We can't get out, there is three feet of snow against the door."

"Well, what are we going to do?"

"First, tip that coal into the stove and open the draught regulator fully and then make breakfast, while I dig my way out with the spade from under the stairs and I'll try to get to the coal bunker."

When she called him twenty minutes later he was cold and wet owing to the snow melting, which had fallen onto his neck, or gone up his sleeves. Forgetting that rationing had started he asked:

"Is there no bacon, Flora?"

"No, we have eaten our ration but I have plenty of eggs, so you'll have to have porridge and then eggs tomorrow."

After breakfast he worked until he reached the coal bunker and filled every bucket he could find and brought them into the kitchen. He was lighting the lounge fire when he heard the noise of an engine being revved up outside, so he opened the window and saw that an Army truck was following a tractor which had an improvised snow plough fixed at the front. He watched the vehicles reach the Drill Hall and the tractor roughly cleared a path to the door, which then opened. Some troops came out and started to unload the truck. Richard closed the window and ran downstairs and told Flora that he was going out of the front door to see if he could reach the Drill Hall to get help in clearing a way into his back yard. The wind had blown the snow past the front door into the yard behind the house but, though it was deep in the garden, there was not more than a foot until he reached the road. When he got to the hall the men were eating their breakfast, which had been brought in the truck from a unit in the camp on the Shipton Road. He told the sergeant who he was and asked them to clear a way to the garage, so that he could get his car out.

It was after lunch that the tractor was driven into the yard and slowly pushed the snow aside, the men working hard digging the snow away from the tractor's path and throwing it up onto the walls at each side. When they had done all they could and the garage doors were open, Richard asked them all into the kitchen and Flora gave them all soup and bread. When they left, Richard gave the sergeant a bottle of whisky and told him to share it out among the lads.

He went into the garage, started the car's engine, and let it run for a bit while he refilled the paraffin heater. In case he had to use the car he put a spade, a strong rope and some sacks into the boot. Then he scattered ashes from the kitchen door across the yard to the garage between the walls of snow and to the dustbin. His next job was to contact the police who told him that the Droughton Road was open for four miles and that a car had got to Seaton, but all the country roads were blocked and most telephones were out of action. He spent the day shovelling snow off all the paths and making a way into Cross Street. There was nothing he could do about the five feet high walls of snow in the yard and in front of the house in Victoria Street.

On Monday morning there had been no more snow and everybody was busy snow-clearing. The Army tractor and an RAF bulldozer cleared a wider path down Victoria Street, followed by Council workmen who were digging a path to each house door and throwing the snow into trucks which were following. When Richard walked to the GPO to send his monthly returns to the Ministry of Agriculture and Fisheries, High Street had now an area of the road cleared for two lanes of traffic and the trucks were going down George Street and tipping the snow on the beach. Workmen loading the horse-drawn Council dust-carts were working in the side streets. When Richard arrived back at the surgery he found Clarence Jones from Little Parkside, who had come on horseback, sent by his father because they had a cow which couldn't calve. Richard drove cautiously because the few inches of snow left on the road had been pressed into ice by the heavy snow-clearing vehicles. It took him a long time to go the four miles, and when he got to the farm gate Stanley was waiting with a horse-drawn sledge, on which he had brought the milk cans to the gate for collection. Richard put his equipment onto the sledge and climbed on beside Stanley. The hard frozen snow was at least four feet deep and the peculiar mounds on the way to the farm were apple trees which were buried. When they reached the buildings, an area had been cleared near the shippon door and a hose pipe led from the kitchen window to a big metal bath. Mrs Jones and the daughter were letting the cows out two at a time to drink, because the trough in the yard was buried. The dead calf's swollen head was protruding from the vulva. Richard cut it off and then was able to reach the forelegs which were turned back and deliver the calf, the placenta coming with it. He put pessaries into the uterus and when Clarence arrived the three of them managed to get the cow to her feet. Having been taken to the car, he drove back to the surgery and went at once to a horse with colic on the docks. By lunchtime he had done two visits and was enjoying his meal when the telephone rang.

"A cow down with milk fever at Leach Farm, Middleton," said the post mistress, "And Jack Clough said it's in a bad way."

"Thank you, I'll try and get there as soon as I can. Do you know if Beech

Hill is open?"

"No it isn't, but the Seaton-Middleton road is."

This meant he had to go on past the two Parkside farms, until he reached the main road, and turn right for Middleton. The single track road ran between walls of snow which were between four and ten feet high. Jack, always in a hurry and brusque in manner, was waiting with a sledge drawn by a tractor—this had a four foot oblong of H angle iron bolted on in front of the radiator.

"I hoped you'd be coming soon or yon cow could be dead, get on."

"I've come as fast as I could, but it's only a single track, you know," said Richard.

"Get on, John, drive a bit faster can't you?"

The deeply unconscious cow was lying on her side in the dung channel and was blown.

"Quick," shouted Richard, "Pull the head up. John, get a bale and ram it under her shoulder."

Her head was pulled up with a rope put round her horns and tied to a boost stake. Richard ran to the house for warm water in which he put two bottles of injection and hurried back into the shippon.

Jack was shouting, "Get those two bales behind her properly!" which John and Robert struggled to do, Jack looking on.

"I wondered where the hell you'd gone to. Get cow injected quick."

"To warm the solution; if I put it in freezing cold it will kill her," said Richard.

"If you don't hurry up soon, she'll be dead."

Richard injected the first bottle very slowly and as he was attaching the second bottle the cow gave a long rumbling belch.

"I think she's going," shouted Jack.

Richard's patience was wearing thin. "I'll bet you ten bob she's not."

"Done," said Jack.

Richard steadily injected the solution; the cow moved her ears and blinked and her head came up. As he finished the injection, she struggled to get her legs under her body.

"Push her back end up and then let her head go," said Richard.

"Leave her head tied, John," said Jack.

"John, let her head go."

"You keep her tied, I want her up in her stall, not in the channel," shouted Jack.

Richard turned to him and said, "I'll have my ten bob and I'll go, you obviously don't need me."

"Ten bob! Go on, I was only joking; don't be so daft."

"Jack, when I am treating an animal I am in charge and I do my very best, so don't interfere. John, let her head go."

He did.

"Robert and John, lift on her tail. Jack, you lift there in front of her stifle and I'll do it this side, now heave!"

The cow got to her feet and they helped her into her stall. Richard at once examined her teats.

"Why are you looking at her bag?"

"Because, Jack, when a cow is trying to get into an upright position she must have her head loose to get her legs under her. If she had to struggle with her head fixed she would probably get a teat under her stifle or her hock and either split it or crush it. She's been lucky, no thanks to you."

"All right, you win; let's go and have some tea." Mary—Mrs Clough—was a very pleasant, friendly, quiet woman, who gave Richard a cup of tea and said:

"It was very good of you to get to her in your car through the ice and snow, thank you very much, Mr Holden."

Her husband in the background grunted his approval, but said nothing. John took Richard back to his car. The freezing wind was blowing snow dust about and the road surface was very slippery. He got into the car and realised the snow dust was freezing on the windscreen. It was almost dark when he got back to the surgery and found a woman who had been waiting with a dog since two o'clock. Richard apologised to the woman when Flora ushered her into the consulting room.

"I am sorry you have had to wait so long. Now, what can I do for you?"

"Will you look at Sandy, he has a lump at the top of his leg."

"Yes, which one?"

"His left one."

After he had muzzled the red setter he and Flora laid the dog on its right side and raised the left leg. Richard recognised a tumour of the axilla and touched it; the dog winced.

"How long has this been coming?"

"I don't know really, but he's been lame for three weeks and getting worse all the time. Can you do anything for him?"

"How old is he?" asked Richard.

"He's seven years old, sir."

"I am sorry, but I can't do anything for your dog. It is a tumour, growing quickly and already painful. The kindest thing I can do, is to destroy him."

The woman burst into tears and sobbed.

"What am I going to do? It's my husband's dog and being in the Terriers he was called up the first week of August and I don't know where he is. Can't you do anything?"

"It is impossible to operate because it is over all the armpit and I am certain it has grown around the artery and nerves there. There is no need to decide now; take him home and think about it. I think you will know when to bring him back."

"How much is it?"

"Nothing," said Richard, and the woman thanked him and left.

Flora said, "I am glad you didn't charge her, she has three children and the Army pays her thirty-eight shillings a week."

"Really, is that all? When she comes back I will destroy it for nothing."

Richard and Flora were almost in tears a week later, when Mrs Shaw and her three children said a very emotional farewell to Sandy. Five months later her husband was killed at Dunkirk.

It was a bitter, freezing night and at 8 o'clock next morning the police telephoned to say that Bill Crook at Oaks Farm had a cow calving and would Richard meet him at the shipyard where he was waiting with a horse and cart. Richard soon found him, and climbed into the cart with his equipment. The big Shire plodded on slowly into the freezing east wind and soon both men were perished with cold. It took a long time to reach the isolated farm and when they walked into the shippon the cow was dead.

"Well, that's a bad do," said Bill, "She was all right when I looked round last night, but she was straining hard to calve when I found her at half past six. What do you think has killed her Mr Holden?"

Richard looked into her mouth which was a pale bluish-white colour. There was no heart beat.

"She has burst inside, Bill, and bled to death."

"Can't we cut her throat and salvage her?"

"It's no use, Bill, she would not bleed. The only thing you can do is drag her outside until Whiteside can collect her."

"Very well. Will you let him know for me?"

"I'll do that, Bill."

Richard felt sorry for Bill; he was only in a small way of business, having twelve milking cows, and the loss of one was a drain on his capital.

The next morning the visit was to a cow down with her calf bed out at Church Farm and again after a slow journey on a horse-drawn sledge the cow was dead on arrival. During that dreadful week most animals died or were dead when Richard arrived and he had difficulty in doing four visits in a day. When he managed to talk to Bob Whiteside later in the week, he learned that there were many dead cattle to collect and hundreds of sheep, and Richard wondered how John Priestley had got on at Chapel House.

At the beginning of the week milk and eggs were in short supply, but now the farmers near to Sandhaven were bringing milk in every day using a pony and trap. Further away, the isolated farms could do nothing with their milk but pour it down the drain or make cheese or butter.

The Council workmen and volunteers worked all day every day snow-clearing. By the middle of February, the milk lorry could reach almost all the farms in the area and Richard could get through a normal day's work and begin to attack the backlog of work waiting to be done for the Ministry of Agriculture and Fisheries.

One day when he visited a farm on the Wilton-Ridgeton road near to the Gillingham Asylum the farmer told him that on the Monday night in the week after the Saturday snowstorm, because he was completely cut off from the outside world, instead of pouring milk down the drain, he and his wife had started making butter and cheese. On the Thursday afternoon he heard the sound of engines and went along the track from the farm as far as he had cleared it. Then by sledge he reached the road and found a small army of men with a bulldozer and vehicles digging a road to the asylum, where yeast and flour were urgently needed so that bread could be baked to feed the thousand inmates. On the Friday they had opened the road to the farm and so he was able again to send the milk to the Board's factory.

In 1938, when electricity had been laid on to some farms, some owner occupiers had water bowls fitted in the shippons and an electric hot water heater fitted in the dairy; a few even had an electric milking machine. Jack Booth at Intack was one of these. One March morning at 6.00 a.m. he rang Richard to say he had two cows dead. On arriving at the farm, Richard found Jack and two men in the long single shippon which had the dairy built on at one end. The dead cows were the first two in from the brick dairy wall, which was shut off from the shippon under the eaves by a triangle of corrugated iron.

"Good morning, Jack, what has happened?"

"I'm not sure, Richard, but I think it's the electric that's killed them."

"Oh, how, Jack?"

"Well you see, I go in the diary about quarter to six and switch on the milking machine and the water boiler. I saw Dave here ride up on his bike and he went into the shippon through the big door halfway down. He flung the dairy sliding door open and shouted, "Quick! four cows are having fits!" As I ran in the first two dropped to the floor, so I climbed in between to loose their chains. When I touched the first one, I got a shock up my arm, so I bawled at Dave to switch off. The other two which were twitching and slavering stopped, and you can see they are better now."

"That's a queer do, Jack. Who put the electric in?"

"Droughton Corporation Electricity Department."

"I think you had better ring them straight away to come and test the wiring, because it will be fatal to turn the electricity on again."

Jack went off to the house to telephone and Richard took blood samples from the ears of both dead cows to examine them for anthrax, though he did not expect to find the disease.

Jack came back and said, "They'll be here at 7 o'clock. I'll put the drive belt on the old engine and get on milking."

"Yes, I'd do that, don't turn the electricity on. I'll go and examine these blood films and then I'll come back."

There were no anthrax germs in the blood films, so Richard went back to the farm and found two workmen from the Electricity Department checking all the electrical equipment and wiring, while Jack was answering their questions. One workman brought a ladder, put it against the shippon wall in the dairy, and climbed up to check a power cable which ran along the ridge beam.

"Mr Booth, who nailed the corrugated iron up here to shut off the dairy from the shippon?"

"I did, why, what's wrong with it?"

"The cable is rubbed through by the rough edge of the iron and the wires are bare. You see, the top edge of the iron isn't nailed to anything and you see how I can move it with my hand backwards and forwards. That's what the wind would do every time you opened the dairy door. The cable should have been in a duct."

"I see. Will you pull the iron down, then, and fit a new cable in a duct?"

"We will, Mr Booth; you know, you could have electrocuted yourself at any time once those wires were bare."

"Yes. I never thought when I nailed that iron sheet up there, I only put it up to stop the draught blowing on to the first cows in this shippon."

"Well, in future if you are doing alterations involving power or even lighting cables, let us know and we will come and advise you."

Richard went home in a sober frame of mind and rang up Bill Wallace to come and fit some more plugs in the dispensary, because the centrifuge, the bench light and the bowl electric fire were all working off one plug; the wires trailed across the floor where they could have got wet or even cut through.

Richard was finishing his breakfast when the phone rang and Flora went and answered it. She came running back, calling:

"Richard, Richard, I must go to mother!"

"Whatever's happened, love?"

"She's fallen down the stairs; that was our Mary; and she's broken her arm and the doctor thinks probably her leg as well."

"Oh, I am sorry Flora, poor Jean; now I'll go and get Marjorie while you get ready. I'll ask her to stay all day and then I'll take you to the station—you'll be in time for that train just before nine."

"Yes, do that, Richard. I'll be ready when you get back."

When Richard went to the Market Café for lunch, he met Dick Williams the abattoir manager, and they talked while they were having their meal. Richard asked him if the rationing of meat had lessened his work, to which Dick replied that he had never been busier since Woolton had become

Minister of Food. He thought however that the scheme of rationing was inequitable because if you had the money you could have lovely meat meals in the hotels and restaurants, while poor people had to manage with their ration. They agreed that at present the system was not having a very great effect on their lives. Richard asked him if any special arrangements had been made to receive casualty animals after closing time and Dick told him the emergency number, which information was very useful later. When Flora returned, the news was better than expected; Jean had broken her left wrist and a rib, but her left leg was only very badly bruised and she only had to stay in hospital overnight.

During March and April many cases of twin lamb disease occurred in which ewes heavy with lamb stopped eating, twitched and tumbled or lay about reluctant to move, and in the latter stages were oblivious to their surroundings. As it was the end of the winter, the ewes were in poor flesh and not fit for slaughter, so the farmer had the double loss both of the ewe and of her lambs. Richard injected many with calcium borogluconate solution. A few responded, but many died, so he telephoned the Department of Veterinary Pathology in Liverpool for advice. The person who answered the phone told Richard that he had the right department, and so he said:

"This is R.B. Holden. I am in practice in Sandhaven and would like to speak to a member of staff."

"And how are you, Richard? This is Norman Robinson speaking. What do you want to know?"

"Well, it is a nice surprise, Norman. I am very well and I hope you are. I want some advice about pregnancy toxaemia of sheep."

Richard got the information he required and also learnt that Norman had qualified in 1933 and was doing research in veterinary pathology. He had not married, though he was almost twenty-nine years old, and he lived in a house not far from the digs of their student days. They promised to keep in touch.

Richard thought, Joe Fowler never alters, when he got the message to go at once to a colt bleeding badly. When he arrived he found the colt had a long wound extending from the shoulder along the chest wall.

"How's this happened, Joe?"

"I was taking him out on a halter when he started playing up. He got away on me and ran into that barbed wire near the Dutch barn. I'm keeping him to see if he makes a good stallion, so I want that sewn up nicely."

"I'll do that, now let's have some help."

"There's only Dave here and me."

"Where's your lad Harold, then?"

"Oh didn't you know, he's married Mary Waring from Beacon Farm and George and me have set him up at Birchnott near Ridgeton. I expect you'll be hearing from him some time. Now what do you want?"

Before long, they had the blindfolds on and a twitch applied. After inject-

ing local anaesthetic, Richard ligated two small arteries and then painstak-
ingly sutured the wound.

"Well, you've made a decent job of that, Richard, I must say."

"Yes, it doesn't look too bad. I'll give him an injection against lockjaw and
then you can get the blinds and the twitch off him. I'll give you the neck
cradle; keep it on all the time so he doesn't lick or bite that wound. Here is
some wound oil, put it on once a day."

He was pleased it had healed very well when he took out the stitches, ten
days later, and Joe at once turned the colt out. Then he injected a cow intravenously with glucose solution because it was suffering from slow fever and
gave Joe a pint bottle of black draught which contained black treacle and ep-
som salts and twelve powders with which to continue treatment. If this didn't
work, Richard told him to turn the cow out in the paddock where the first
grass of spring was showing green.

With the spring the amount of work lessened, and Richard operated on a
big gelding with fistulous withers in April. It belonged to the Cooperative
Society, was skewbald in colour and loved any titbits people gave to it. The
operation went well and as soon as the news leaked out, a regular procession
of children took lumps of sugar, bread and apples to their favourite horse,
Brownie. The local reporter wrote a short note about the horse's progress
every week until it appeared on the streets again in the summer and
Brownie's "doctor" was often mentioned. Richard never discovered who
among the veterinary surgeons in the area reported this to the Royal College
of Veterinary Surgeons. He received a letter from the Registrar, Fred
Bullock, asking for an explanation why his name had appeared in the press
regarding the horse, because this amounted to indirect advertising and was
not permitted. He replied that he had never given permission for his name to
be mentioned, nor met the reporter, but that the friendly horse was a great
favourite with children, as was his driver, and so the need had arisen for the
public to be kept informed as to the progress of the case. In reply, the Royal
College told him in future to preserve his anonymity and not to reveal the
location of his practice, and he was warned as to his future conduct.

He could scarcely believe that a year had passed since he took over the
practice, when George Duke telephoned to say he would be collecting all the
books, receipts etc. the next day. A fortnight later he and Flora were
delighted to see that the Income and Expenditure account showed a good
profit and that the total at the bottom of the balance sheet had increased by
£260.

During the month he examined herds in the morning and the evening and
finally wiped out the backlog of work waiting to be done for the Ministry of
Agriculture and Fisheries. He was appalled by the number of tubercular
cows he found, and by the advanced state of the disease in the animals when

he made the post mortem. He had two herds to examine in the tiny village of Marhey. The big one was at Old Hall Farm and after examining all the cows and the bull he had to tell Tom Lee that the only thing he had found wrong was a slight mastitis in two cows' udders, to treat which he gave Tom a packet of powders. He then went to 4 Meadow Bank. This was the last of a row of cottages which had been built for farm workers at the end of the last century. Behind each cottage was a long garden. They were about half way between Marhey and Teston, and George Smith who lived at Number 4 worked on a farm in Teston. He kept two cows at Meadow Bank and was waiting for Richard when he arrived.

"Are you the vet from the Ministry?"

"Yes, I'm Mr Holden, and you are Mr G. Smith?"

"Yes."

"Good, where are your cows?"

"In the shed at the back of the house, follow me."

The path wound round the cottage which was in a ramshackle state and the cowshed was even worse. There Richard examined two cows, one in fair condition which was going dry and another which was very thin which George said had been calved six weeks. It had a tuberculous hind quarter.

"How long has this quarter been like this?"

"Since she calved, she had a bit of mastitis and it left it hard."

"This is not the result of the mastitis, it is a tuberculous quarter so I must give you this Form A at once. You'll see it says you must not dispose of the animal and any milk from it must not be used for human consumption."

"But I sell milk to the three cottages."

"Listen, I have just told you, that milk has to be thrown away."

"Things are hard enough; I've my little girl in hospital and now I've no milk to sell and you're going to take my cow. How much are you going to give me for it?"

"Ten pounds," said Richard.

"Is that all? I won't take that."

"If you don't accept my valuation, an independent valuer will be sent, who may give you less."

Richard felt no sympathy for a man who for a few coppers was exposing his own family and his neighbours to the deadly disease. In the end George Smith signed the valuation form. Examined microscopically the milk sample showed many TB germs and at the post mortem the cow was found to be an advanced case, so Smith received £2 10s. 0d. From the new doctor in Wyreham, Dr Kershaw, Richard later learned that George Smith's daughter had a TB hip and another child from the first cottage had glandular TB. Both children recovered after a long time in the Children's Hospital, though Betty Smith walked with a built-up boot on her left leg for the rest of her life.

As he had been so busy that week Richard had arranged to castrate one cat and spay another on Saturday afternoon after the surgery had finished. It was late in the afternoon before he began operating, helped by Flora. He operated on the female cat first, using ether oxygen for the anaesthetic, and had just finished dealing with the tom cat when, in his breezy manner, John walked in to receive his instructions, pulled out his lighter and flicked it on to light his cigarette. The bang of the explosion stunned Richard for a second and as bits of glass fell to the floor, the remains of the anaesthetic apparatus blazed furiously, sending off dense black smoke.

Richard grabbed a towel, threw it over the blazing mass and picked it up, shouting, "Open the front door, quick, John!" and he ran to the front steps and threw the lot in the front garden.

"Get a shovel, John, and throw soil all over it."

As he walked back into the surgery he was aware of a loud buzzing in his ears, but went up to Flora who was leaning on the table,

"Flora, are you all right?"

"Yes, Richard, I was just bending down putting the cat in its basket when the bang came. I'm OK, but what about the windows?"

Richard then noticed that a side window had been blown out and the lower half of the big bay window was shattered. John came in, very contrite.

"Oh, I am sorry, Mr Holden, I didn't know it would blow up like that."

"Of course you didn't. It's my stupid fault. I should have had a notice on the door long ago to say no smoking and no naked lights. I'll get two printed in red on Monday. For now, John, get on your bike and go to Tom Wright, you know, the plumber in Shipton Street and tell him to come at once and get those windows repaired."

John was off in a rush, and Flora and Richard cleared up the broken glass inside and out and threw it along with the ruined anaesthetic apparatus into the dustbin. The windows were replaced before it went dark and neither cat took any harm. Nevertheless, he decided to use Nembutal intravenously in future if possible. It was pentobarbitone and came in yellow capsules containing 1½ grains of the drug, a white powder. This he dissolved in sterile water before use. He bought some very fine hypodermic needles and soon became expert at giving intravenous injections in the dog and cat. But he obtained another ether-oxygen anaesthetic apparatus which he used for very vicious or wild cats, which were difficult to restrain. The red "No smoking" notices were plain to see, and spent matches, fag ends and empty Woodbine packets disappeared from the waiting room floor!

On Thursday 9th May at 11 o'clock Richard had just got into bed when the phone rang. He picked it up.

"Holden, Veterinary Surgeon."

"This is Harold Fowler at Birchnott near Ridgeton. Duchess, our big mare, can't foal. Will you come at once?"

"Yes, Harold, when did she start?"

"About half an hour ago; the bag's burst, but nothing's happened."

"Right, Harold, I'll set off right away. I'll want some hot water, soap and a towel and a strong box or a bale to stand on. I'll see you soon."

"How far is that place?" asked Flora.

"About twenty miles, so I won't be back till three or four."

He put everything he thought he might need in the car and set off on the lovely moonlit night. He was glad of the moonlight because the cowled headlamps gave so little light.

When he stopped the car in the farmyard, he lowered the window as a figure approached. It was Joe Fowler.

"Good evening, Richard. I'm glad you haven't taken long. She's one of my best mares."

"Right, Joe, take this bag; I'll bring the rest of my stuff."

Standing on a strong box, he disinfected the mare's vulva and began to explore the position of the foal. The foal's head was turned back towards the mare's tail and all Richard could feel was the base of the neck.

"What's wrong, Richard?" asked Joe.

"Head's right back."

"Hell that's a bad do, what can you do for her?"

Richard explained how he wanted to reach the eye and fix a blunt hook in it to see if he could pull the head round. He tried for a long time but when he had hold of an ear of the foal the mare strained and squeezed his arms so hard that he had to let go.

He now explained to Joe that he was going to take the foal's leg off at the shoulder and then put sharp hooks in its neck and pull the head and neck nearer the vulva. After working for half an hour he had cut the leg free on the inside, but he could not work to cut the skin away behind the shoulder because the mare strained so hard. He withdrew his arm and said to Joe:

"There's only one thing I can do and that is to chloroform her to stop her straining. It's risky, but do you agree?"

"If that's the only way to foal her, I agree."

"All right, let's have a thick bed of straw down first, and Harold, can you go and get two more men to help. Joe, let's have some more hot water. When they come back, I'll put the hobbles on, then the chloroform mask and when she starts to wobble we will pull her down. I want her lying on her near side if possible."

Everything for once went according to plan. Joe was in charge of the chloroform. Harold pulled on a rope attached to the leg and Richard quickly cut through the skin with the embryotomy knife and out came the leg.

Richard watched the mare's breathing, which was very regular, got down on his knees and soon fixed a sharp hook in the foal's neck. "Pull steadily, Harold."

Richard pushed the foal's chest away and slowly the head came towards him until he could put a sharp hook in the eye. He removed the first hook and when Harold pulled again Richard got his fingers in the foal's nostrils and pulled the head towards him and downwards.

He told Joe to take the mask off, took a rope and fixed it to the remaining leg, made certain the hooks were fast in both eyes and they and the two men all pulled together. Out came the foal steadily; and then the afterbirth. Richard had never felt such a sense of triumph and relief before. He made Joe and one of the men hold the mare's head down and he put two pessaries and two handfuls of sterile sulphanilamide into the uterus. Then he took the D out of the chain and let the hobbles fall off. The mare was recovering rapidly and when they couldn't keep her head down they pushed her into an upright position.

Richard took off his overall, washed and dressed and they made the mare rise. Richard went to the foal and turned the head back to the position it had been in inside the mare; it was as long as his arm.

"I can see now why you couldn't reach it," said Joe, "especially with her straining like that. Harold, put a rug on her and clear up. I'll help you put your tackle in the car and then we'll go in the house for a drink of tea."

Richard felt exhausted when he sat down by the fire and slowly drank the strong, sweet tea. Joe and Harold came in with the two men, for their mugs of tea.

"I can't thank you enough, Richard, for getting that foal. Do you think she'll be all right?"

"Yes, she's not torn; and I checked that cleansing, it's all there. So I'd give her a drink of aired water and some hay, and I'll be off home."

Richard walked into Cross Street at half past five, to be met by Flora wearing her dressing gown.

"I've just taken a message from Brian Halhead at Meetham Lodge. He has a cow down with milk fever in a bad way. Do you want a cup of tea?"

"No, I've had a mug and some cake at Fowler's. I'll go and get this done and then I'll be ready for my breakfast and a rest."

When he got to the Lodge he had to go on a tractor down a green lane and across a field to reach the cow. He injected two lots of solution intravenously. When he left her later she was sitting up, but would not get up. When he got back to the buildings, Brian came out of a box and said:

"Hello, Mr Holden, how is she?"

"She's sitting up and quite bright, she should get up soon."

"Good. Can you have a look at this cow in the box; she can't calve."

When Richard put on his wet overall Brian said:

"So you've calved one already this morning."

"No I haven't, I've been at Fowler's at Birchnott all night foaling a mare."

As he corrected the malpresentation he realised how his arms ached, but soon he delivered a live calf. When they came out of the box the cow which had had milk fever was standing at the shippon door waiting to go in. Richard said "Don't milk her."

As he walked into the kitchen at Cross Street Flora came running through and said, "I've just been listening to the eight o'clock news. Hitler has invaded Belgium and Holland and the Army is moving to help Belgium."

Richard said, "So the balloon's gone up, what a night! I'll never forget it."

He never did, the memory of that night of struggle and tiredness followed by the dramatic ending of the "Phoney War" with the coming of morning, was never erased by the passing of the years. They listened to the news at one o'clock, which said that Brussels and Lille had been bombed.

"Richard what are we going to do? That's only about four hundred miles away. They might start bombing us soon."

"Really, Flora, I've been so busy I've never thought about it, but I wouldn't like to have to run to one of the shelters in George Street or on East Promenade if bombs were falling. I think I'd rather stop here."

"I agree, but where would we go? We haven't got a cellar, and I don't feel like being under the stairs with all the house on top of us."

They finally decided to make a shelter in the stable block because the ground floor was eight feet high, and a big beam in the ceiling ran the length of the building, strongly supported in the centre where the stairs went up to the loft. The news that Winston Churchill had been made Prime Minister didn't affect Richard much at the time, but his speeches cheered him up no end, and he made a point of listening to every speech he could. The building of the air raid shelter was postponed for a bit.

Richard had to foal only two mares that season, but the foals were a source of trouble. He treated sleepy foals which would not suck; constipated foals; and others with joint ill. He was very disappointed when a foal developed joint ill after he had vaccinated the mare with joint ill mixed bacterin, and the owner had some harsh words to say about the efficiency of vaccines! There was even more grumbling about mastitis in cows, which was increasing in frequency and severity and not responding so well to sulphanilamide treatment. This was often because the invading organism was the staphylococcus and the use of machine milking on more farms was one of the agents causing its spread. A few farmers were interested in the Panel Scheme which had been agreed between the NFU, the Ministry of Agriculture and Fisheries and the National Veterinary Medical Association which had been started for the control of bovine mastitis, contagious abortion, Johne's disease and infertility. It also provided for bovine pregnancy diagnosis; a free diagnostic service, and cheap sulphanilamide. During the year three farms joined the scheme and Richard began to make the required quarterly visits to the farms.

When Anthony Eden broadcast an appeal for Local Defence Volunteers, Richard was very keen to join and some days later went to the drill hall to an inaugural meeting. There were about forty men present and it was decided to appeal for more men to come to a meeting in a week's time to be enrolled. This was held in the sports pavilion at the Grammar School, Albert Road. Col. Laycarte-Porter and Major McNicoll, both retired officers, were in charge, and it was business-like. Forms were filled in, but they declined Richard's offer to serve because his movements were so unpredictable. With the news going from bad to worse and the evacuation from Dunkirk, Richard began to think that in the near future he would be defending his own home against German troops parachuting down, and yet it all somehow seemed unreal as in the lovely weather he drove along quiet country roads doing the job he loved so well.

But the news reels at the Palace on Saturday night rammed home the fact that every day the tide of war was flowing nearer, especially with the fall of France. What brought the reality of it home to Flora and Richard was the fact that eggs though rationed were in very short supply! What next?

Jean Dickinson came to stay for a few days. She was completely recovered from her fall, except for a lump just above her left wrist, which was stiff. She brought the news that Bill had got his calling up papers and so had Richard's cousin Harry Holden at Alresford. Uncle Harry was in the LDVs in the local platoon, which was part of a company commanded from Winchester, and the route march there and back to the village had nearly finished off half of them, who had got out of the habit of marching!

Nearer home, at Sandhaven, they drilled on the King George V playing fields, the Memorial fields for the king for whom they had fought in the first world war, and many of them wore a row of medals. They placed their chief observation post on the top of Beech Hill and after dark often stopped Richard to check his identity. When they had a night exercise they manned the pill boxes on Middleton Road and Droughton Road and soon afterwards all the road signs were taken down and signposts removed. Richard often had to run back to his car to immobilize it, by taking out the rotor arm. Soon he had to apply to the Regional Office to get supplementary petrol coupons because as he did more farm work his original allocation was not enough, and he always had a can containing a gallon of petrol in the car to use if the tank was getting empty. He made certain that every night he called at Hindle's garage and had the tank topped up and did this for the rest of his life.

In July the weather was hot and one or two colic cases happened every week among the horses belonging to the docks, the railways or to the various trades which used horse transport. Early one evening he went to treat one of Uncle Tom's horses and then went on to the steel works to treat one of theirs. A tank factory had been built, next to the vehicle works, and near to the steel works, ten miles south of Droughton. It was the first time he had visited the works, but as it was daylight he easily found the huge complex and after two identity checks reached the stables. The head horseman Tommy Atherton was waiting for Richard, holding a great 18.1 hands black Shire gelding by a rope attached to his head collar. He treated it for spasmodic colic and while they waited to see if the four gallons of medicated water would stop the colicky spasms, Richard looked at the other five Shires in the stable, and gave Tommy such medicines including horse balls, liniments, and powders which Richard decided he should keep by him for first aid treatment. The horses were in very good condition and the stable, loose box and tack room all very well kept. Richard left when the horse was quiet after about half an hour. He checked the milometer reading on leaving the works and on arriving home; it was twenty-three miles. With more people keeping pigs there were more outbreaks of swine erysipelas, and Richard treated two sows at George Whiteside's Seedhill Farm.

At Marhey on the main Sandhaven-Droughton Road, the big bend had been straightened out by making a wide new road across the base of the triangle. As a result, Old Hall Farm was half a mile up the old road, but only two hundred yards if you left your car on the main road, climbed the stile, and followed the path over to the farm. Richard was with Tom Lee in the shippon at Old Hall one morning in August examining a cow which was ill, when one of his men came running in and said:

"Boss, that new Dr Kershaw is coming across the front pasture."

"He can't be, George. The damned fool, is the bull in with the cows this morning?"

"Yes, you told me to turn him out to see if those two cows are bulling today."

"Aye, I did. You go and get both shotguns from the house, and a box of cartridges and bring them to the yard gate quick. Come on, Mr Holden, bring that pitch fork with you. Frank, Frank come here quick!" he shouted. Frank came at the double and they all ran to the yard gate and there half way between the main road and the farm was Dr Kershaw, carrying his black bag and blithely walking along, not knowing that the Friesian stock bull, a huge animal, was about thirty yards behind him, stalking him. Two men came with pitch forks, and Frank with the guns.

"Frank, give me one loaded gun and you have the other. If the bull rushes forward fire one barrel over his head. Keep the other barrel until we can hit him. George, go and get Bracken and keep hold of him; if we have to fire let him go, he'll worry that bull as he hates him. You three spread out along the hedge and be ready to jump through and divert him as he comes forward and grab the doctor."

They took up their positions, and with mounting tension and excitement watched as the doctor came nearer and the bull closed the gap between them. He would be about twenty paces from the hedge when the bull charged.

Tom bellowed, "Quick! Dr Kershaw, run like hell towards me."

The doctor did, Tom opened the gate, Frank fired into the air and Bracken in a flash was at the bull which turned away. The doctor almost collapsed into Tom's and Richard's arms.

He was shocked and white-faced.

"Mr Lee, I can't thank you enough for what you have just done for me. I didn't know you turned the bull out with the cows; he could have killed me. Thank you so much. I've never lived in the country before."

"Yes, it was lucky George here spotted you. Come along to the house. George, get that damned dog back and Frank, unload those guns. Come on, Mr Holden."

Tom gave the Doctor a whisky and water, and Richard drank tea, which he preferred, while he listened as Dr Kershaw told them that he had been born in London and after qualifying as a doctor had lived for five years in Birmingham. After the death of his father-in-law he had come to Wyreham six months ago and until this episode had been very happy to live and practise in this lovely rural area. He then picked up his bag and said to Tom:

"Now, where is the patient?" and together they left the room to go and see Mrs Lee.

Richard excused himself and drove away to get on with his day's work. A policeman stopped him as he reached Ryton and told him that there was an air raid alert, asked him to take cover and directed him to a shelter down the road. As he reached it the "all clear" sounded, the second false alarm in a week. Richard had followed the course of the aerial battles in the south in the newspapers and seen the photographs of shot-down enemy planes and captured pilots. This made him determined to make their air raid shelter ready, because it was now obvious that sooner or later they would be bombed. For two nights that week, with Dick Hoggarth, he worked bolting two lengths of telegraph pole to the main beam in the stable, giving it maximum support. The brick wall for the loose box was very substantial and an old door closed off the other side of the space under the stairs. Inside they put up shelves, and soon a teapot, cups and saucers were brought in by Flora, together with a whole pile of things she thought might be needed in the refuge room: two old chairs and a table; later she bought two camp beds, and by then the room was fairly full. In the house, Flora was finding cooking more difficult, with meat, ham, butter, fats, and now tea rationed and even eggs in short supply. She asked Richard to try and get eggs, butter or cheese on the farms, but he refused to ask, saying it was not professional to try and take advantage of his position. This attitude irritated her, but one bright spot was that the mortgage had gone down again, they were paying it off steadily.

This hot August weather brought more work, with pigs ill, cows with summer mastitis, and a condition Richard had not seen for some years. George Meadows at Boundary rang up in the afternoon to report a cow dead in the field. As with George he walked towards the cow, Richard asked:

"Has she been having cake?"

"No. The milk has gone up since I turned the cows in here at the beginning of the week. I took a hay crop off it and that shower of rain really has brought it on. She was all right this morning."

As he took a blood sample from the ear, Richard noticed that there was a mound of foam around the cow's nostrils and that the carcase was fairly blown.

"I think this will be negative, George; if it is, I'll ask Whiteside to meet me here and open her; is that O.K.?"

"Yes, Richard, do that while I go and get on milking."

The blood smear was negative and Richard met Bob Whiteside at seven o'clock after being told it was negative for anthrax, George had dragged the carcase using a tractor into the farm yard. Bob quickly opened the carcase and got out the lungs which were huge. When cut into, froth slowly oozed out of them.

"George, you've got fog fever here."

"Well, what is it? I've never had it before."

"We don't really know, but it always appears where the aftermath has grown up very thick and lush—really foggy like this pasture has."

"But I always put the cows in here about now, because this grows up strong, being a water meadow really, with the boundary brook running down that side."

"Well, in the present weather conditions it is obviously not safe to leave them in here. I would ration them for a few days. You know, put them in for an hour first day, then two hours the next and so on."

"Right, I'll do that if it's the answer, but my milk will go down."

"George, I'm not saying it's the answer, we don't know the answer, but it is the best thing to do if you don't want another."

George was short of pasture, because he had ploughed up land for potatoes and oats, so he used the meadow for two more days, when a second cow was found dead. He, cursing the War Agricultural Committee, then did what Richard had advised and that was the end of the outbreak. When a heifer was found dead at Sykes, the next farm, Richard wondered if there was a connection, until the post mortem showed husk. He had to treat fifteen strong animals, a tiring job on a hot autumn day. Again, he had to go to

Uncle Tom's to treat the same horse which had had colic three weeks before. He took a gag and some tooth rasps with him. After administering the medicine, he got Tom and Frank to stand each side of the horse's head and hold the gag while he examined its mouth. He then saw that it was an old horse and its molar teeth were in a badly worn condition.

"You know, Uncle, this horse should have been attended to sooner; its back teeth are badly worn. It must have been dropping its food or quidding for some time."

"Richard, you rasped its teeth at the beginning of the year and it's always been a dirty eater. It's really old age, isn't it?"

"Yes, it is."

"Then I'll put it out to grass, and when it's fattened up a bit, I'll sell it for meat. What with coal rationing and this hot summer, I can do with a mouth less."

"I think that's probably the best thing to do; you see, it's gone a lot easier already. I think these colics are all caused by badly chewed-up food."

"Put it in the box, Frank, and come on, Richard, we will go and have a cup of tea."

Auntie Nellie made the tea, and as Frank came in she said:

"Richard, did Frank tell you he has been called up?"

"No, you didn't, Frank, when did this come?"

"Two days ago. I've to go for the medical next Thursday."

"What are you going to do, Uncle? This will be the second man to go. If it goes on like this you'll have Auntie driving one of the lorries."

"That's probably what it will come to. I don't mean you, Nellie, but Billy Leigh's wife, she is hard up on her Army allowance. I saw her a week ago; she can't go and leave her little lad, so offered to work part time."

Richard put his cup down and said, "I must go, thank you for the tea," and, turning to Frank, "Well, Frank, I wish you all the best and when you get leave come and see me and Flora, won't you."

"Yes, I'll do that." They shook hands, and they all came to see Richard leave. He for some strange reason felt he would not see Frank again, and momentarily felt intensely sad.

He arrived home to find a very worried Flora—Tommy had got out and disappeared. He always followed her about, and when she had answered the bell and opened the front door, he had brushed past her, run round the caller, then jumped over the front gate and run into Victoria Street. As an hour had elapsed since he ran away, Richard walked to the police station to inquire if he had been taken there. He had not, but one constable said that he had seen a group of dogs fighting on the beach and he was certain one was a brown and white one. He walked along the East Promenade, but there were no dogs in sight, so he went home. Tommy was there with a bloodstained bandage round his head and Flora in tears.

"Now, what's happened? Did someone bring him back?"

"No, he was whining at the back door a bit since and his white ear is all chewed and torn. I've bandaged it as well as I could."

"There's no need to cry, love, come on and hold him."

He picked up Tommy and carried him into the surgery. When the bandage was removed he saw that half of the ear flap had been torn across and was hanging by a thread, and the rest was badly lacerated. Richard anaesthetised him by injecting a small dose of Nembutal intravenously, cut away the torn cartilaginous part and was able to suture the inner and outer layers of skin so that they covered the cartilage. The flap was now about an inch long, just covering the aural canal. After that there was no mistaking the vet's dog which had one brown ear on a white head. He persisted in escaping, which Richard attributed to his sexual appetite, so he castrated him. This operation appeared to cure him, but soon he began to escape again and one afternoon came back on three legs. He had a bad overriding fracture of the left femur. When Richard examined him under a light anaesthetic he could feel three separate pieces of the femur, and there was damage to the hip joint. Tommy lived in the hospital room for six weeks and the femur's fractured pieces roughly united, but the leg was an inch shorter than the other hind leg. In spite of this he still escaped often by jumping over the gate, and they could not understand the reason for this until, over a period, people's remarks about Tommy gave the answer to the riddle.

The first clue was provided by Frank Wood the butcher, when Richard called in the shop to treat his big old cat.

"Hello, Richard, you've just missed your dog."

"What do you mean, Frank?"

"Don't you know? he comes here two or three mornings a week and sits outside and howls until I throw a bone to him when he picks it up and runs off down Bath Street to the Beach."

"No! Really, I didn't know that, Frank. Look, if he's a nuisance, ring Flora and she'll come and take him home. Honestly, we didn't know where he went to and I think if you don't feed him he'd soon pack up coming."
the same trick there, Walter's told me."

"Well, that takes the biscuit; anyway, thanks for telling me, Frank; we will try and keep him in more."

Later, Richard drove along the Promenade and could see Tommy happily chasing seagulls all on his own. He went to Wilkinson's the ironmongers and bought a steel dog chain, and when he arrived home he fixed it just inside the kitchen door. When Tommy came home he was fastened to the chain by his collar and sulked until Flora took him for a walk after tea; and Richard began to take him for a walk before breakfast, whenever he could.

When autumn approached, the weather was even finer as the news became worse and more laconic. When the news reader said: "Enemy planes attacked targets in south England today and damage was caused. Four enemy planes were destroyed", Richard felt frustrated by the lack of detailed information, yet exhilarated because we were winning the battles with enemy planes. But the seriousness of the situation was underlined by petrol rationing becoming very strict and he sent a diary of visits he made and the mileage with his next application for petrol coupons. He received three quarters of what he had applied for, and was told to apply for supplementary coupons if required. It was for making a useless journey which wasted petrol that caused Chris Robson the cattle remover to have a row with Richard.

Bob Barker at High Moor sent a message that he had a cow down. When Richard arrived he found the cow a week calved, eating cut grass with relish, very bright and alert, but she would not get up out of the dung channel, where she had been overnight.

"Well, Bob, this channel is so slippy I'm not surprised she won't get up. I'll give her an injection for milk fever while you get some sand or ashes."

"But she hasn't got milk fever."

"It looks as though she hasn't, but if the calcium level in the blood is only slightly down they often won't get up. I also want a bucket of warm water, soap and a towel."

By the time the cow had been injected, two buckets full of ashes, the water, towel and a sliver of soap had been brought. Richard examined the cow *per rectum*, while Bob's son Tom moved the cow's uppermost hind leg about, which she resented and almost kicked him. The ashes were thrown in front of and under the cow.

"Come on, Bob, you lift on the tail, you that side Tom, and I'll be this; altogether now, heave."

The cow raised her hindquarters two feet up from the floor, maintained herself there for probably a quarter of a minute then sank down again. She wriggled about until she was comfortable.

"Well, the idle bitch, she could do it if she tried. What do you think, Mr Holden?"

"I am sure she could; I can't feel anything wrong with her bones inside; she should get up."

"Then we'll leave her. When will you come again, Mr Holden?"

"In two days time if I don't hear from you. You must turn her over twice a day."

On the second visit, the cow was still in the same position. Richard got Bob to move the stall division and with much pushing and pulling, they got the cow out of the dung channel and into the stall. Again she half rose and then sank back. Bob tied a gate at both ends, so the cow would not fall back into the channel. Richard gave to Bob a bottle of medicine which was *Liquor*

Strychninae, with instructions to give her a dessertspoonful of the liquid in half a pint of water once a day. Three days later, Bob sent a message to say that the cow was still down, but they had got her in a box. Richard rang John Barker, Bob's brother, and asked him to pass on the message that he would go to see the cow at eleven o'clock next morning, would take the horse slings and that he would need six men to help.

With John, Bob and Tom, and men from other farms, seven men had assembled. Soon the pulley block was fixed to a strong beam over the cow and the big belly band passed under her; the breast piece and breeching were strapped on, and the steel bar hooked on to the belly band's steel rings. Then the pulley hook was put through the hole in the centre of the bar. Four tightly-packed bales of straw were brought and instructions given that when the cow was high enough off the floor they had to be pushed under her belly to stop her sinking down again. Two men pulled on the chain, one held the halter to keep her head still and the others stood each side of her, ready to pull a leg to each "corner" when the bales were placed underneath her. But when this was done, she hung limply in the slings and resisted all attempts to put her legs under her to take her weight and stand on them. Bob shouted and hit her round her head with his cap; cold water was poured in her ear and her tail was pulled out straight and rubbed between two sticks. But all to no avail and at last Bob shouted:

"Let the damn cow down!"

When this was done she began to eat hay.

"How did you get her in here, Bob?"

"The six of us rolled her onto a gate and then the horse pulled her in here."

"I think it's no good, so will you ring Chris Robson and tell him to collect her and take her to the abattoir."

"Yes, I'll do that, but there's no earthly reason why she can't get up."

Just as Richard reached the main road Chris Robson drove past. Richard turned to follow him and when he could pass, waved him to stop.

"Hello, Mr Holden, what do you want?"

"I've a job for you, Chris. Bob Barker at High Moor wants you to take a cow to the abattoir."

"Why there?"

"Because she's been down a week; she's a good cow, you know, and seven of us have struggled for half an hour with her in the slings, but she won't stand."

"I can't go now, you know, being auction day. I'll have some customers waiting for me there."

"It's up to you Chris, he did say he wanted you to move her, and you could not be nearer. She's a big Friesian in the box at the end of the shippon."

"Aye, I suppose I'd better go for her, I'll turn round. Thanks, Mr Holden. Cheerio."

On Monday, Richard was at Bill Meadow's Whingate Farm, examining a riding pony, when Chris Robson drove his cattle wagon into the yard. He climbed out of the cab, came across to Richard, and in a threatening manner loudly said:

"Who do you think you are? you daft devil, making me waste me' time and petrol running to Barker's, and nowt wrong wi' his cow."

"What are you talking about?"

"Look, Holden, I got there, there was no one about; there wasn't a cow on the place, except a big Friesian in a box."

"Right, that was the one. Didn't you go to the house and ask Mrs Barker where the men were? They had probably taken John and the men home."

"No I didn't; there was no need to. The bloody cow was looking at me over the door of the box."

"Get away, that's fantastic! I couldn't have believed it. Robson, you're making it up."

"I'm not, I tell you the bloody cow was up, so don't send me on any more wild goose chases again."

Richard was getting annoyed.

"Listen, Robson, I didn't send you anywhere; as Bob is not on the telephone I was his messenger. The cow had been down a week and was still down when we left her, so get that in your head."

"Now, you two, calm down," said Bill. "It's obvious she suddenly got up, it does happen. One of my cows did the same trick on me a few years ago."

"Maybe," said Robson, "but I haven't all day to waste. Help me unload your cow, Bill."

"Yes, and Richard, go in and Liz will make you a cup of tea."

Liz was listening to the news and as it was just ending, she switched off the wireless set.

"Hello, Richard, how nice to see you. Do sit down while I brew the tea. How is Flora?"

"She is very well, Liz, except for Tommy."

"Oh, what's he been up to?" she asked. Richard had begun to tell Elizabeth the story of Tommy's mishaps, when Bill came in. Richard was still annoyed with Chris and said so.

"There's no need to take it to heart, Richard," said Bill. "I've known him a long time and he can be very bolshy if anything annoys him, but his heart's in the right place."

"Maybe it is, but I'm not going to be told off for something which was not my fault."

"I'd forget it Richard, there is enough trouble in the world without having grudges and making enemies."

"I'd say there is," said Elizabeth, "the news reader just said that enemy planes had bombed London again today, inflicting casualties and damage. The poor things must be in a dreadful state after all these days of bombing."

"Yes, I agree," said Richard who had now calmed down, so he drank his tea, thanked them and left. How lucky to live in Sandhaven!

The October weather was wet and cold, but began well for Richard when Bill Bainbridge from Duckworth Hall rang up and asked Richard to go to a cow calving. When he arrived, Bill explained that he wanted Richard to do his work, because he had sacked Tommy Knowles from Wilton after two cows had died while he was treating them.

Richard soon calved the cow and the heifer calf was alive which pleased him, while the bitch he had done the Caesarian operation on nearly a year before followed Bill everywhere. But later in the week at Jack Clough's Leach House things went wrong. The cow could not calve because one of the calf's legs was bent backwards. Richard had attached a calving rope to it, and two men pulled but the leg would not move.

"Why won't it move?" asked Jack.

"Because it's a deformity—it's grown that way and I will have to cut the leg off before the calf can come."

"Right, let's get on with it. What do you want me to do?"

"I want you to hold this thinner rope which is attached to my embryotomy knife and do as I say."

Richard introduced the knife, and slowly cut through the skin and muscle behind the shoulder blades. With Jack pulling on the rope, the knife quickly cut along the top of the blade and then downwards in front of it. Richard was joining up the cut behind the shoulder with the one in front, and Jack pulled steadily. Suddenly there was resistance as the knife cut into cartilage.

"Wait a minute, Jack, the knife has jammed; don't pull."

Richard pushed the knife back until it was free and only cutting through skin. He held the knife in his right hand, the blade towards the calf, and used his left hand to guide the knife's direction.

"Now pull gently, Jack."

Instead Jack jerked as he pulled and the knife instantly cut Richard's left hand from the base of the thumb towards his wrist.

"Stop, let go! You're cutting me, Jack!" and as Richard withdrew his arms and the knife, blood flowed freely from his left hand.

"Now look what you've done, I told you to pull gently."

"I'm sorry, Richard, what shall I do?"

"Go and get the brown leather case off the back seat of the car." When he came back with it, Richard told him the dressings he wanted, and Jack used them to bandage Richard's hand. At once Richard returned to the job; soon the leg was pulled out, then he delivered the calf. Jack said, "Thanks, Richard," and walked off, leaving his men to clear up. At the Memorial Hospital, Richard went into Casualty where the Doctor put ten stitches in the wound in his hand and bandaged it. This was followed by an anti-tetanus injection.

At the Home Farm there was an outbreak of husk and five eight-months-old heifer calves died, much to Bill Griffin the manager's annoyance, because they were all full pedigree Friesians.

The injured hand was a hindrance, but Richard did all the work as it arose. The wound was slow to heal, so the stitches were not taken out until the tenth day. A few days later he went to Seedhill, and with George Whiteside's help calved a cow which was two weeks before her time. He went back three days later and tried to remove the afterbirth, but it was impossible, so he put pessaries and sulphanilamide powder into the uterus. He carefully washed the greenish coloured sticky slime off his arm with disinfectant. The cow parted with the afterbirth after a week, and began to lose her appetite. Richard found that she had a temperature, and a sticky, brownish discharge from her vulva. He prescribed sulphanilamide powders by mouth, to be followed by tonic powders. He told George that he would take a smear of the discharge and examine it. He did not expect what he found: TB organisms in the smear. He immediately acted under the TB order. At the post-mortem the cow had an advanced TB peritonitis and metritis. Richard was thankful that he had disinfected his arm well.

The month ended in a tragedy which saddened all the Lawson family and Richard. Flora's cousin Mark was the eldest of three sons of Uncle Jack and Margaret who lived next door in Holme. He had been in the Army for nine months, and was driving a truck near Bromley, south of London, delivering urgently needed supplies, when an air raid developed almost overhead. When he saw an air raid shelter he stopped and told his mate to run to it. Mark (having secured the tarpaulin) was still in the driver's seat when a bomb burst in front of the truck. The little two feet square windscreen smashed into thousands of pieces and blinded Mark in both eyes, as he and the truck were hurled backwards. He was badly injured but survived after months in hospital. Mark had been Flora's favourite companion of her childhood, so she went with Jack and Margaret to see him. When she came back Richard met her at the station, and he put his arms round her as she began to cry, and said:

"Oh, Richard, I hardly recognised him, you should see Mark's poor battered face. Whatever will become of him–it's dreadful." He led her to the car, holding back his own tears; he always became very upset whenever Flora cried.

Later that evening, going to the Home Farm to a cow down with milk fever, he found himself whistling the tune "A Nightingale sang in Berkeley Square." How stupid, he thought, to write that lyric; with all the bombing, there would not be a nightingale within twenty miles of London.

There had been two air raid alerts in October, followed soon by the All Clear. But one evening in November the alert began at 9 o'clock and Richard and Flora went to their shelter with Ming in a cat basket and Tommy on a lead. Soon they heard aeroplane's engines "jinking" overhead.

"They are German aircraft," said Richard.

"Be quiet," said Flora.

"Why? They can't hear us up there."

"I know, but I'm listening to the sound of the plane's engines. It is dying away, they are going over, another false alarm."

No sooner had Flora spoken, than there was the sound of a dull thud in the distance, soon followed by a loud crash.

"Oh Richard, they are bombing us, I'm scared."

Richard put his arms round her and held her close, as the scream of a falling bomb was followed by a terrific explosion. The floor trembled slightly and the electric light went out. They clung to each other in the darkness and listened to two more explosions which were further away.

"Make a light, Richard, please." He found the matches, struck one, and lit the oil lamp. He got two mugs off the shelf, filled them with hot sweet tea from the Thermos, and gave one mug to Flora.

"I wonder where that bomb fell when the lights went out. It must have been very near."

"It must have been within a hundred yards," said Richard, "You could feel the ground shake."

Some time later, enemy aircraft passed over again but did not drop any more bombs. It was almost midnight when the All Clear sounded. Using their shaded torch, they came out of their shelter, and went back into the house. As no water came out of the tap when they turned it on, they did not have a cup of cocoa, and by torch light went to bed. Flora had put the hot water bottles into the bed before the air raid started, so it was warm and they quickly fell asleep. Next morning the water and electricity supplies had been restored and Richard took Tommy for a walk. The bomb had fallen on a big house at the corner of Cross Street and George Street and it had been reduced to a heap of rubble. One wall was still upright and this was being demolished. A temporary water main had been laid on the pavement, and people picked their way over it and the rubble in the road, as they made their way to work. It had been a near-miss for 2 Cross Street. Two windows facing the street had been shattered and a chimney pot was lying smashed in the road. Nearer to the corner with George Street some houses were badly damaged. The wrecked building used as offices had been unoccupied and so no one was killed, but some people had been hurt who lived in the houses opposite which also were badly damaged. The bombs had fallen in a straight line from the river near the shipyard, one fell on the golf course and the last near Far Parkside Farm.

When Richard came home for lunch, he found the bottom of Victoria Street closed, because a large water main had burst, making a deep hole in the road and had undermined the pavement. Many men were labouring non-stop to repair the damage in George Street before darkness came. The buses had been re-routed down Ship Street and Corporation Street to reach High Street. Everybody Richard spoke to was relieved that Sandhaven had sustained so little damage, but were afraid of what might happen in the next few months. After supper Richard completed several forms and wrote out an order for drugs, while Flora wrote to her cousin Annie, whose wedding they had attended three years before. A baby boy had been born to her and Tom. Though the Holdens had been invited to the christening, they had to refuse as it was impossible to go under war-time conditions. At ten to nine Flora said:

"Come on, Richard, hurry up; I want this letter to catch the nine o'clock post."

"Right, I'm off now. I'll catch it easily if I run all the way."

It was a very dark night, but he ran over Cross Street and down Victoria Street and noticed the gleam of red lights where the water main had burst. They distracted his attention and he ran into the wooden wall which had been erected round the collapsed pavement and the dangerous building beside it. For a moment he was stunned, the letters fell from his hand. He felt the blood pouring from his nose, and switched on his torch to find the letters. The Town Hall clock showed two minutes to nine when he posted the letters. Flora was upset when he arrived home. His nose and one eyebrow were cut, and he had a black eye. She bathed his face gently with Dettol and water and later washed the front of his jacket and his shirt. His face was sore for three days and ever after he always used his torch because even with a shade it helped.

Flora's sister Mary had a great friend, Rosemary, and they went everywhere together, having almost identical interests. Mary, like Flora, had been very distressed by her brother Mark's blindness, and this was probably the reason why she volunteered for the Auxiliary Territorial Service (ATS). The two girls joined up together and were sent to Hereford for driver training. On receiving the news, Flora was worried about her mother, alone in the big house in Holme, and at once went by train to see her, to try and find out what she intended to do. Her journey was useless, because Jean firmly stated that she had no intention of leaving the house she had lived in since the day of her marriage. She would only leave it, and come and live with Flora, if Hitler reduced it to a heap of stones. Until then she was quite happy where

she was, and relied on Jack and Margaret next door. Their Anderson air raid
shelters were near each other at the top of each garden at the back of the
houses and during a raid she was not alone because Mr and Mrs Wilson, her
other neighbours, shared it with her. In spite of the rebuff, Flora was pleased
she had gone to see her mother, and arrived home in good spirits during an
air raid alert.

As they walked into the surgery John came through and said:

"Mr Holden, I've just taken a message from Tom Walker at Fell Top,
Icken. He has a cow with her calf bed out,"

"What did you say?"

"Well, I said you were out, but would be back soon and it would take you
a while to get there, because there was an alert on."

"What did he say to that?"

"'Aye mebbe, but tell him to get here soon, she's a damn good cow.'"

"Thanks, John. I'll be off, Flora, and I'll be quite a time before I'm back,
its eighteen miles there."

When he got to the top of Victoria Street, on to the Middleton Road, a
Warden stopped him and told him to turn off his headlights, because aircraft
had been heard passing over. Though there was some moonlight it was difficult driving under these conditions, but he could see the reason for it when
he got to the top of Beech Hill. Over towards Droughton he could see search
light beams moving about the sky. He stopped the car and listened, but could
not hear any aircraft, only the faint noise of gunfire. He drove on through
Middleton up the Higher Carden road and it was a good bit later when he
drove up the bumpy road and into the yard of Fell Top Farm. As he got out
of his car a gleam of light showed for a moment from the direction of the
house and three figures approached him.

"Evening, Mr Holden, It is you, isn't it?"

"Yes, it is, Tom. Where is the cow?"

"At the far end of the long shippon. Follow me."

At that moment a lit oil-lamp was produced from inside an overcoat, and
the light appeared very bright to Richard's eyes, accustomed to the semi-
darkness.

Tom shouted, "Dad, put that bloody lamp inside your coat, you'll get us
all killed!"

"Eh, what's that?" said Grandfather, who was stone deaf. Tom grabbed
the lamp from him, put it inside his coat, and walked towards the shippon;
the other three men followed his illuminated clogs. In the shippon the lamp
was hung up and Richard could see that half the lamp glass had been blacked
out but it showed the pulley blocks hanging from a beam.

"I see you have put the blocks up; won't she get up, Tom?"

"No, so I wrapped the calf bed in a sheet and put it on a clean sack. The water is hot in the big bucket."

"Good, before we hoist her, I'll remove the cleansing."

He was doing this when they heard the sound of aircraft engines, which was followed by the scream of a bomb falling and the explosion. They all ran for it; Grandad was first out of the door and first into the cellar under the house. Richard arrived last, having been impeded by his overall.

"By Jove, Tom, your Dad can sprint."

"Aye, he can, but he was better when he was younger. He was a fell runner then, and won prizes."

After about five minutes they went back to the cow. Her hindquarters were raised, a bale put under her belly and Tom and his son John held up the uterus on the sack. Richard struggled and pushed, and had got the uterus about halfway back when an aircraft was heard overhead again. They all stood motionless, hardly daring to speak, until they heard the bomb falling and the explosion.

Again they all ran for it—Grandfather leading—leaving the cow to her fate. After a short while in the cellar, Tom went up the stairs and listened. "Come on, it's gone," he said, and they returned to the shippon. Richard soon replaced the uterus, then put into it sulphanilamide powder and antiseptic pessaries, after which he put on the strappings, the bale was removed and the cow's hindquarters lowered. He was giving her an injection of calcium solution when the sound of an aircraft was heard faintly and then it died away.

"That one's gone over," said Tom.

"Yes, thank God for that. I was getting worried about your cow, leaving her hoisted up like that,"

"Aye, so was I, but she looks not so bad after all, I'll just go and..." The rest of the sentence was lost in the noise of a most terrific explosion and they all flung themselves down on the floor. The door flew open; the lamp went out, and in the darkness the noise was indescribable as debris rained down on the shippon's corrugated iron roof, and some of the cows bellowed with fright.

The noise subsided and Tom shouted, "Is everyone all right?" They all shouted yes, and he walked over to the vaguely outlined doorway, and shut the door. He struck a match and, finding the lamp, lit it, while the other three got to their feet. Richard found himself trembling and his ears were hurting; he couldn't hear well when Tom said, "Hellfire, that bomb was close."

"I don't think it was a bomb," said Richard, "It was something much bigger than that—probably one of those land mines like they have dropped on London, because there was no noise when it came down, and the aircraft had been gone some minutes."

"Aye, I hadn't thought of them. Anyway, it made the cow get up!"

He fastened her up, and then tied a sack round her. He dosed her with a pint of stimulant medicine and John brought a bucket of water which the cow drank, then he threw some hay to her.

"That's it, Mr Holden, come on to the house."

Richard was surprised to find Mrs Walker in the blacked-out kitchen, never having taken shelter, and she was very calm when she said, "Tom, the bedroom windows on the quarry side are smashed in, so we will have to use the big bedroom tonight. The tea's brewed." Richard drank the cup of tea and, feeling very weary, set off home.

When Richard went back to the farm the next day, to collect the strappings, the cow was fully recovered. John, who was nailing boards over the broken windows,told him that the mine had fallen in the quarry, and brought down a great heap of rock, and apart from breaking most of the windows, had blown off all the chimney pots and damaged the roof. That evening the final edition of the *Post* said that a city had been bombed in the north of England and some bombs had been dropped in country districts. Richard later got to know from Chris Robson, that a farmhouse near Kendrick had received a direct hit, and six people had been killed, among them a cousin of Tom Walker. Dr McConnell examined Richard's ears, assured him that the ear drums were not damaged and that the ringing noise would soon die away.

Late one afternoon Richard went to visit cows at two farms, telling Flora that he would be back about six thirty. He was delayed at both farms, so did not get back until well after seven o'clock, and Flora was annoyed.

"Richard, I'm getting fed up with you giving me a time when you want your meal, and coming home three-quarters of an hour later. It's hard enough to think up meals with the little meat we get, but then keeping it hot dries it up and spoils it. I'm tired out with sleeping badly with you out half the night and all the work there is to do. Can't Marjorie come more mornings in the week?"

"I'm sorry I'm late, Flora, but at Park Hall the cow had a bad mastitis, and then I had to see another with a chaff in her eye. When I got to Blacklands, as well as a cow with pneumonia they had one with slow fever which I had to inject, I couldn't be any quicker."

"Well, in future we will have dinner at 6 o'clock, and the cows will have to wait. Can Marjorie come more often?"

"All right, but why?"

"Because I've so much to do, Richard. I'm up early, often just after six with the damned phone, and there is the cleaning, washing, ironing, the door and the surgery; dispensing, and helping Marjorie check all the entries and totals. Then there's the shopping and all the rest of it."

"Yes. I know that, but the practice is getting busier and often I'm dog tired."

"Don't I know it, you just fall into bed and you're fast asleep. Can I see if Marjorie will come each morning from Tuesday to Saturday, because if she can and with John it would be a lot easier."

"Yes, you do that."

"I will. Anyway, let's get our meal before it's ruined."

Marjorie could only come on Tuesday, Thursday and Saturday mornings, which was agreed. Flora had made up her mind to get more help, and set off to see if she could find Mrs Shaw. The latter was doing anything to supplement her allowance from the Army, so Flora asked her to come five mornings a week to work in the house cleaning and dusting, and also to answer the doorbell and the 'phone. Annie Shaw agreed at once, because her sister who had a weak heart had come to live with her, and she would have the children's lunch ready each day when they came home from school.

Flora did not beat about the bush.

"Richard, I've got Mrs Shaw to come five mornings a week."

"We don't need her as much as that do we?"

"I do, I'm the prisoner in this house. I get out only a few hours each week. It's different for you, out all day meeting people."

"It's not all right, Flora, it's hard work, wet and cold. It's not like being in a warm house all day."

"Oh damn the house, I've engaged her, and you can pay her from the practice, it's a legitimate expense."

"I don't know if George Duke will allow it."

"He'll jolly well have to, or we get another accountant."

"I'll ask him, then,"

"No, you won't, you'll tell him what we want because we pay his bills."

"I'll do that then, but calm down, Flora."

"No,I won't, you go on wrapped up in your vet work oblivious to what's going on. We rarely go anywhere. John can come on Sunday morning, then I can go to church with Isabel Lord, because you never attempt to go."

"You have got it all worked out, haven't you?"

"No,I haven't, but if I don't do something you won't. Another thing, what are we going to do about children? I told you after the abortion I wanted another baby and Jean would love a grandchild. Can't we go and see Dr Bill and get his advice?"

"Do you think it's necessary?"

"Yes, of course, over two years have gone by, and during that time Betty Meadows has had a baby boy for their Brenda, and even Isabel who was so ill when she came here, had a baby boy a month ago."

"I didn't know that, funny, Jim didn't tell me."

"Of course you wouldn't know, I bet you never ask him how she is, do you?—because you're just not interested."

"Oh I am, but somehow there is so much to do and remember that things like that get crowded out of my mind, because to me the job's the main thing."

"No, it bloody well isn't. Our life together, and I mean really together is the most important thing. I know we have got this far by concentrating on the practice, but there is a lot more to life than vetting and don't you forget it."

"All right, I damn well won't. I'll go and see Bill McConnell today and ask his advice."

"You'd better; it's time we did something about our future together."

He saw Bill that afternoon, who advised that they had an appointment with Mr Graham the gynaecologist. That night before he fell asleep, he remembered to make love to Flora, but it was a half-hearted affair.

It was a frosty night early in December when he went to Tom Nuttall at Bridge House, Higher Carden to a heifer which could not calve. With the light from the moon in the first quarter, it was not too difficult driving. Tom was a well known breeder of dairy Shorthorns and was a very capable farmer. The very light-roan heifer was tied up in a box and well bedded with clean straw, and the soap, towel and bucket full of hot water were quickly produced when Richard arrived.

"Hello, Tom, how long has she been calving?"

"I don't really know, Mr Holden. She's a week over her time, and every now and then gives a heave but nothing happens, but she has passed some water." Richard was surprised when he examined her to find that he could just get his hand through the vulva and four inches into the vagina, but no further. It was completely blocked by a wall of tissue except for a little hole at the bottom of the wall, through which he could get his finger, but he could not feel anything.

Realising that by now Richard should have most of his arm inside the heifer, Tom asked:

"Is it a twisted calf bed, Mr Holden?"

"No, Tom, it isn't. I'm just going to examine her through the rectum and then I'll explain it to you."

This examination revealed that the anterior vagina was a round tube of hard tissue, beyond which he could feel a calf, which did not move when he pressed down on it. "Tom, I want a pencil and paper."

John, Tom's son was sent for some while Richard took off his overall and got dressed.

"What you've got here, Tom, is a case of White Heifer disease or to give it its technical name, Atresia Vaginae, which means the passage is very narrow or blocked by tissue. This one is blocked by tissue with a little passage through it. It feels about eight inches long and there is a big dead calf beyond it. There is no way it can be born naturally, it would have to be a Caesarian operation."

"Well, that is a devil. What do you advise?"

Richard said, "The operation is only about fifty per cent successful. The calf is dead, the heifer will never breed again and she is in good condition. I would have her killed at once."

"At this time of the night? I wonder who would kill her?"

"Who's your butcher?"

"Tommy Horlick in Higher Carden; he would kill it, but he's not on the 'phone."

"Oh, I can go for him and I've got my humane killer in the car. Have you got a gambit and some pulley blocks you could hang on that beam?"

"Aye, I have."

"Right, then you get the blocks up there. We will want two clean four-gallon buckets and a clean sheet, and plenty of hot water. I'll go for Tommy."

"Aye, I will, I'll do owt to save a good carcase of beef, come on, John."

When Richard found the butcher's shop in Higher Carden, he knocked hard on the door and after a short time got his twitch from the car and hammered on the door. Suddenly the bedroom window above was opened and a gruff voice shouted:

"Who's that? What the hell do you want at this time of the night?"

Richard explained the position, Tommy said he would come and slammed the window shut. Richard was getting very cold in the freezing car by the time the butcher finally appeared, still wearing his woollen night cap.

Back at the farm, Richard shot the heifer, and Tommy soon showed that he was a master butcher, as he expertly dressed the carcase. The pluck was put in one bucket and the head in the other. The gambit was put through under the strong tendons above the hocks, then the gambit was hooked onto the pulley block and the carcase raised.

When Tommy had finished dressing the carcase he washed it down with hot water. The intestines were put into a clean sack and Tommy washed and got fully dressed.

"Now what are you going to do with it?"

"Take it to the abattoir in the morning."

"I know you'll do that, but it's very warm in here with it being joined to the shippon. To set properly, she'd be better outside with it freezing."

The carcase was lowered onto a strong gate which was covered with sacks and the horse pulled it into the orchard. There the carcase, wrapped in a clean sheet, was hung from a tree. Richard went back to the house, wrote out his certificate for the abattoir manager and, having told Tom Nuttall to take everything belonging to the carcase with it to the abattoir, drove off home at almost midnight.

The Home Guard had a post in Higher Carden which was on the main Mereside-Southall road. The lads who had done the first turn were stood down at midnight; five who lived in Wilsdon mounted their cycles and in a group rode off down the Middleton Road. By the light of the half moon, Bridge Farm could be seen on the right side of the road, and as they approached it one of them said:

"Hey, what's that white thing in Tommy Nuttall's orchard?"

"Nowt. Tha' seeing things in't moonlight."

"No I'm not, look it's there, it's white by that big tree."

"Hell, it's a bloody ghost."

That did it, they were gone in a flash and it was a fast race to reach Wilsdon.

There was some scoffing and jeering at them that evening in the Wheat-sheaf pub from those who had not been on duty the previous night.

"How do you know it was a ghost? You should have gone and challenged it."

"You can't challenge a ghost, you daft devil."

"Ghost my foot, it was probably a Jerry parachutist wi' his parachute caught in t' tree."

"It couldn't have been, the post would have got a signal if any aircraft were about and there weren't any."

"Anyway, it boils down to this, five gallant soldiers were frightened by Tommy's grey mare."

"It weren't his mare, it was a ghost. We all saw it and we didn't stop to argue, I can tell you."

"All right forget it, we'll have a good look when we're coming home next time."

They did and of course saw nothing. Meanwhile the carcase was passed top grade at the abattoir.

A week later it was a still frosty night with the countryside illuminated by the light from the full moon. When Richard answered the 'phone, Tommy Nuttall said:

"Mr Holden, I've got the twin heifer to that other one and she can't calve, she's got one of the calf's legs out but can't shift it."

"Right, Tom, don't pull on it, and I'll come straight away."

When he arrived at the farm, examination of the heifer revealed almost the same condition which he had found in her sister a week before. The only difference was that the hole through the fibrous mass was larger, and through it one foot of the calf was protruding.

"Tom, it's just like the other one, so she will have to be killed."

"It's a pity, but as there's nowt else for it let's get on."

When Richard arrived at Tommy Horlicks, he said:

"Aye, of course I'll come, but he's making a bloody habit of it. How many more times is this going to happen?"

"Oh, I'm certain this is the last one."

"I hope so," said Tom.

By eleven o'clock the carcase, wrapped in a clean sheet, was hanging from a branch of the same tree in the orchard.

It was a different guard which stood down at midnight, but three lived in Wilsdon and were the leaders of the opposition to the tale of the ghost. As they approached Bridge Farm they were only thinking of getting home and into bed to get warm.

When Ted Bamber said, "I think Tom Crane were right about that ghost after all," they jerked alert.

"How? Where is it?"

He pointed to the orchard.

"Over there by the big tree, and it isn't a horse."

"By gum, it is a bloody ghost. Let's go!"

And they did. No challenges were made; it was just a very rapid retreat by the three brave soldiers. That night in the Wheatsheaf the argument about the ghost got so heated that it almost got to blows, until burly Ben Belcher intervened—he was a landlord whose word was law, having been an amateur heavyweight boxer in his youth.

John Nuttall went to the pub for the Christmas draw which was run by the Cricket Club. In the course of the evening he explained it all to a spellbound audience, and so the "ghost" died.

Again the carcase had been an excellent one.

On the evening of 21st December the air raid alert began early, and Flora was pleased that Richard was at home. She was very frightened if she was alone and an air raid began. Later Richard had to go to Ryton Lodge and treat a cow for milk fever.

The cow was staggering about and when Harry Helm nosed her she went down, which made it easier to inject her intravenously, which Richard did slowly. Soon after he had finished she rose to her feet, and the calf immediately began to suck, so it was taken away from her. As he walked to the car he said to Harry:

"By the pink glow in the sky, it looks as though Liverpool is catching it tonight."

"Yes, poor devils, Jerry obviously means to smash up the docks. I hope he doesn't come back to Sandhaven."

"Yes, so do I. Goodnight Harry."

When Richard got home, the pink glow in the sky had turned red, and he was sad that the city where he had been so happy years before was being bombed so heavily. He joined Flora in their air raid shelter, and it was very late before the "All Clear" sounded.

Next day, it was just before lunchtime when the door bell rang, and

Richard went to answer it. He opened the door, and a man was standing there whom he felt he should know, but could not identify. His face was filthy with soot, his blood-shot eyes were half closed, his hair black and singed, as was the front of his coat; he was dirtier than any chimney sweep. In a tremulous voice, the figure said: "Richard, it's me, Norman."

"Good God, Norman, whatever happened? Come on in, where's your case?"

"I haven't got one, all I've got is what I stand up in."

He followed Richard through the house and into the kitchen where he was introduced to Flora.

"Sit down, Norman, what do you want? What can we do for you?"

"Can I have a mug of tea, and a bath?"

"Of course you can. I'll get you the tea, and Flora will run your bath and get you a towel." Flora went upstairs to get the bath ready.

"So you were in Liverpool's bombing last night? It must have been dreadful."

The reply came slowly. "Yes it was, three of us were fire watching, but as the bombing got worse we left the roof, and went down into a deep shelter. When it ended we came up and there were fires everywhere, and dust. A lot of Bedford Street North is a heap of rubble, the digs and the pub are too."

"How did you get out?"

"Well, I decided to get out of the city, before a follow-up raid came. I climbed over rubble, and past wrecked and smouldering buildings. It took me a long time because the city centre is still burning. I walked up the middle of Tithebarn Street and buildings were burning on both sides. I waited a long time in the station with other people, and then a train came."

"By Jove, you have been lucky."

"Yes I was," said Norman and finished his tea. Then he said, "Richard, can I borrow some clothes?"

"Yes, I'll get some ready while you have your bath."

At lunch Norman had recovered a bit. His wavy blond hair was clean, though dark in places where it had been singed, but his face was very pale.

"When did you last get to bed?"

"Oh two days ago, but that doesn't matter. All I want is to get to my cousin's in Skipton because my mother is there; she was bombed out of Manchester, you know."

"You're sure, Norman, because you can stay as long as you like, and go to bed right away."

"No thanks, Richard. I do want to go if you'll take me to the station, and I'm all right for money."

"I'll do that and after Skipton you'll go back to the University?"

"Not on your life. I'm joining the RAF so that I can fight the bastards."
He got up, thanked Flora for lunch and went with Richard to the station.

Norman gravely thanked Richard and said he would return the clothes. When they shook hands and said goodbye, Richard was near to tears; fate saw to it that they never met again.

Back at the house Flora said that Jean would come the next day by train with Mary who was on leave and had sold her car. So that evening they decorated the house and put all the Christmas cards on display, including one from Ted and Mary who sent their best wishes. Flora also arranged the following night to meet up with Tom and Betty Hayes; Jim Lord and Isabel; Gordon Hindle and Pat; and Tommy Bishop and Joan at the Royal Hotel, instead of having a party at home. She was very happy to see her mother and sister, who had brought food and presents, but Jean was adamant that they were having the night off, and took them all for dinner at the Porter Arms. In spite of rationing it was an excellent meal, and later it was a very jolly two hours they spent with their friends in the Royal Hotel lounge. Just as Christmas lunch was ready, Richard had to go twenty miles to Chapel House at Rushworth to calve a cow, so he had his meal at 4 o'clock, just as he had at Christmas 1939. He was thankful that St. Paul's had escaped destruction in the great air raid on the following Sunday night. When he got his Monday morning's paper and saw the photograph of the Cathedral surrounded by fires, he realised what a miracle had taken place.

Richard was stopped at the top of Beech Hill, by an Air Raid Warden and a member of the Home Guard and ordered to drive on side lights only because there was an alert. When he got to the Cock Inn in Middleton, Tom Sharples came out of the back door of the pub carrying a lighted oil lamp.

"Tom, put that lamp out, don't you know there's an alert on?"

"Eh hell, so there is; you know, I just lit it and came out without thinking."

He put the lamp inside his coat and ran across the yard into a box. Richard followed him, closed the door and injected the cow for milk fever. They pushed the cow into a sitting position and put her calf behind a gate which was across a corner. They heard noises in the yard, followed by a loud bang on the roof. Tom blew out the lamp, and opened the door and found two incendiary bombs burning in the yard—the last of a scattered line which extended across the field as points of burning light.

"Quick, Richard, run round the front and see if any are on the roof."

Tom smothered the two in the yard with a shovel full of sand, as Richard returned to say none had dropped on the pub's roof. The sound of aircraft engines died away and when they went into the box, by the light of his torch he could see the cow had got up.

"You were lucky, Tom; if that lot had dropped on the roof you would have been in trouble."

"I would that. I'm glad I've a slate roof, I'd be worried if I had a thatch one like Ben at the Wheatsheaf."

When Richard arrived home, the stirrup pump, shovel, and the buckets of sand and water were put near to the back door. He was becoming worried that their turn might be coming, when Jerry would bomb them again.

The snow which fell towards the end of the month was not as deep as the year before, but it froze hard and became ice on the roads and pavements, making them very dangerous. Richard arrived at Cross Roads Farm at Wyreham at tea time, got out of the car and, using his torch, walked across the hard, level snow towards the buildings. He had just gone past the muck heap when the snow gave way under him and he found himself up to his thighs in the liquid muck which had drained from the heap, or been washed off the yard into the pit. Cursing himself for not taking the track in the snow instead of a short cut to the shippon he pulled himself out. He walked to the dairy and went in. Bill Harrison looked round.

"What's happened to you, Mr Holden?"

"I fell into the pit by the muck heap; the ice and snow gave way under me."

"Well, get your rubber boots off, and your pants, and I'll get you a pair of bib and brace overalls and another pair of boots."

He opened the door which led in to the shippon and told young Tom to go and get the clothes. Bill gave Richard a bucket of hot water, soap and a towel, and he washed his legs and feet, dried himself and put on the overalls and boots. After this the cow got attended to.

He put his muck-soiled trousers and boots in a sack and when he got home washed out the boots and put the trousers to soak in disinfectant. Later they were washed, dried and ironed, but it was useless because they had shrunk so much he could not wear them.

After a week of the snow and frost the Corporation sent out workmen who threw shovelfuls of salt and sand onto the road from the back of a moving lorry.

Each shovelful fell at intervals of about six feet and during the day slowly melted the ice, and this made trenches across the road. After a few days, the conditions became so bad that the buses had to be withdrawn, and with picks and shovels men cleared the treated streets, a slow laborious job. Many of the buses broke springs and so did other vehicles. At night it was dangerous to drive a car, as Richard found out at the end of the week.

He had gone through Shipton on his way to Ryton and in places the snow was piled in heaps at the roadside. It was an unfenced road and sheep roamed freely. He was just approaching Rose Farm when what appeared to be a heap of snow suddenly ran across the road in front of him. He jammed on his brakes, but hit the sheep with a thud and, sliding, crashed into a heap of frozen snow. He got out and shone his torch but there was no sign of the sheep. Grumbling to himself he got back into the car, started the engine and started to go back. There was a dreadful rubbing noise, so he stopped and got out, to find the bumper was bent on to the tyre of the front wheel. He could not move it, so he walked into Rose Farm to find Harold Marsden. He knocked on the kitchen door and Harold opened it.

"Hello, Mr Holden, what's the matter?"

"Two things Harold. The first is, I've hit one of your sheep which looked like a heap of snow until it ran in front of the car; there was a pretty solid bump so it could be injured."

"Then I'll have a look for it in the morning."

"The other thing is, the bumper is bent onto the front tyre, so could I borrow a hammer and a crowbar?"

"Yes, I'll just go and get them and I'll come and help you."

They soon hammered and bent the bumper almost straight, so the car could be driven and Richard thanked Harold and continued on his way to Ryton. It was a pot-holed road down to Sands House, and rough at the best of times. Now it was terrible; the car bounced up and down and crashed through the ice into deeper holes, the steering being almost wrenched out of his hands.

Leslie Howarth said, "I'm glad you've come, Mr Holden. It's a big calf and we can't move it."

After he examined the cow, Richard laughed and said:

"Leslie, you could pull until you were blue in the face and you wouldn't move it."

"Why not?"

"Because it's twins, and you've roped one leg of each twin."

He quickly repelled one calf and delivered the nearer one, and then the other. One was dead but the other was alive.

"I'm sorry I was late getting here, Leslie, but it's hard driving at night," and he told him about his accident near Rose Farm.

"I'm not surprised. Harold's sheep don't give way to traffic, they are a danger on that road."

"Yes, and your lane is getting worse again and terribly rough."

"I know, we'll have a day filling up the holes when the snow's gone."

Later, Richard wished he had filled them up earlier because as he was going down the lane he broke a back spring.

Next morning he went to Dock Garage and Gordon Hindle told Richard that only one leaf had broken. He fixed a wooden block above the axle, so the car could be driven more safely. In the afternoon, when he arrived back at the garage, the blacksmith had made a new leaf, and in an hour the repaired spring was refitted to the car. Gordon also checked the steering and found the alignment was correct, but the wall of the tyre was almost cut through, so the wheel was changed so that the damaged tyre could have a gaiter put inside to strengthen the wall, and allow the wheel to be kept as a spare, because tyres were getting more difficult to obtain. Richard had only two left from the store he had bought eighteen months before.

After a night of severe frost, freezing mist still hung in the air, so Richard was warming glycerine, which he carried with him and rubbed over the windscreen to stop it freezing up. It was just before 9 o'clock that morning when he answered the 'phone.

"Holden, Veterinary Surgeon."

"Is that Mr R.B. Holden speaking?"

"Yes, what do you want?"

"This is the County Police, Droughton, Inspector Lee speaking. For family reasons we're trying to find a Miss Flora Dickenson who married a veterinary surgeon some years ago. That is all the information I have to go on, so I am ringing all the vets in the county to try and locate the lady."

"You've found her, she's my wife, but what do you want her for?"

"For a private family matter. May I speak to the lady, who is now Mrs Flora Holden, I presume?"

"Yes. I'll get her. Wait a minute."

When Richard told Flora that the police wanted to talk to her, she panicked.

"It's our Bill, Oh Richard, I know it is, he will have been killed."

"Wait, love, come on to the 'phone and then we'll find out."

Flora was trembling when she picked up the 'phone.

"This is Mrs Flora Holden speaking. What? Yes I was Miss Flora Dickenson and my father's name was Tom."

Richard's fears were mounting that Jean had had some accident.

"Yes, that's right," said Flora. "She's my Auntie Winnie and the number is Ward 8, Morton Royal Infirmary. Oh I will, thank you very much, Inspector. I know she rarely wrote to anyone and was a bit of a recluse. Thank you again. Goodbye."

"Well, what was all that?"

"Auntie Winnie has been living on her own for some months in that big house. Her neighbour had not seen her for some days, and the milkman could not get a reply, so the police were called. They got in and found her lying on the floor in the dining room having had a stroke. She was very cold and they've taken her to MRI and she wants to see me as soon as possible."

"Right. I've nothing urgent for this morning, so I'll tell Marjorie where we are going and she can hold the fort, then we can go at once."

Auntie Winnie, sitting propped up in bed, was being given tea from a feeding cup by a nurse when they reached the bedside. She waved the nurse away and Flora leaned over and kissed her. Though Winnie's left arm and leg were paralysed, she could speak almost normally, and wanted to know all about the family. Then she asked Flora to go and see that her house in Morton was secure, and pay any bills which might have come. Flora promised to do this, and to come again, but Winnie interrupted and told her the name and address of her solicitors. The nurse now asked them to leave, so Flora kissed her again, and as they came out of the ward the Matron was waiting to talk to them. She wanted all Winnie's particulars and then said that the doctor did not expect his patient to survive, so Flora left her address and telephone number with the Matron. When they left the Infirmary, they went to the offices of Winnie's solicitors, and found out that they were also her executors. It was almost lunchtime when they arrived back in Sandhaven so, after a quick meal, Richard set off on his day's round, and it was late when he had finished.

Winnie died two days later, and the funeral was in Morton on a bitter morning at the end of the week.

Flora and Jean met many relatives of Winnie's late husband who they had never met before, and at the lunch, gaps in the family tree were filled in. The solicitor told Flora that she was a beneficiary under her aunt's will and that she could obtain the keys to the house from their offices; he also gave her a copy of her aunt's will. When she got home and read it she found she was to receive the residuary estate. This she did not understand, so she went to see the solicitor. He explained that, as Winnie and her husband Harry had no children, he in his will had left all his money and house in trust for named nephews and nieces. In her lifetime his wife Winnie had the income from the capital sum, and could live in the house rate and rent free. He also explained that, apart from the lounge and dining room furniture, which Winnie had left to her favourite niece Elsie Laffan, all the rest of the contents belonged to Flora. He expressed the wish that Mrs Holden would remove the contents at her earliest convenience and gave her the keys to the property.

On a day of freezing mist and bitter cold, Richard and Flora went to the house, which was a depressing sight because ice hung from below the bathroom window down the wall to ground level. In the hall everything was thickly coated with dust, especially in the dining room, where it was obvious Auntie Winnie had lived. A trail of ashes led from the fireplace over the lovely Persian carpet through the kitchen and out to the dustbin in the yard. The water had not been turned off at the main, and a window had been left open in the bathroom which had caused the pipes to freeze and burst and there was ice on the floor all round the toilet. Richard told Flora to stop worrying about the state of the house, because it was not their concern; all they had to do was remove the contents. To try and get a little heat in the house they lit the gas fire in the morning room and the water was turned off. Flora then decided to start in the kitchen. They found the cupboards full of tinned food which must have been bought before the war started, and many utensils which would be useful. The tins were taken out and packed in the car, along with crockery and cutlery. Richard opened a drawer and found it full of used white and blue paper bags, with which he made a fire in the kitchen grate, having first made certain that the hot water boiler was behind the diningroom grate. When he emptied the drawer, at the bottom he found a layer of pennies, halfpennies and farthings. In the next drawer Flora found shillings and sixpences; in another florins and half crowns; but the prize was in a drawer which contained serviettes, tablecloths and teatowels. Underneath these there was a thick layer of ten shilling, one pound and five pound notes, in packets held together by paper bands. They decided that when the first day of the month had arrived, Auntie had put any money left over from the previous month into the drawer, and then gone to the bank to draw her new month's allowance. All the money was put into a suitcase which Richard found in a bedroom, so that it could be counted later. Together they ransacked the house but could not find any silver, so gave up looking, and turned their attention to the pictures and small antiques. In the hall, Flora noticed the grandfather clock had stopped and opened the door of the case, out of curiosity to see if the weights and pendulum were there. They were—with the silver—all of which was wrapped in newspaper. They soon were admiring the candlesticks, tea service, jewel box and silver cutlery, along with serving and tea spoons, all of which were packed into another suitcase. When the 'phone rang it was Marjorie to tell Richard that there was a cow down with milk fever at Ryton Lodge and could he go soon. The two suitcases were put in the car, and the house locked up before they left in the gathering darkness.

They sat up late that night counting the money, which came to £287 14*s*.7½*d*.

By train and bus Flora went alone to the house two days later, taking a Thermos flask of hot coffee and a packed lunch with her. After lighting the gas fire, she went out to the coal house to find some wood, and also found about five bags of coal and an equivalent amount of coke. With the wood and coal she soon had a fire going in the kitchen, and completed emptying all the cupboards and drawers. She then went into the hall and then, after taking everything she wanted, locked up both that room and the lounge ready for Elsie to remove her furniture. She then systematically went through the house making a list of everything she wanted, and moved them into the kitchen, which soon looked like an Aladdin's cave filled with pictures, boxes of soap, sheets, towels, pillows, eiderdowns, carpets, electric lamps, trays, bottles of wines and spirits and so on. She knew that her aunt had trained at an Art College in London and was a good painter but had given it up when she married. In one bedroom she found a large wooden steamer trunk, and in it found the top tray full of palettes, tubes of paint, brushes, and knives, together with many canvases. Underneath the tray was a wedding dress with all white matching accessories, and two hats, all wrapped in newspapers of

1904. Flora decided to keep three of the paintings, and dispose of the box and its contents. She now had three lists, one of things she wanted; the second of everything which would go to the sale room; and the third of whatever remained, to go to the Salvation Army.

And so it was done, everything was brought to Sandhaven by horse and cart, except the coal and coke which Uncle Tom put into sacks and delivered some time later. The last part of the windfall came in the form of a letter from the bank manager, which said that the solicitors of the late Mrs Winifred Thurgood had paid the money from her bank account to Mrs Flora Holden, and it amounted to £2,400. Flora was overjoyed, she had never had enough money to have an account and now she had been left a small fortune.

Richard admired the mahogany standard lamp in the lounge, and the antique oak roll-top desk which was put in the office. Flora kept the mink fur coat for herself, but gave a good cloth coat and Chilprufe underwear to Mrs Shaw, who was glad also of the dresses, aprons and curtains, which she could alter to use to clothe her growing children. When the pink Persian carpet was returned from the cleaners and laid on the lounge floor, the furnishing of the room was complete.

The freezing fogs continued, coating everything with ice, and on the Beech Hill the telephone wires were so coated that they were as thick as one's arm, and hung down between the posts almost to the ground. Somehow the Post Office kept the service going though farmers a long way away, having no phone, usually sent a telegram. Richard never forgot the morning when he went to Above Beck at Wilsdon to cleanse a cow. Though sand and ashes had been scattered on the hill, he only arrived at the top with difficulty and was glad to get into the relative warmth of the shippon and treat the cow. Disaster struck as he was coming down the hill in second gear. He was about halfway down when he realised the car was sliding down the incline and was gathering speed. He cautiously pressed the brake pedal and the car skidded across the road, but he managed to straighten up as the T–junction was approached at a fast speed. The far wall of the T–junction was part of the stone-built bridge. In a flash, he decided to try to turn left for Middleton and turned the wheel, but the car was continuing straight on, so he wrenched the wheel round. With a shudder the car half turned left and crashed into the bridge. Richard's face hit the steering wheel, his knees the dashboard, and blood began to run from his eyebrow and nose. He sat there for a short time, half-stunned, while behind him the smell of medicines grew strong, leaking from the broken bottles.

He wiped the blood from his eyebrow and eyelashes, and climbed out of the car through the passenger door.

The car was a mess. The offside front door was buckled, and the running board broken; the windscreen and window broken; the offside front tyre had burst; and the headlight, bumper, sidelight, and wing were broken and bent. Though his knees were hurting, he had set off to walk the quarter of a mile to Wilsdon to get help, when he heard a lorry coming up behind him, the engine grinding away in a low gear.

He turned and saw it was Chris Robson. He stopped his cattle truck beside the car, so Richard walked back.

"I thought it was your car, that's why I stopped," said Chris. "By gum, your face is a bit of a mess."

"I know," said Richard, "I've been lucky, but my knees hurt, they hit the dashboard. But the car's a right mess."

"Aye, it is, but I think if I get my tools and we smash off that bent part of the bumper, and knock the wing up, then we could jack it up and get the wheel changed. Have you got a spare?"

"Yes, I have, I can get it out."

"Well, that's what we'll do and then I can tow you to Dock Garage."

After this had been done, the car was towed to Hindle's Garage; Chris, characteristically, would not take any payment.

"Forget it, Richard, I couldn't leave you stuck there; you'll be able to do summat for me one day, I bet."

Richard phoned Flora while Gordon Hindle prepared an old Hillman Minx for Richard to use and then helped him put everything into it which could be salvaged from the Austin. After Flora had dressed his face, he had a meal and then rested all afternoon, although in the early evening he had to go to two cases. Next day Gordon Hindle told him that the chassis was twisted and that it would be better to dispose of the car. Tom Whittingham, the agent for the Insurance Company, had examined the car, and agreed with the estimate of the cost of the repairs. On Richard's behalf, Gordon had applied for an Austin utility saloon to replace the old car, but did not expect to be allocated one.

Some nights later, the air raid alert had just begun when Tommy Atherton, horse foreman at the steel works, rang to say one of the horses had colic and was in a bad way. It took Richard a long time to get there, driving on sidelights only, over the slippery frozen roads.

"Good evening, Mr Holden," said Tommy, "I'm glad you're here because he is getting worse."

"When did he start?"

"About six o'clock. With two drivers helping me, we got a pint of red medicine and half of the black one down him, but it had no effect, so that's when I rang you."

Richard followed the dim light from the shaded torch into the box and closed the door. Tommy switched on the light—the low wattage bulb just made things visible. The huge horse was lying on his side, sweating hard, and the steam rising from him showed plainly in the freezing air.

"Can you get him up?"

"Yes," said the foreman, and hit the horse hard with a broad leather strap a few times, until he suddenly sat up and then got up. His eyes were reddened, the pulse fast and thin, and he tried to crouch, while looking towards his flanks. Richard threw a towel over the horse's loins and listened for noises in his abdomen on both sides, but there were none. Tommy held up a foreleg while Richard examined the gelding *per rectum*, which the horse resented. The bowel lining was sticky, and clung to Richard's arm as he withdrew it.

"It's a bad do. I am certain he has either got a blockage in his small bowel or else it is twisted. Let's get him dosed, that should tell us which it is."

The stomach tube was passed and a double dose of chloral hydrate in four gallons of saline was administered. The horse at once lay down and began to roll.

"Let's get out of here before he kills us."

As they came out of the box gunfire could be heard in the distance.

"Sounds as though we have two chances of that, with Jerry coming this way," said Richard.

As they sat by the fire in the feeble light in the tack room, they were disturbed when every now and then with a crash the horse's hooves hit the box wall as he rolled about. The noise of gunfire was getting louder when they next inspected the horse, which was just the same, though he was beginning to injure himself. Richard dosed him again; and as they went into the tack room, the noise of a bomb exploding was heard, though it was far off. The horse continued to roll, and after a very loud crash, Richard went to have a look at him but found his condition unchanged. He decided to wait another half hour and, if no signs of recovery were obvious, to shoot him. Near to the works the guns had begun to fire, and more explosions were heard. More noise was heard from the horse as a stick of bombs fell, and Richard and Tommy flung themselves on the floor. Each explosion got nearer, and with a scream one bomb fell and exploded near to the yard side of the stable, followed by the crash of the horse rolling. The scream of another bomb falling ended with a terrific explosion which put the light out and deafened Richard, as it landed nearby on the railway lines. There was a terrific crash from the horse, followed by the noise of falling debris and the tinkle of falling glass.

"Are you OK, Tommy?" shouted Richard,

"Yes!" bawled the foreman, "But some of the roof's gone."

In a quarter of an hour the gunfire had almost stopped, and in the firelight Tommy said, "I think he must be dead. He's not made a noise for a bit, shall we go and look?"

"I wouldn't be surprised if he is, but I'm not going out yet, there could be mines coming down."

They waited a little longer and then went into the box where, by the light of their torches, they could see the horse standing quietly. The sweating was obviously less, and as Richard felt the horse's pulse Tommy went and got a bucket of aired water from the tack room and held it up to the horse's head. He drank all of it.

"By God, he's getting better, Mr Holden,"

"Yes, he is. I think the bomb exploding made him roll so hard from fright that it untwisted his guts."

"Well, would you believe it, that bloody Hitler's cured him."

"It could be, it was either the bomb or the medicine, though I must say the medicine wasn't having much effect."

Next morning the horse was normal, but the damaged skin around his head, hips and hocks bore witness to the pain he had endured, and took some days to heal.

In spite of rationing and a general shortage of food, people still kept their dogs and cats, and the surgery was a very warm and bright place to work in after the dark and cold outside. Winter was releasing its grip, and frost-free brighter days had a tonic effect on everybody. Richard realised that, after four years continuous use, he would have to replace some small animal equipment and he was becoming increasingly aware that he lacked much that was vital for a correct diagnosis. This fact was underlined the afternoon that Flora ushered Dr McConnell's sister Fiona into the surgery. She put a wicker basket onto the table and when she raised the lid a lovely seal point Siamese gave Richard that confident unwavering stare characteristic of the breed.

"I didn't know Bill had a cat."

"He hasn't, it's mine and he's called Muang."

"And why have you brought him, Fiona?"

"Because he will not eat."

"Really, since when?"

"For two days now, and he usually eats like a horse."

"Lift him out, please."

Richard examined the cat and found everything normal.

"It's strange, Fiona, everything is normal. What symptoms is he showing?"

"He just walks up to his plate and takes a mouthful, gives a gulp, miaows and walks away."

"Right, I'll try and see that he is not choked by giving him this sugar-coated pill."

Fiona held the cat's forelegs and Richard gently administered the pill. The cat gulped and miaowed loudly.

"Well, that's down but he did not like it, so there is a painful condition in his oesophagus, that's the food pipe here in the neck."

Richard gently palpated the area and though he could feel nothing out of the ordinary, the cat suddenly growled and tried to scratch.

"It's in cases like this when I wish I had an X-Ray machine, to rule out something like a single small lead shot. Would you leave him with me, and ask Bill to ring me to see if we could have an X-Ray taken at the Memorial Hospital."

"Yes, I'll do that."

Bill soon arranged this. The cat was laid on his side, Richard holding his head and Fiona his hindquarters, while one film was taken. Then he was X-rayed sitting up, with his neck and head extended. When the radiographer brought the wet negatives back later, both Bill and Richard studied them carefully, but could see nothing abnormal.

Bill said, "I'll go and find John Leigh, the radiologist, and let him have a look at these films, because he is the expert."

John came and examined them, and said:

"The left-hand wall of the oesophagus has a darker outline than the right. Did you take this from above to below?"

"Yes we did."

"Then I would like one taken with the cat lying on his back."

When this was done and the film developed, a very thin sewing needle about an inch and a quarter long was revealed lying parallel to and beside the oesophagus.

"There's the foreign body which is causing all the trouble, and it should be easy to remove."

"Thank you very much for your help, Dr Leigh. I don't think I would have found it on my own," said Richard.

"Probably not, you see positioning the patient is very important in X-Ray work and when properly done will confirm your diagnosis; but if incorrect it will be of no help at all. It's worth remembering."

"I won't forget that, and many thanks again."

That evening, under a general anaesthetic, Richard removed the needle and vowed to have an X-Ray machine and an endoscope in the near future. Naturally, as dog does not eat dog. Richard did not send Fiona an invoice for his services, as she was his doctor's sister.

With the coming of April the spring work began, with Vic Whitehead from Far Parkside ringing at 7.00 a.m. to say he was bringing a ewe to the surgery because she could not lamb. By the time Richard had lambed her, Tom Walker from Fell Top arrived with two ewes in a trailer, so by breakfast time three live and one dead lamb had been delivered. As he walked into the kitchen Flora said:

"I hope you haven't forgotten your appointment with Tommy Duke this morning, Richard."

"No, I haven't, but thanks for reminding me; all the same, I think we should go together."

"Yes. I'd like that. Come on, your breakfast is ready."

He had almost finished eating, when Eric Sugden at Boundary Farm had a cow down with milk fever. Fortunately it was not too far away and so Flora and Richard were on time for their appointment with the solicitor. Tommy was pleased to see them, and took the cheque which completed the payment for the practice.

"I must say, Richard, that you have done very well, paying off the capital owed in the eight quarterly instalments as was required."

"Yes, it's been hard work for both of us, but it's worth having one millstone taken off our necks. It will allow us to concentrate on paying off the house mortgage. Could you tell us if we can pay it off before the end of the ten years?"

"Yes, you can, but I'd check with the building society."

"Thanks, Tommy, we will do that."

"And how is Edna?" asked Flora.

"Very well. I'll tell her you were enquiring."

"Well, Flora, that's one milestone reached," said Richard as they walked to the car. "Yes, really the two years have flown. It only seems yesterday we were thinking we might be doing the wrong thing, but it is turning out right after all."

They arrived at the surgery to find a Corporation 'bus stopped on the corner and the lady conductor standing at the front door talking to Marjorie.

"Hello, looks like a run-over case," but it was not; the conductor wanted the fare for Tommy, who had got on the bus at the West Road stop and run upstairs and hidden under a seat. As no passenger owned him the conductor looked at the address on the disc on his collar and so stopped the bus at the corner of Cross Street. Tommy had jumped off and run around the back of the house, so the conductor had rung the bell to collect the fare. Richard apologised for the inconvenience, and paid up, wondering what his dog would get up to next. With that he began a full day's work which ended with him farrowing a sow at eight o'clock that night. It was while kneeling behind the sow that he realised that his knees were painful. When he got home he immediately had a bath and saw that both were slightly swollen. He decided that he had got a mild synovitis from doing so much kneeling on stone floors, and this was aggravating any damage caused by the car crash. But in spite of this he did all the spring work of castrations, dockings and foalings of the heavy horses and all the different parturition cases with their attendant troubles, but was not sorry when cows were turned out at the end of the month, and work became less.

Mr Graham, the consultant gynaecologist, examined Richard first at the hospital and asked him to strip. He examined him carefully and *per rectum*, after which he asked Richard to provide a sperm sample in the contraceptive he provided. He then left the cubicle and, calling for a nurse, went off to examine Flora. After some minutes his assistant took away the sperm sample and Richard dressed. Some time later, the nurse asked him to go to Mr Graham's room and join Flora. He told Richard that he found him very healthy apart from his knees.

Sexually, everything was normal, and the sperm count and wave motion were very good.

Turning to Flora, he told her that again everything was normal, but in view of her earlier abortion and irregular periods he advised a dilation and curettage as soon as he could arrange it. But even without this, he could find no reason why Flora had not conceived again.

She went into hospital a week later, and the operative procedures were carried out; she returned home two days later. After this they made love very often, both hoping with all their hearts that a child would be conceived and with its birth their happiness would be complete.

But any thoughts of love he might have had vanished when at 7.00 a.m. on a glorious May morning he received a call from George Meadows at Boundary Farm, just as Flora poured his second cup of tea.

"Morning, Richard, can you come at once? I've a cow here looks as if she is going to have a fit."

"Yes, George; be as quiet as you can with her and tie her up with a halter. It's probably staggers. I won't be long."

As Richard drank the tea, the 'phone rang again. It was Harry Allen from North End which was two miles beyond Boundary. He milked thirty cows and fed a lot of pigs. He was worried,

"Mr Holden, will you come at once. I've two cows ill, and my milk's down to nowt this morning."

"Harry I'm just off to a staggers case. How ill are these cows?"

"Oh, they're badly, and slavering and smacking their lips."

"They're what? Good Lord, that's something I didn't want to hear."

"Why? What is it? Do you think it could be the foot and mouth?"

"It sounds very like it, and it's no use my coming because I can't do anything; it's a Ministry job, you know. You must report your suspicions at once to Tom Long, the copper in Middleton—that's the law. You telephone him, don't go off your place and don't let any one on; lock the gate until the Ministry have been. I'll let them know now. They will be along pretty soon."

He put down the phone and, turning to Flora, said:

"Look Flora, I must go, I've a staggers at George Meadows at Boundary.

Ring the Ministry of Agriculture and Fisheries at the office in Droughton; you'll be put through to the Duty Officer. Tell him I think there's a suspect outbreak of foot and mouth from a conversation I have had with Harry Allen at North End Farm, Middleton, and that I've told him to inform the police."

"Right, I'll do that at once."

George's younger brother Mick was delivering milk and just turning out of Wyreham Road when Richard roared past almost causing the horse to bolt. The farmyard gate was open, so he drove right up to the shippon door where George was waiting.

"That's near enough, me lad," he said, "I'll want that door tomorrow."

"I know, but I've been delayed on the 'phone. It looks as though it's going to be one of those days. Tell Mick I'm sorry, I nearly made his horse bolt as I cut the corner."

"I will. The cow's here."

Richard noticed that the cow was twitching and blinking rapidly.

"Yes. It's staggers all right, George. Did you milk her out?"

"No, I took the cluster off, because it was upsetting her."

"Good, let's get her injected; I don't want her to go into a fit, so move slowly and quietly."

Richard injected 200 cc. of dextro-mag solution intravenously and followed this with 100 cc. of a 25% solution of magnesium sulphate. When he had finished, he said to George:

"I'd wait a bit, and see what effect that has. You know, it's lucky you didn't milk her out, it makes them far worse if you do. They look as though they are milking well."

"They are that, Richard, my milk has fairly gone up since I turned out."

"In that case, to try and prevent further cases I'd get some iodised mineral salts from Boots in Droughton, and feed it in their ration every day."

"I'll do that."

Betty came into the shippon.

"Hello, Richard, Flora says you've to go to Barkers at High Moor to a cow down with milk fever."

"I must be off then. I'll call back and have another look at this cow; don't turn her out."

At High Moor, the cow was down in the field, with her newborn calf besides her. Though he injected 500 cc. solution intravenously, the cow would not get up, so they left her sitting up and Bob said he would let Richard know if she did not get up by midday.

As he stopped outside the post office in Wyreham, the post mistress came running out to tell him to go as quickly as he could to Joe Fowler's at Abbey Stud.

Driving at full speed, he took the Middleton Road, and soon arrived outside the box in Joe's yards where Joe and two men were awaiting him. Everything was ready and soon Richard was standing on a table examining the Shire mare which could not foal. The foal was alive, but one leg was turned back. Using a carrier he pushed the rope towards the elbow. Each time he attempted to reach the loop on the rope's end the mare strained with all her strength and he had to withdraw his arm. On the fourth attempt, using his left arm he grasped it, threaded the rope through it, and pushed it down to the knee. As Joe pulled on the rope Richard pushed the foal's shoulder upwards, and the knee came forwards. He pushed the rope down to the foot, and then pushed the shoulder up with one hand; with the other he turned the foot towards himself.

The mare strained, and both feet of the foal pushed against his chest.

"Quick, Joe, grab that other foot and pull."

But before they had time to pull, the mare forced the foal out and the two men gently lowered it out onto the straw.

"Look out, Mr Holden, get outside; she's a bad devil once she's got her foal, she'll come at you."

While Joe fended her off with a brush, Richard got outside, followed by the men carrying the table and buckets.

"Go on, you bad old bitch, get licking your foal. It looks a good 'un, Mr Holden, with its four white legs, and it's a filly, just what I wanted out of her."

As he fastened his watch on his wrist—the last present his mother gave him—he was surprised to see that it was ten thirty.

"Time's flown this morning—I must be off. Joe, make certain she gets rid of all that cleansing. If she doesn't, let me know in the morning, first thing."

Back at Boundary Farm, Richard injected the 100 cc. left in the bottle; the cow was quieter, and was over the crisis, much to George's relief.

He was ravenously hungry when he reached the surgery, and glad to eat the lunch which Flora quickly produced. She read out a list of visits waiting to be done, among which were a cow with a broken horn which was bleeding; a mare and a cow to cleanse; and a horse with a thick leg.

"At this rate, Flora, I'll be lucky if I'm back before five."

He was spooning sugar into his cup of tea when Flora stopped him.

"Really, Richard, don't use so much sugar. You know, for three weeks we've been getting less than the ration at Field's; it's really short and I've not much left."

"I didn't know it was as bad as that, Flora, but I'll tell you what I'll do. I'll see if Jim Lord has any saccharine tablets—you know it's a sugar substitute."

"Are they safe to use?"

"Oh yes it's a chemical substance that is very sweet and has been used for years in the food trade, making jams and cakes."

When he answered the 'phone it was the Divisional Veterinary Officer of the Ministry of Agriculture and Fisheries, who told Richard that the suspected outbreak of foot and mouth disease at North End Farm had been confirmed so a standstill order was coming into operation for the area within a radius of five miles from the farm. Bob Dawson also advised him to be thorough in his questioning on the 'phone of any farmer who reported lame pigs or suddenly-ill cattle before he visited the farm; if he had any suspicions to ring the office at once, and not to visit the farm.

Everywhere he went that afternoon the farmer had two or three animals to be treated. At Harold Marsden's he had to inspect his laying birds, and soon diagnosed fowl coryza. Thus he just had time to gulp down his tea, and attend to the animals brought to the evening surgery. The last one was the spaniel bitch belonging to Bill Griffin, the manager of the Home Farm. It was an acute case of pyometra in the seven-year-old bitch, and so Richard operated on her that evening, even though he was very tired. When he went to bed at 11 o'clock he was pleased to see that she was coming round from the anaesthetic.

When farmers learned the next day of the foot and mouth disease outbreak, they became cautious and Richard had only one visit that morning. It was lunchtime when Gordon Hindle telephoned to say that the new car he had been allocated had arrived. It was a Utility black Austin car, DTJ 19, of which Richard took delivery at the weekend and he was pleased to leave the old Hillman Minx with Gordon. He was very grateful to Gordon because, apart from the greater reliability of the new car, it had eased his worries over tyres; he now had five new ones on the car, and two in store which were of the same size. Flora was thrilled with the new car, but insisted that if he could have a new car, she could have a new suit.

He agreed at once when she said she would pay for the suit, which comprised a jacket and skirt in a powder blue colour. He bought her a blouse with matching accessories and was very proud when he drove her to church for Communion on the next Sunday morning. He didn't tell her, but secretly he thought she had never looked lovelier. Richard himself never bothered about clothes, but had plenty of jackets and trousers in saxonies and tweeds, and a very good grey suit. He wished he had bought another suit two weeks later, when clothes rationing was introduced on 1st June.

It was a little later that Mrs Shaw annoyed Flora when at lunchtime on the Friday she said that she was starting work on the Monday morning at the Government factory on Dock Road. Flora paid her the week's wages due, and wished her all the best in her new job. When Richard arrived home, Flora really let off steam.

"You know, it's not good enough to leave at a moment's notice the way she has done; and to think of all I've done for her, giving her a steady job and clothes for herself and the children and even furniture from Auntie Winnie's."

"I agree with you, it's really thoughtless, but the problem is who will take her place? Have you anybody in mind?"

"I haven't but I thought I would ask John when he comes tonight what his nephew's widow is doing? She might be able to come."

"Sounds a good idea. If she is anything like John she would be first class."

Mavis was living at home looking after her mother who was becoming disabled with arthritis, while her father worked as an engineer in the shipyard. She agreed to come, provided she could begin at half past eight each morning and go home to Old Lane at 10 o'clock to make her mother a hot drink, and finish work at 12 o'clock, so that she would be home to give her father his lunch on time. Flora readily agreed and when she began work in July she turned out to be an excellent worker.

Two miles from Sandhaven was Oaks Farm of 100 acres in extent. The owner was Mrs Crook, helped on the farm by her two sons. Actually it was Bill, the elder one, who was the driving force and the brains in the enterprise. He was a tall, fair-haired strongly-built man, twenty-two years of age, who, on the sudden death of his father had left the Grammar School, and at sixteen years old had begun to run the farm helped by his mother and a hired man. They had all worked hard and Bill, who was interested in science, had kept up to date in his farming methods. On Richard's advice he had made his cattle into a closed herd, which would soon have become Attested if war had not broken out. Another milk round in Sandhaven had been run by Joe Brockbank from premises in Broad Street. In 1940 he became terminally ill, so Mrs Crook bought the round and put Tom, her younger eighteen-year-old son in charge of it, so that she got a better price for the farm's milk than she could have got from the Board. Richard had made few visits to the farm, and was a little surprised one lovely summer afternoon to have to visit two cows with milk fever.

At the farm Bill came up to the car and said:

"Don't get out, Mr Holden, the one that is really bad is down in the field and you can drive right up to her."

"Get in, Bill, that makes it quicker; when did she calve?"

"Seven weeks ago, that's what I don't like about her. I've never had one have milk fever as long as this after calving and she is right bad."

"Oh, it does happen sometimes."

As they drove up to her Richard said,

"By jove, she is bad, lying flat out like that and she's a bit blown. Get out quick and pull her head up. I'll just get my stuff and give you a hand."

Before Richard could do this Bill shouted: "It's no use, Mr Holden, she's dead."

Looking at her Richard said:

"To me she's gone too quickly for it to be just milk fever. Anyway, I must take a blood smear and a swab before I let Bob Whiteside know, and we can find out what has killed her."

When he had taken his samples they drove back to the farm, where the other cow was in a box with her new born calf.

"Bill, take the calf out, it can have a suck later."

He examined the cow, and as it was a case of milk fever he gave her an intravenous injection of calcium borogluconate solution, and before they left the box she got to her feet.

He was puzzled when he examined the stained blood smear and the black rods of the anthrax bacillus came into focus. You don't get the disease in cows at grass.

"Yes, Bill, it's suspect anthrax; but the question is, where has it come from? Are you feeding any cattle cake?"

"No, Mr Holden, they haven't had any; I'm trying to build up a stock for the winter."

"Well then, for the present, Bill, keep them out of that pasture."

"I can't do that, because I kept them on the 20-acre until they had eaten it bare, so that the contractor could get on putting in the new water main to the Government factory. That's at the bottom of the field I am using now, it's the only grass there is available."

"Look, Bill, either put them back on the bare field or fence that area off until the Ministry have been. I'll let them know straight away and the police."

"Everything is happening in your parish lately," said Bob Dawson, "First you have foot and mouth and now anthrax. Send the diagnostic smear and the swab to Weybridge at once, won't you."

"Yes, I'll do that."

"Good, Richard. We'll deal with the carcase."

It was late evening when Bill Crook rang again. "Mr Holden, can you come right away, I've another cow real bad."

"Bill, I'll be there in ten minutes."

Having put his rubber boots and his oilskin coat, Richard drove very quickly to the farm and, taking a large bottle of disinfectant and his bag, walked with Bill into the shippon. Bill explained, "You know, at milking time she gave very little milk and her bag was hot, so I thought she was starting with mastitis. I got some mastitis powder and with Tom's help I drenched her with it."

The cow was unsteady on her feet, and blood-stained liquid dung was running down her tail and some was in the channel behind her. Before Richard could take her temperature, she began to bellow, and then collapsed into a sitting position, rolled over onto her side, and died.

"Well that's a bad do, Bill. It looks like anthrax again, but I will have to take a smear and confirm it."

"Mr Holden, I've lost two good cows in four hours. Tell me, how many more will we lose?"

"I don't know, Bill, it depends on how many have picked up the germ. Were many of the cows round that first one down the field.?"

"Yes they were—sniffing and licking."

"Then you could lose some more."

"Then can't you do something to stop it spreading like this?"

"Bill, I think Prontosil injections and the mastitis powder might help, but what they want is anti-anthrax serum."

"Right, let us get it into them right away."

"I can't do that; you see, it doesn't keep and as you very rarely need it, you only order it for an outbreak like this."

"Then get it ordered right away."

"I will, but first of all I've got to stop this germ spreading everywhere. Will you shout for your Tom to bring two buckets of hot water, and a sack and some hay and leave them outside the door."

Richard took a blood smear and a swab soaked in blood from the dead animal. When the water arrived he poured plenty of Cresol disinfectant into each bucket. He soaked the sack in disinfectant and placed it outside the door and then rolled up some hay into a tight ball and stuffed it into the drain blocking it. He soaked his hands in disinfectant and then splashed it on the floor in front of them all the way up to the cow and round it. He pushed hay up her nostrils with a stick and then blocked her anus by pushing in a ball of hay. The rest of the disinfectant he poured over the cow's hindquarters and the dung behind her. At the door they both washed their hands and clothing and boots with disinfectant and then crossed the yard to the house.

Mrs Crook was seated at the table in the kitchen. Looking up, she said:

"Mr Holden, you will have a cup of tea, won't you?"

"Yes, I will, thank you, but I do want you to listen to me while I explain about this outbreak of anthrax you have here."

The three men took their cups of tea and sat down, and Richard continued, "I am sorry to tell you that another cow has just died of the disease."

"Oh, Mr Holden, not another, that's two today." said Mrs Crook. "Can't you stop it?"

"I am certain it can be stopped, but I think you will lose more cows before we can get serum from London with which to treat them and that will cost a good few pounds."

"Do you know how much it will be, Mr Holden?"

"I don't until I can get in touch with the firm and I only hope they have not been bombed out. Why I said you will lose more cows is because we don't know where they are getting the germ from and until that is found and shut off, the cows will still eat the germ and will die. I hope the Ministry's men tomorrow can find the source of the outbreak."

"So do I, Mr Holden, but will you get all the serum we need for the cattle right away."

"I will; how many cattle have you?"

Bill got his herd book and soon told Richard the number. Richard said that he would get twelve doses extra, so that he would have some serum with which to treat any animal which showed symptoms after the first dose.

Mrs Crook looked at Richard and said, "Mr Holden, will you please get whatever you think you'll need to save the herd. Since we came here sixteen years ago, we have slaved to get where we are today, and I am not going to lose it all for a few pounds."

"I will do that, and I'll give Bill some more mastitis powder and Prontosil to give to any cow that is becoming ill, but I hope the serum comes before you lose any more. I'll be off now. Goodnight, everybody, and thank you for the tea, Mrs Crook."

The blood smear was positive, but he got no reply when he telephoned the serum company that night.

At 6.30 a.m. Bill rang to say that he had found another cow dead in the field, and one cow had staggered part way to the buildings, then collapsed and died. When Richard got back to the surgery and examined the smears, both cases proved anthrax positive. He then rang the serum company and gave his order, explaining that he wanted the serum very urgently, stressing that it must be put on the first available express passenger train. The Manager promised to do this and to let Richard know the train on which he had put the parcel so that he could meet it at Sandhaven.

"You've got three more cases, Richard?" said Bob Dawson, "That's some outbreak. Have you any idea where the infection is coming from?"

"Yes, in my opinion, it's come from the soil from a trench which is being dug across one of the biggest pastures on the farm."

"Thanks, I'll have a good look at that this morning when I get there."

At lunchtime Flora got to know that the train would arrive at eight o'clock that night and Richard hoped that it would be on time because now every minute saved was vital. At 4 o'clock Bill rang to say another cow had died and wanted to know when the serum would arrive. Richard, to be on the safe side, said probably about 9 o'clock. Bill went on to say that the officers of the Ministry had found some cattle bones in the soil from the trench and thought that the disease had come from there, so all work in the trench had been stopped and a fence was being erected across that end of the field.

As Richard drove to the station just before eight o'clock an air raid alert began and he spent an hour impatiently awaiting the train's arrival. He ran down to the guard's van, collected the parcel and signed for it and then tore out of the station and drove away at full speed, Bill was waiting for him and said that he had drenched two cows which had given very little milk earlier. Richard gave both a large dose of serum intravenously and then continued injecting every animal subcutaneously. It was very late when they finished and neither of them had much sleep that night, because at 6.00 a.m. he was back at the farm and again injected the two cows which had been ill the night before. Bill told Richard that he had noticed that if a cow's udder was very hot to the touch all over, she was beginning to develop the disease. During the next hour three cows gave less milk than usual, so he injected these. Both men were pleased when no more deaths occurred. Richard was more than relieved, especially when he learnt that the restrictions had been removed from Harry Allen's farm.

In that high summer of the second year of the war, everyone Richard knew was doing something to supply themselves with food. In the evenings, they were working in their gardens, or on allotments. The cottager's pig was becoming more important; more people were keeping pigs because, on giving up some of the points for meat in their ration books, they could keep half the pig when it was slaughtered. In the hot weather the number of cases of swine erysipelas increased and Richard, viewing his rapidly dwindling stock of anti-serum, realised he could not wait for more to arrive in the Willows hamper. So he ordered a special delivery of serum from the serum company in London, and was pleased when it arrived very quickly and ended his worries. The practice had not gone quiet in the summer, so he found he had to delegate more work to his staff. Dispensing, trimming dogs, tending to the garden round the house, decorating inside it, and more secretarial work was all done by Marjorie, Mavis and John, supervised by Flora. Richard was devoting all his time to his professional work, almost to the exclusion of everything else and this showed in the increased income of the practice. His building society book showed that the capital still owing on the house was under £800. George Duke said that he was pleased to see Richard's hard work was paying dividends. The profit and loss account showed a good profit on the year's work and the balance sheet was healthy.

Richard's pleasure was short-lived, because a few nights later in the *Evening Post* were two notices of "Death on Active Service". The first was of the death of one of his closest school friends—Hugh Howard, who had qualified as a dental surgeon and been killed while serving in the Army Dental Corps. The second was about Tom Seddon, a pilot officer listed as "Missing presumed killed". Tom, a fair-haired, blue-eyed, big chap had played in the soccer team with Richard, though he was two years behind him in school. Richard at once wrote a letter of sympathy to Hugh's father, this being the second tragedy for the latter because his wife had died two months before. The deaths on active service disturbed Richard and he began to question the morality of his right to enjoy life and build up a successful practice while his friends were dying in defence of his country and of himself. These doubts increased when he received a letter from Norman in which he described his life to date. He gave a detailed description of the great crowd of chaps with whom he was taking the flying training course in the RAF. When he and Richard had first met, Norman had said that he was really very interested in mathematics and would have liked to make his career in that subject; his father however had persuaded him to study veterinary science, in the hope that eventually Norman would join him in the city horse practice. In the letter he said that his interest in maths was very useful now in navigation and that he was sure that he would obtain his "Wings" soon.

Further up the estuary from Sandhaven were extensive marshes where local farmers, for a fee payable to the Trustees of the Marsh, were allowed to graze their dry cows and in-calf heifers in the summer. One day at the end of August Richard went to treat a dry cow at Low House Farm near Ryton, the home of the Marsh Ranger, whose duty was to inspect all the animals on the Marsh once a day and to get them on to high ground when high tides flooded in. The cow belonged to Harry Carter from Seaton and Richard found an obviously ill animal, hollow from not eating, which had a temperature of 104.5°F. It was an Ayrshire and he found all the white areas raised above the level of the surrounding skin and painful to the touch. Harry said he had dosed the animal with powder for mastitis about a week before, but the udder was now normal. Richard decided that the condition was an allergic reaction to something the animal had eaten. He injected it with adrenaline solution and gave Harry a pint bottle of concentrated fever medicine with which to continue the treatment. A week later the cow was bright and eating well, but the skin of the affected areas was dead, looked like old leather and was peeling away from the underlying flesh, so Richard gave acriflavine emulsion to the Marsh Ranger for application to the raw areas twice a day.

After some months, when he treated the new calved cow for milk fever, the dead skin had been shed and the hairless pink areas made the cow look as though she originally had been burnt. Though he doubted his diagnosis, Richard dismissed the case from his mind and worked non-stop through the busy autumn days. Because he had so much work in the country, he changed the surgery hours back to the evening, so that he could drive about mainly in daylight. In late September he used to stop the car and for a few minutes relax picking blackberries from the hedges, or he would leave Flora to do it while he went to a nearby farm and then picked her up on his way back. At night he helped her make blackberry and apple jam for which part of the sugar ration had been carefully hoarded and more saccharine bought from Jim Lord.

Between Wilton and Catley the canal wound through some idyllic scenery, with the trees lovely in their autumn colours. The fields of some farms ran down to the edge of the canal towpath, as at Hill Crest Farm where one field was on a steep slope. Bob Whittaker and his two men were repairing gaps in the hedges made by the cows which had now been housed for the winter. At the top of the slope was the Fordson tractor, behind which a trailer was hooked on, containing posts, wire and sledge hammers. Bob was a wealthy progressive farmer who had a large herd of pedigree dairy Shorthorns, which would have been Attested by now if the War had not intervened. He had one son, George, twelve years old, big for his age and his parents idolised him.

On this bright morning in late October, Richard was driving down the road to the farm when, on looking to his right, he was pleased to see the tractor being driven down the slope and three figures walking behind it. This meant that he would not have to wait for Bob to come to the shippon, so he drove past the house and through the farmyard to turn his car round. On looking ahead he was horrified to see the tractor careering down the slope out of control, with George in the driving seat and the three men running behind it waving their arms. At the moment he realised what was happening, the tractor crashed onto the towpath and, rolling over onto its side, skidded into the canal, dragging the trailer with it and sank beneath the water. He at once drove as quickly as he could to the place, but even then Dennis, one of the men, was swimming about and diving into the muddy water while Bob and the other man stood on the path. Richard jumped from the car, pulled off his coat and jacket and was about to jump into the water when Dennis swam to the side, pushing George before him. Bob and Richard pulled them both onto the path and Bob, frantic with worry and carrying George in his arms, shouted:

"Richard, quick, help me into the car and drive like hell to the house!"

He did. Bob ran with his son in his arms into the house and within minutes Richard was driving like mad to Goswick to find Dr Horrocks. As he roared into Catley village he saw the doctor's car standing outside the post office. Richard stopped, rushed into the shop and gabbled his story. He was soon left behind by Tom Horrocks driving very quickly in his big Austin Six car. Richard arrived back at the farm to find the other labourer standing beside the doctor's car.

"How's George? Do you know anything?"

"No I don't," he replied, "The doctor's inside, but I think he were dead when Dennis found him. Why the hell he didn't jump off I don't know, when we were all shouting at him to get off the damn thing."

"I didn't know he could drive a tractor," said Richard.

"Oh, aye, he could. Bob let him drive it in the yard, but yon Fordson was too big for him. I told Bob so, but he wouldn't listen."

It was obvious from Dr Shorrock's manner as he came out of the house and gently closed the door, that the worst had happened, but Richard still asked:

"Is he going to be all right?"

"No, he is not. I'm sorry, Mr Holden but he has just died, from a severe injury to his head. It is a dreadful tragedy for them."

The picture of Ezra and Martha when John died flashed through Richard's mind and he was near to tears. He walked to the shippon, treated the cow and left medicine for it. Driving home he wondered how he would have reacted if he and Flora had lost a son like that. He thought, "I think I would go crazy if I saw all my hopes dashed at one stroke." As he walked into the kitchen, Flora took one look at his face and said:

"Richard, whatever's the matter?" He slowly told her the story and then cried in his misery, "Hugh, and Tommy Seddon and now this, I'm really so upset, love, I don't know what to do."

Flora brought him a glass of brandy and soda and made him drink it. She sat beside him, stroked his hair and kissed him, and he slowly felt better. Then she made him have his lunch, but in her mind she was worried that he was working too hard, with never a day off and no relaxation.

Within a year Bob became an apathetic alcoholic, but Dennis ran the farm helped by Mrs Whittaker, when she had overcome her grief; she was a much stronger character than her husband. It took Bob two years to get over the loss of his only son, and begin to work again.

When George Duke did the half-year audit, he found everything was going well and completed the PAYE forms for the month, watched by Richard who then signed the cheque for the amount owing. This new tax on the wages of some of the staff had been introduced some months before, but it was the first time he had seen the forms filled in. In was another war-time burden, which had to be endured, like the cut in coal and fuel supplies just as the winter was beginning. He began to buy logs where he saw them for sale, and stored them in the garage, because he still had bags of coal and coke which he had brought from Auntie Winnie's store in the disused outside lavatory. As Christmas approached, Flora grumbled that more things were disappearing from the shops, and when onions became hard to get Dick Hoggarth brought some big ones he had grown in the garden at the end of the yard. Richard now got together all the gardening tools Mrs Walker had given to them, and those from Auntie Winnie's, and got John to clean and oil them ready for use next spring, because Flora had decided to grow vegetables like everybody else. She had borrowed two books on gardening from the public library. It was about this time that milk became rationed, but Mick Meadows told Richard that if ever they were short of milk to call at the farm and get some.

After a hurried lunch, Richard had gone to Marhey to a cow choked. The animal had been let out with others into the yard, so they could drink at the trough before they had a feed of cabbage. The affected animal, finding the barn door open, had gone in and had been gorging herself on potatoes before she had been chased out. She had swallowed the potato unchewed and it had stuck in her throat. Richard found the cow partially blown and salivating copiously. He fitted the ratchet gag into the cow's mouth, with Tom Bolton holding one side and his son George the other. Richard opened the gag to its widest extent, and then pushed his arm into the animal's mouth. With the gag up to his elbow he could just reach the potato with his fingers, but could not move it. It was large and would not go down, so obviously it must be brought back into the mouth. The cow was struggling and blowing saliva into Richard's face. He withdrew his arm and explained the position of the potato to Tom, and asked him to press with his thumbs behind the potato. It could be felt in the neck, and would have to be pushed forwards and upwards. With George holding the cow's horns, and Tom with his hands in position, Richard pushed his arm into the cow's mouth again.

"Push up hard, Tom," said Richard as his fingers touched the potato, and slowly he was pushing them round the potato.

"Harder, quick, Tom." Tom did as he was asked, and suddenly Richard had his fingers and thumb round the potato and withdrew it. The cow gave a long belch and coughed more saliva all over him.

"That's a good do, Mr Holden, I'm right glad to see that out without you having to help her to let the gas out."

"So am I, Tom, but I hate these jobs; look at my arm all scratched with her teeth. Let's have a bucket of water, some soap and a towel."

He washed his arm, face and hands and dried them, then rubbed his antiseptic cream all over the arm. It was almost dark and the bitter wind was driving the sleet before it as he stopped at the village post office. There was a message for him to to go Fred Noblett at Highgate Farm at Ryton to a heifer calving. He was glad it was on the way home, because he felt tired and his indigestion was making itself felt.

Fred and his wife had no children, so Fred ran the farm with the help of two men while his wife was in charge of the eggs, butter making, and the cream separation. Winifred only did the latter for themselves and their friends. Fred had sixty milking cows of assorted breeds and Richard found that the heifer was a Shorthorn which had been served by a Friesian bull. This was a cross Richard hated, because always it caused a difficult calving.

The heifer was down and well bedded, but the floor of the box was made of cobblestones and was badly drained. Richard asked for more straw to be put down and then tried to make the heifer rise but she would not. So he got down on his knees and examined her, to find the calf's head was turned back to the side on which she was lying.

"Come on, Fred, she's lying on the calf's head, we will have to turn her over."

When the three men had done this, Richard knelt down and then lay down on his stomach, so that he could reach the calf's head. The heifer strained powerfully.

"Will you pinch her back, Fred, as hard as you can and one of you hold her nose to try and stop her straining so hard."

Finally, after a struggle, Richard got hold of the calf's lower jaw, roped it, and pulled until the head came round into the correct position.

Richard got to his feet and said, "By jove, Fred, these cobbles hurt like hell, let's have some more straw. I've got the head turned round, but as it's a big calf I'll put strong ropes on it. Bring a good halter, Fred, and tie the heifer to that ring and also bring three milking stool legs."

Richard got down again on the new straw and fixed the loop of a calving rope through the calf's mouth and over its poll. He then attached a rope to each leg, after tying it to one of the stool legs, and gave one to each man. Still kneeling, he supervised the pulling on the ropes and very slowly the calf began to move. When the calf's nose was showing at, and the feet were protruding through the vulva, they all stopped for a breather.

"I think she has been calving all night, Fred, that calf's as dry as a bone, so I'm going to put some lubricant in her passage." Knowing that he should have sent for Richard earlier, Fred kept quiet. After Richard had liberally applied the antiseptic cream to as much of the calf's head and legs as he could reach they began to pull steadily but it was at least ten minutes before the calf's head came out. Then the leg ropes were tied to a fencing post and two men using it as a lever pushed on it as hard as they could for quite a time before the big, dead bull calf was delivered. There was a little laceration of the vulva and vagina which Richard dressed with antiseptic emulsion after putting sulphamilamide into the uterus.

They left the beast in a sitting position but it was two days before she got up. Later that evening Flora wanted to know why Richard was limping.

"Oh, my knees are sore after kneeling on that cobblestone floor at Fred Noblett's. It was a rough do, and I feel really tired tonight; what with a sore arm, sore knees and indigestion I feel jiggered."

"I didn't realise that you felt as rotten as that, I'll put the hot water bottle in the bed, and then make you some Horlicks, and then you are going to bed right away."

"I will that, but I'll have a bath first, and I'll use more than five inches of hot water too," He did and he slept well; as there was no strenuous work on the Sunday he rapidly felt better. The news on the wireless on the Monday morning did not depress him; he felt that the bombing of the American Navy at Pearl Harbor would bring the Americans into the war and probably shorten it. But when he saw the News at the cinema that week he was astonished at the destruction and loss of so many ships and men.

Ming began to walk round the house giving her mating call,

"I know one thing, Flora, we won't get much sleep with that cat making that row. I'll take her to Tom Billsborough's cat tomorrow."

"I wish you would, she's never stopped howling all day, and I would like a kitten."

As luck would have it, Richard had a cow to see in Marhey the next morning, and he left the cat at Billsborough's, saying he would collect her at the weekend. Uncle Tom rang up and asked for various medicines and dressings to be delivered, so this gave Richard a reason for being in Droughton, if he should be stopped by the police. He collected Ming after her successful mating, and went to the stables. Tom was pleased to see him, and wanted all his news about the family. Auntie Nellie made tea and while they were drinking it she said that they had just received a letter from Frank in which he said he had been promoted to Sergeant in the Royal Artillery and wished them all a Happy Christmas, but he did not tell them where he was.

Richard arrived home to be met by Flora who said that an announcement on the wireless had stated that two British ships, the *Prince of Wales* and the *Repulse* had been sunk by the Japanese in the Far East. A wave of sadness swept over him, and he was near to tears when he bent down and let Ming out of the basket. When the phone rang Flora answered it, and came back to say that Jean would be coming on Saturday 22nd December by train, and had written to Bill and Mary and told them to come to Sandhaven if they were given leave.

"So there could be five of us at Christmas. Now what can I give them?" asked Flora.

"Don't worry, I'll go round to Frank Wood this afternoon and ask him for a turkey."

"You'll be lucky if you get one."

"No harm in trying, Flora."

Frank said he could not promise anything but would try to get any poultry he could. Failing that he was certain he could supply the meat ration to all his customers. He did give Richard a parcel for Flora, and when she opened it she was pleased to find that it was beef suet, so now she could make mince-meat and plum pudding with the dried fruit she had hoarded.

They decided to have a party on 22nd December, and, as alcoholic drinks were in short supply, to ask all their guests to bring a bottle of whatever drink they had, so that a punch could be made. In the meantime, Richard's arm had healed; his knees were less painful, but his indigestion was worse. He did not consult Dr McConnell, but made up a prescription containing *Bism. Carb., Mag. Carb. Lev., Sodii. Bic., and Tinct. Belladonna,* and this gave him a lot of relief.

A day earlier than expected Jean arrived, bringing with her a loin of pork, for which Flora was very grateful. Together the next day they decorated the lounge and put out all the Christmas cards. The letter with Uncle Harry's card informed them that Flora's cousin Harry was now a Captain in the Army in Egypt. The card sent to Richard from his father and signed "Mary and Ted", still ignored Flora's existence. Richard did not tear up the card, but, becoming reconciled to the fact that the gulf between him and his relatives was impassable, he put it among the other cards on the mantlepiece. The two women went to Bishop's and got meat pies, and spent the afternoon making pork and stuffing sandwiches. The big brass jam pan was well scoured inside, washed and put ready for the making of the punch. In addition to inviting their usual friends, they invited Dick Harrison the bank manager and his wife Marianne, making nineteen people altogether, until Mary arrived at half past eight.

After everybody had drunk a glass of warm punch, the alcoholic content of which was not high, according to Bill McConnell, the party went with a swing, and all agreed it had been most enjoyable, though the Revd. Evans and Edna had to leave early. Dr McConnell and Richard together were able to be most attentive to the guests, because neither had to leave to visit a patient.

Frank Wood produced a small turkey on Christmas Eve, and Flora and Jean were making it ready for cooking when the door bell rang, and Mary ran to answer it.

Her cry of delight when she opened the door brought them all running to see who it was. It was Bill, and Richard saw before him an uninhibited expression of the love and affection all the members of his wife's family had for each other, as Jean and her three children hugged and kissed in the joy of being together again. When they returned to the kitchen they found Ming crouched on the floor eating the turkey's gizzard which she had stolen from the table, but as it was Christmas she was forgiven. Bill was now a corporal in the Tank Corps, a big, tough-looking, pipe-smoking man, who had thumbed a lift from Catterick Camp, and taken nine hours to reach Sandhaven. After a late dinner, they all went to the midnight service at St. Luke's, which had now been completely blacked out so that evening services could be held.

When Christmas lunch was ready to be served, the phone rang and Richard had to go to Waterford Farm at Runfold to a cow with a prolapsed uterus. So, leaving the family to the feast, he drove through deserted lanes to the case. Bill Pickles was standing in the yard waiting and said:

"I'm glad you've not been so long, Mr Holden, because when I got back from the village on my bike, the next cow had walked on the calf bed and burst it."

"Quick, let's get to her."

Bill led the way and Richard found the organ torn, with the coils of intestines coming through the tear, and blood running steadily down the dung channel.

"Bill, I'm sorry, but it's hopeless."

"Aye, I thought so, too,"

"Anyway, she is bleeding well, so I'm not going to shoot her, but will cut the calf bed away so that she bleeds out completely."

Richard ran to the car, and got his razor-sharp post mortem knife, and ran back to the cow, which was obviously dying, having fallen onto her side. He quickly cut the uterus away; blood and intestines poured out, and as they watched, the cow died.

"Bill, is John Snipe your butcher in the village?"

"Yes he is, Mr Holden."

"Right. Well she will have to be dressed soon, so I'll go for him. You put a pulley block up on that cross beam, so we can hoist her. Get plenty of hot water ready, and a clean sheet to wrap the carcase in, and some clean buckets for the head and pluck and liver."

John was half asleep by the fire when his wife ushered Richard into the living room, but he was instantly ready to help Bill Pickles and went to change into his working clothes, and get his knives and steel. Back at the farm John speedily dressed the animal, while Richard told them about the two heifers which had had to be killed at Higher Carden twelve months before.

"Aye, it's lucky it happened now and not tonight, because the missus and me are going to our Fred's at Wyresham, and you would have been stuck."

"Oh, I don't know John, I'd have gone for Frank Wood. Anyway, thanks a lot for coming and doing the job."

"Aye, thanks, John and both of you come to the house for a wash and a drink."

Richard ate the piece of cake offered, and drank their health, and set off home through the gathering darkness, grumbling to himself that only once in the last three years had he eaten his Christmas lunch with his family.

After Jean, Mary and Bill had left on Boxing Day, work came in steadily, keeping Richard busy for the rest of the week, so he hoped for a quiet New Year's Eve. It was not to be, for at 8 o'clock he got a call to go to Shepherd's Farm at Goswick to a cow which could not calve. He was loathe to leave Flora, but as it was a cold evening he put a Thermos flask of tea in the car, and after wrapping up well set off.

When he arrived at the farm Tom Jackson said that he was sorry he had

had to send for Richard, but the cow had been trying to calve since tea time.

The examination revealed a twisted vagina.

"Tom, she can't calve because she's got what you call a twisted calfbed, so she will have to be rolled. How much help have you got?"

"There's only me and the missus."

"I'll need another at least. We will have to go for your man, what's his name, Bob?"

"Yes, he lives about half a mile away, in the village."

They collected him, and after casting the cow, Mrs Jackson attended to the head, and the two men to the legs. After three rolls, the twist was undone, and Richard then delivered a big dead calf. He washed and, putting on his top clothes, politely excused himself and drove off. It was a very black night, and after a few miles because his eyes ached and he was cold he stopped the car, and drank two cups of tea. The silence was absolute; there were no signs of life; it could have been a cold dead world, and Richard felt depressed and apprehensive as he sat there. Suddenly he thought of Ben Lawson and Frank Bradshaw, and felt vaguely uneasy, and prayed that whatever was prompting him to think of them would not come to pass. He drove off to get away from his fears, and did not mention them when he got home. He was glad to have supper with Flora in the warm kitchen, and as soon as he had written up the day's work in the Day Book, they went to bed and were sound asleep when 1942 came at midnight.